VETERINARY LASER THERAPY IN SMALL ANIMAL PRACTICE

VETERINARY LASER THERAPY IN SMALL ANIMAL PRACTICE

First edition

María Suárez Redondo DVM PhD CVA
Complutense University of Madrid – Veterinary Clinical Hospital (HCVC)
Integra Vetersalud Centro Veterinario

Bryan J. Stephens PhD
SOUND Technologies, Inc

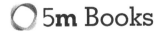 5m Books

First published 2019, reprinted 2021, 2022

Published by
5m Books Ltd
Lings, Great Easton
Essex CM6 2HH, UK
www.5mbooks.com

A catalogue record for this book is available from the British Library.

ISBN 9781789180053

Book layout by Servis Filmsetting Ltd, Stockport, Cheshire
Printed and bound by CPI Group (UK) Ltd, Croydon, CR0 4YY
Photo credits as indicated in the acknowledgments

Contents

Preface

For me, I am driven by two main philosophies: know more today about the world than I knew yesterday and lessen the suffering of others. You'd be surprised how far that gets you.

— Neil deGrasse Tyson

 When we first started writing and thinking about this project, we pictured at least two kinds of situations in which the book could be used. The reader might have some time to sit down and enjoy learning more about laser therapy; but the book should also be useful when a patient has just come in with a severe otitis, a bite wound, or a dehiscence after a fracture repair. Or maybe it is Mr. Whiskers who did not seem to improve after his last session and you want to modify some parameters to get the clinical response you expect.

Clinical results will probably be obvious shortly after you first implement laser therapy in your practice. But as treatments progress, you will also be faced with more challenging cases. In such situations, it becomes even more important to have a good knowledge of the parameters you can modify. This, together with a good review of what has been published and reported, will allow you to make more well-founded, customized choices for such patients.

I hope you enjoy performing laser therapy and offering that option to your patients. You are relieving their pain, speeding up their recovery, and improving their quality of life. At a molecular level, that is literally happening at the speed of light.

— María

 We struggled with the two extremes of books that currently exist on this topic and in this profession: textbooks written by academics and guidebooks written by laser users. The academics obviously understand best what is fundamentally happening with light's interaction with biological tissue, but their experimentations are often in cell culture, or at best on mice. That is where you go to learn the principles and where to start. The laser-user authors are clinicians who have, for one reason or another, purchased a therapy laser from one of the dozens of companies selling lasers of all types and with all sorts of output parameters, begun to have clinical success using the parameters in those manufacturer-preset protocols, and then started lecturing and writing about their success stories.

Neither of these types of writing are terribly useful. We imagine you are reading this book to answer questions like, "what parameters of laser have the best chance of working on this Rottweiler's aching hip, what kinds of biological effects should I expect on the treated tissue, how long should I expect to wait to see clinical results, and what techniques could I use to maximize my consistency and efficacy." The answer shouldn't be to point you to an *in vitro* study of 25 mW exposure of 808 nm light on genetically modified strands of *E. coli* to measure the rotation rate of the flagellum as an indicator of their enhanced transmembrane proton potential (don't laugh, this is serious stuff). But neither should the answer be to show you before-and-after pictures of a pug who had a bruised elbow and who after being treated with one commercially available laser was "feeling better" according to the pet owner (again, don't laugh; those of you who have been to laser lectures even at reputable conferences have undoubtedly heard this).

Instead, you will hear clinical advice from the clinician: a soft-tissue surgeon who teaches at university, has engaged in her own micro- and macro-studies, but also founded an integrative veterinary practice and treats with laser on a daily basis. You will also hear science from the scientist, someone who is formally trained in radiation and who has developed laser hardware, software, and treatment protocols. But only when necessary to give you a basic understanding and the basis you need to formulate your own opinions of why to use which parameters and when. And sprinkled everywhere throughout, you will be introduced to relevant literature that connects the dots between these two realms.

You WILL be a more consistent and effective laser therapist after reading this book.

— Bryan

Acknowledgments

Being a vet brings many joys to your life; I am so lucky to work for my amazing patients every day. They are our true masters and I keep learning from them in health and disease. Their displays of gratitude and their clinical improvements make me deeply happy, and they are the main reason behind this book: I want as many patients as possible to benefit from laser therapy.

Another joy of being a vet is when you get the chance to work with great colleagues, and I have that opportunity at the university, in private practice, and as a laser therapy consultant. I am very thankful to my fellow vets who showed their trust in me by referring their cases, and to the owners of these animals who decided to choose laser therapy for their beloved animal companions. At the hospital, students, interns, and residents have helped a lot with the cases; they are a daily inspiration, and I am thankful and very proud of them. Dr. K. Gámez Maidanskaia even translated Russian articles for me! Some of the figures have been supplied by kind permission of the Complutense Veterinary Clinical Hospital in Madrid, Spain (see below for details). All the other photographs were taken at Integra Vetersalud Centro Veterinario. This practice is where my colleagues Dr. S. Salgado – who was also essential in helping with goniometry – Dr. M. Bravo, and Dr. P. González are the greatest team to work with and share the same enthusiasm and dedication for our patients, and they absolutely are part of the therapeutic team in the cases.

I would not have dived into laser therapy when I did if I had not met Bryan Stephens; he is to me the brightest mind in laser science, and over the years has always helped me with every technical question I could possibly have, in the most clear and straightforward way. Working with him is such a pleasure, and I would not have wanted to start this project without him. Mr. S. Francisco always gave me his trust and I am so thankful for that. Thank you also to Dr. S. Barabas for the support and the insight into daily practice in the UK.

Being a vet also poses many challenges, and an almost constant one is to find some kind of balance between your dedication to your profession, which is not just a job, and your family and personal life. Writing this book made that even more difficult, and I thank my dear parents and especially my husband Jose, Señor Perales, for their patience, unconditional support, and understanding of so many stolen evenings, weekends, and holidays. My four-legged family is as important and dear to me, and this book is dedicated to them, the ones that sleep by my side and the ones that await downstream.

Another very patient person was our wonderful editor, Sarah Hulbert; I would like to thank her for the support and for always being so understanding, charming, and professional.

It has taken years to build up the knowledge and courage to write this book. There are of course too many people to thank on this page for all the guidance, knowledge, experience, perspective, interactions, and support through those years. But my biggest thanks go to two beautiful boys ... my best friends in this world: Quinn and Cooper. Daddy loves you, and is lucky to have you.

About the images in the book

- Case no. 8 in Chapter 7 (with Figures C8.1, C8.3, and C8.6) and Case no. 17 in Chapter 9 (with Figures C17.3a and C17.4a) were first reported in *Veterinary Times*.[1]

- In Chapter 9, Figures C13.1a, C13.1b, C13.2a, C13.2b, C13.3a, C13.3b, and C13.4 in Case no. 13; and Figures C17.1a, C17.1b, and C17.2 in Case no. 17 are courtesy of Dr. I. García Real and Dr. P. García Fernández, Complutense Veterinary Teaching Hospital Madrid, Spain; with permission.

- In Chapter 9, Figures C20.1, C20.4, and C20.6 in Case no. 20; and Figures C22.1, C22.6, and C22.7 in Case no. 22 are courtesy of Dr. I. García Real and Dr. J. Rodríguez Quirós, Complutense Veterinary Teaching Hospital Madrid, Spain; with permission.

- Figures 3.3 to 3.6 in Chapter 3; Figures 7.1 to 7.4, 7.6, 7.8a, 7.10, 7.13, 7.14 and case study Figures C3.2, C5.1, C9.1 to C9.5, C11.1, C11.2, and C12.1 to C12.7 in Chapter 7; and case study Figures C17.3 to C17.8, C22.2 to C22.5, and C24.1 to C24.3 in Chapter 9, were taken at the Complutense Veterinary Clinical Hospital in Madrid, Spain; with permission.

- All other photographs in the book regarding clinical cases, therapeutic procedures, and goniometry were taken at Integra Vetersalud Centro Veterinario, Majadahonda, Spain.

Abbreviations

AA	arachidonic acid		IGF	insulin-like growth factor
ALP	alkaline phosphatase		IL	interleukin
ALT	alanine aminotransferase		IL-1RA	interleukin 1 receptor antagonist
ATP	adenosine triphosphate		iNOS	inducible nitric oxide synthase
BDNF	brain-derived neurotrophic factor		IRIS	International Renal Interest Society
bFGF	basic fibroblast growth factor		IVDD	intervertebral disk disease
BRONJ	biphosphonate-related osteonecrosis of jaws		LCADSS	Localized Canine Atopic Dermatitis Severity Score
CBPI	Canine Brief Pain Inventory		LED	light-emitting diode
CCLR	cranial cruciate ligament rupture		LOAD	Liverpool Osteoarthritis in Dogs
CNS	central nervous system		LOX	lipoxygenase
CE	Conformité Européenne		LPVAS	Localized Pruritic Visual Analogue Score
CO	carbon monoxide		LT	laser therapy
COAST	Canine Osteoarthritis Staging Tool		LTX	leukotrienes
COI	Canine Orthopedic Index		LTB$_4$	leukotriene B4
COX	cyclooxygenase		MC	male castrated
CT	computed tomography		MFS	Modified Frankel Score
CW	continuous wave		MMP	matrix metalloproteinase
DC	duty cycle		MNC	male, non-castrated
DJD	degenerative joint disease		MRI	magnetic resonance imaging
DNA	deoxyribonucleic acid		MSC	mesenchymal stem cells
EGF	epidermal growth factor		NAALT	North American Association for Photobiomodulation Therapy
eNOS	endothelial nitric oxide synthase			
Ep	energy per pulse		NGF	nerve growth factor
FDA	Food and Drug Administration		NMES	neuromuscular electrical stimulation
FGF	fibroblast growth factor		nNOS	neuronal nitric oxide synthase
FLUTD	feline lower urinary tract disease		NO	nitric oxide
FMPI	Feline Musculoskeletal Pain Index		NOS	nitric oxide synthase
fp	pulse frequency		NRS	numerical rating scales
FS	female spayed		NSAID	non-steroidal anti-inflammatory drug
GABA	gamma-amino butyric acid		OA	osteoarthritis
IBD	inflammatory bowel disease		*Pa*	average power
ICAM-1	intercellular adhesion molecule-1		PAH	pulmonary arterial hypertension
IG-E	immunoglobulin E		PAF	platelet activating factor

PCR	polymerase chain reaction		TLT	transcranial laser therapy
PDGF	platelet-derived growth factor		TNF	tumor necrosis factor
PGE2	prostaglandin E2		TP	trigger point
PGI_2	prostacyclin		TPLO	tibial plateau leveling osteotomy
PLA_2	phospholipase A2		TTA	tibial tuberosity advancement
PMF	pulsed magnetic field		TU	therapeutic ultrasound
Pp	peak power		TSCIS	Texas Spinal Cord Injury Score
PRP	platelet-rich plasma		TSH	thyroid stimulating hormone
RNS	reactive nitrogen species		Tx	treatment
ROM	range of motion		TXA2	thromoboxane A2
ROS	reactive oxygen species		UV	ultraviolet
SIRS	systemic inflammatory response syndrome		VAS	visual analogue scales
SSI	surgical site infection		VCAMs	vascular cell adhesion molecules
TBI	traumatic brain injury		VEGF	vascular endothelial growth factor
TCM	Traditional Chinese Medicine		WALT	World Association of Laser Therapy
TCVM	Traditional Chinese Veterinary Medicine		WSAVA	World Small Animal Veterinary Association
TENS	transcutaneous electrical stimulation			
TGF	transforming growth factor		WHS	Wound Healing Society

Some of what you will see

His vs. hers

As you've read in the Preface and you will see throughout the book, we (each author) have written our chapters somewhat independently. We've obviously collaborated on this book (as well as in real-life laser cases), but we've each got our own little niche, and so were keen to give autonomy to the other. That said, you may see these little icons appear from time to time when one of us has a comment on the other's work that we think at that point in the text will help you keep the balance of scientific and clinical perspective. Hopefully you can guess which is which. And no, Bryan doesn't look anything like his icon.

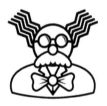 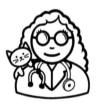

Colored boxes

You will see some colored boxes at places in the text where there is something important to say, but not necessarily directly in the flow of the surrounding text. They could be example calculations or case studies or asides.

As another way to keep some balance, each of us has written a short summary of the other author's chapters. These are not meant as *"Cliff's Notes" that bullet-point all the ideas of the chapter. Instead they are some take-home points from each chapter that (we hope) will help transition to the next. Chapters 10 and 11 don't have these summaries since we co-wrote them.*

Introduction: light as a healing tool

One brute fact on which the rest of this book builds is that light can cause physiological changes in the body. The extent of these changes will be explored much further, but if you have trouble with this basic premise, try reconciling our ability to see without first accepting that light can initiate chemical reactions that lead to electrical impulses (and as it turns out, vice versa) that deeply affect our living selves.

A long time ago, however, people realized that the human eye only sees a fraction of the light around us. Among other things, this usually obstructs our understanding that different kinds of light can penetrate through things that visible light cannot. Eventually the field of radiography was born, and now we take this idea as a given. But you picked up this book to learn about a different flavor of light (the infrared) and what kind of physiological changes it can initiate that can help your patients. The hallmarks of laser therapy (LT) are how it helps in different stages of healing, as well as its anti-inflammatory and analgesic properties. These are interrelated, since tissue healing involves a certain degree of inflammatory response, and more inflammation usually means more pain (not this simple, but we will discuss this in detail later).

Tissue healing involves hemostasis, inflammation, a variable amount of debridement/resorption, proliferation, and remodeling or maturation. Briefly, what we see in practice is that LT makes tissue leave the inflammatory phase to go into the repair (anabolic) phase faster, progressing to its own homeostasis. In an acute injury this means faster healing; chronic inflammation leads to non-healing ulcers, degenerative diseases, and chronic pain, to mention a few, so exiting that state is also a basic and general therapeutic target. This anti-inflammatory effect is based both in the metabolic improvement of the tissue (more oxygen, more ATP) and the decrease in inflammatory mediators.

Of course different tissues exhibit their particularities in the healing or repair process: wound healing is different from bone healing. Tissue proliferation may take days to weeks, and may be achieved by primary or secondary healing. Both involve fibroblast recruitment, extracellular matrix deposition, and angiogenesis; LT influences all of these processes, from new blood vessel formation, fibroblast proliferation, differentiation, and migration, to osteoblastic activity as well as collagen production.[2]

Laser increases platelet-derived growth factor (PDGF) and basic fibroblast growth factor (bFGF), among other growth factors, which have a stimulating effect on the growth of fibroblasts.[3] The magnitude of this increase is about threefold to sixfold compared to control cultures in some studies.[4] There will be more fibroblasts, and they will be working more efficiently, producing more collagen.[5, 6] Not all collagen is the same, though. In the earlier stages of tissue healing the synthesis of type III collagen is higher, but then a lot of this is gradually replaced by type I collagen fibers, which are more resistant, better organized, and also predominate in normal intact tissue. LT improves tensile strength by increasing the amount of type I collagen.[7, 8] This remodeling phase starts while proliferation is still happening, but can go on for months. More extracellular matrix is synthesized, but at the same time degraded, and cellularity and vascularity decrease. There is further contraction in the case of wounds, and if the process happens correctly, the resulting tensile strength increases because of a proper alignment of collagen fibers, thickening of the skin layers, and cartilage and bone mineralization, depending on the tissue type. LT has been proven to influence these processes, speeding up the rate at which they take place and improving the final result.

This brief list of positive effects is intended to get one thing off the table right away: we know that laser works. That was a good question about 10 to 20 years ago. We have enough evidence (a lot of which we will show in the coming chapters) that it works to promote healing, modulate inflammation, and decrease pain. Of course experimental animal studies are more abundant and additional clinical studies should be carried out, but there are actually high quality trials, reviews, and meta-analysis of LT that support this. Our goal from here on is to dig into how we can do things better.

Note about the terms laser therapy and photobiomodulation

In this book we use the term "laser therapy" (and its abbreviation "LT") almost exclusively in reference to this beneficial, non-destructive, light-based modality. The more robust and increasingly popular term is "photobiomodulation," which does admittedly tell the story better since it is a story of light (from a laser, LED, etc.) enhancing the body's natural healing mechanisms. The reason we use LT instead of PBM is that, as you'll be able to tell very quickly, the tone of this book is very conversational. And as such, we want you to hear us talking through the words. We don't want you stumbling over the mouthful that is the internal pronunciation of photobiomodulation. Laser therapy is much easier to say (even in your head) and so we'll stick with that.

PART 1

Light's actions in the body

CHAPTER 1

Light is just the catalyst

"Goodbye," said the fox. "And now here is my secret, a very simple secret: It is only with the heart that one can see rightly; what is essential is invisible to the eye."

— Antoine de Saint-Exupéry

After reading that last section you should feel like Harry Potter with the Elder Wand in your hand as you wield your laser. It is a powerful tool. But now it's time to burst your bubble and tell you that light doesn't do ANY of that. If you shine light on a vial of growth factors, you will get a slightly warmer vial of growth factors, nothing more. The body can, however, be triggered to synthesize more of them. In fact, all of the effects we just highlighted are simply enhancements of the body's ability to regulate itself in a positive direction. And light can be that catalyst in a completely non-invasive way. In order to do so, it has to be absorbed, and by something that is somewhere early in the chain of interactions that causes the body to release those growth factors. The really cool part is that the body is so good at communication within itself that the initial trigger of these eventual events can be seemingly unrelated to the desired effect. More on that later, but first, what does it even mean for something to absorb light?

When you spill water on the table, you use a paper towel to "absorb" the water. But that is not the same. The water molecules are still completely intact, they have just bonded with the particles in the towel. Then you simply move them somewhere else, by either throwing them into the trash or wringing them down the drain. With light, though, the story is different. Light comes into an interaction, but does not come out. So what is light and how can this be explained?

1.1 Electromagnetic radiation

Light has some very cool properties, both classical and quantum-mechanical (in fact, both at the same time), and can be described in a bunch of different ways. But before you get scared off by the scary "quantum" word, let's simplify this pragmatically. Light is simply an oscillating electric and magnetic field. We call the distance between any two peaks of this oscillation the wavelength of light. One important, but somewhat obvious feature of light is that it always travels at the same speed (in a vacuum; we'll get to what happens in a medium later). That said, another equivalent way to define light is by the frequency, i.e. the number of oscillation cycles per unit of time. (NOTE: This is not to be confused with pulse frequency or repetition rate. That has to do with turning light on and off periodically. We'll get to that later.) Since we know the wave's propagation speed (distance traveled per unit of time), if we know how many times it oscillates, we also know the distance between oscillations, and vice versa (Fig. 1.1).

The ONLY fundamental difference between the different flavors of light is this one-dimensional scale of the oscillating wave, whether you are referring to it as wavelength or frequency. In fact, depending on the region of the full spectrum of light (fittingly enough, called the electromagnetic spectrum), one or the other of these quantities is preferred. My favorite AM sports radio station when I was growing up broadcasted using light at 660 kHz (frequency); I heated up my coffee in the microwave this morning with light at 2.45 GHz (also frequency); but my favorite color is 450 nm (wavelength of blue light). Indeed these are all just different colors of light; the human eye only evolved to contain

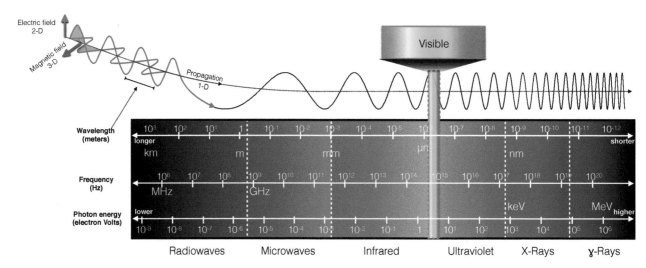

Figure 1.1 Structure of light as an electromagnetic wave (top). You can also see the scale of photon energy across the full electromagnetic spectrum.

cones that can detect wavelengths from about 390–700 nm, which is what we call the visible part of the spectrum. The near-infrared spans from about 700–1100 nm. I'll bounce between these descriptions (wavelength and frequency) many times, but either one of them tells the whole story.

This is the full, classical picture of light as it pertains to the kinds of therapy discussed in this book, i.e. non-ionizing (and in particular, visible and infrared) light incident on living biological tissue. There is so much more interesting stuff to learn about light, but not much of it will help you in the clinic, so we will not cover it here.

OK, one more tidbit because it's cool and head-spinning and it will affect how we talk about light a little later on: it turns out that the energy of light is directly proportional to its frequency (and therefore inversely proportional to its wavelength). To compound this, the amount of energy any "piece" of light carries is discrete or "quantized." These individual packets of light are called photons and make up the quantum picture of light.

The main question remains: why does frequency, this one characteristic of this phenomenon we call light, determine such a broad range of implications, i.e. from destruction to manipulation, from imaging to therapy?

Oddly enough, that question boils down to a different kind of question: what happens when something that wiggles bumps into something else that wiggles? We've already established that light can be described as an oscillating field. Well, matter is made up of atoms, groups of them called molecules, and big groups of them called tissues. Inside the atom, electrons are orbiting the nucleus in a cloud that has some structure to it and has an equilibrium state. Molecules are atoms connected by bonds, which are made up of some sharing of these electron clouds and which also have an equilibrium state. And most of the equilibrium states of these entities are electrically neutral. This doesn't mean that there are no charged particles, but rather that there are as many positively charged things as there are negatively charged things.

But light is an oscillating electromagnetic field, and charged particles in this kind of field experience a force. So shining light on matter exerts a force on these equilibrium states, and as it passes by, the matter creates some recoil force, much like a spring (warning: we physicists use the concept of springs to explain everything). The force experienced by the matter is proportional to the energy of the field (frequency of the light) and the mass and charge of the particles (atomic/molecular structure) of the matter.

So matter, in effect, is just a bunch of charged atomic nuclei tied together with a bunch of springs. The types of interactions you get, then, are simply regulated by the frequency of oscillation of the light and how this corresponds to the frequency of oscillation of the bonds of the things they bump into.

1.2 Absorbing light

Absorption happens when the frequency of light is close to the natural frequency of the thing it interacts with. Just like pushing a child on a swing, if you push in sync with the natural rhythm, you can transfer the most energy of your push to the child. But as I mentioned above, light is "quantized," so this energy transfer is an all-or-nothing kind of thing: you don't absorb a piece of a photon. If a photon of light transfers all of its energy to the incident matter, we call that an absorption event.

On the atomic scale, the transitions between electron energy levels correspond to light's frequency in the X-ray region of the spectrum, which is why X-rays interact strongly with atoms, so much so that individual electrons can be knocked completely out of orbit in what is called ionization. This kind of process leads to all sorts of sporadic and dangerous effects, because when an atom is missing an electron, it does whatever it can to steal one from another atom, and the chain continues. Molecular bonds can be broken and whole molecules can be destroyed this way. In fact, more than two-thirds of all light-induced mammalian DNA damage happens when water becomes ionized into what's called a hydroxyl radical.

On the molecular level, though, the bonds are much more flimsy, i.e. they have much slower natural frequencies (which makes sense because bigger things move more slowly), and so light in the visible and infrared range takes over the interactions. And because lower frequency means less energy, the interactions are often not as catastrophic to the matter. Instead, the molecular bonds that absorb the incident light's energy wiggle and twist and stretch and contract. Though smaller in magnitude, these types of molecular manipulations lead to all types of changes in chemistry (more on this in section 1.3).

Absorption, even of visible and infrared light, is not always calm, though. If matter has a particular bond with a natural frequency that coincides with the incident light, and a lot of light is used, the absorption events lead to re-enforced vibrations that create heat and can literally shake molecules apart. This is why putting things that contain water (e.g. most of your food) in the microwave, which uses light with a frequency (and therefore energy) that is 200,000 times less than visible light, heats your food much better than holding that day-old pizza next to your desk lamp, however bright it may be. The bonds in water have a huge absorption peak (a resonant frequency of bending/twisting) in the microwave region of the spectrum. This same idea is used in surgical lasers to ablate tissue in a very efficient, localized way.

In general, then, targeting something in tissue with your laser means finding something in the cells of that tissue that does something productive when it absorbs light, determining the resonant frequency of that something, then using the color of light that coincides with that frequency. Simple. So what in the body absorbs light and what happens once it does?

1.3 Light's bio-targets

Here I need to remind you that this is not a textbook on light. Instead it is a useful guide to laser therapy. For that reason, the following discussion is limited to the interactions of light in the visible-to-near-infrared portion of the spectrum, where therapy lasers (all of them) live. And the focus is on things that are present in sufficient quantity in the body to be worth mentioning. Luckily for us, there are only a few.

The most prolific substance in the body happens to be one of the main absorbers of infrared light in the body: water. Volumes of textbooks have been written on water and its role in the sustenance of life, but the fact is, the molecule itself is actually very simple: two hydrogen molecules bond (i.e. share electrons) with one oxygen molecule. If you can get this pair of bonds bouncing and wiggling around, water can do some wonderful things. We'll explore more of this soon, but for now, target number one is water.

Absorber number two of light in the body is melanin. This is the pigment in the skin and hair/fur that gives it the appearance of color. In the visible region of light, the amount of dark or light you see tells you which kind and how much light that material absorbs or reflects. Let me explain. Black is not really a color. To the contrary, black is the lack of color. So if you see something that is black, that material is absorbing most of the visible light shining on it, and therefore reflecting very little of it back for your eye to see. White is the combination of all light. So when you see something white, much less of that light is being absorbed; rather most of it is being reflected back to your eye. How about something in the middle?

Grass is green. That is to say, it has lots of chlorophyll that needs to absorb light for photosynthesis. So would shining green or, say, red light be better for plant growth? Well, if the grass is green, then it reflects most of the green light back to your eye, which means it doesn't absorb green very well. If you used red light instead, a greater proportion would be absorbed. Why are greenhouses green then? Probably because that's more aesthetically pleasing to the eye. But in principle, a green-tinted glass would act like a filter of green light, allowing through a greater proportion of what is left (white light minus the green), which would therefore be a more efficient illuminator of the chlorophyll.

Well, the same holds with melanin. Darker skin contains more melanin, which absorbs visible light more strongly, and also, as it turns out, near-infrared light. This is no accident. We have evolved skin to protect us from the sun's light. Again, it is no accident that the majority of the sun's light is in the visible and near-infrared range. In fact, only about 6% of the sun's light is in the ultraviolet (UV) range. The reason we care so much about this is that UV is ionizing light, meaning that with a single photon it can break a chemical bond and cause cellular damage, or worse, a genetic mutation. That is worse because if one of your cells dies, you have 10,000,000,000,000 more to back it up. If one of your cells mutates, however, that can lead to a whole mess of altered cells that multiply faster than normal cells and spread through the bloodstream to other places where they multiply further. This is called cancer.

But back to the infrared. We've evolved with melanin to protect us from sunlight, but that protection wanes as you creep from the visible to the infrared, and by the time you get to about 900 nm and greater, absorption by melanin disappears and the skin is virtually invisible. So, for the shorter wavelengths, melanin acts like a barrier to light passing through the body, but as wavelength increases, its effect becomes negligible.

Absorbers #1 (water) and #2 (melanin) absorb best on opposite sides of the spectrum: water on the longer wavelengths (> 950 nm) and melanin on the shorter wavelengths (< 750 nm). This creates a valley in the spectrum where the body is most transparent. Light in this region can make it past the skin without burning a hole and into the body without "searing the meat." For that reason, we call it the "therapeutic window."

Regardless of what other absorbers we talk about next, their action outside this window is pretty much pointless, because even if their absorption led to the growth of magic pixie dust in your cells, you really couldn't get enough light there to initiate the magic. Fortunately for us, targets #3 and #4 do in fact absorb well in this window.

Hemoglobin is at the heart of red blood cells. It is comprised of an iron core and four "claws" of folded proteins. Combined, they can quite literally "hold" molecular oxygen (four molecules of O_2). It is this iron core that absorbs light very well, mostly because iron is a very heavy element compared to the organic chemistry (mostly carbon and oxygen) around it, and so it acts as a nice contrast agent, especially in the near-infrared close to its peak of absorption at 905 nm.

Lastly, an enzyme called cytochrome c oxidase located on the membrane of the mitochondria inside your cells absorbs near-infrared light. Much like hemoglobin, this enzyme absorbs principally because of its relatively heavy core of copper. Also like hemoglobin, this enzyme "carries" molecular oxygen, but this time within the cell as it works through the respiratory chain in the process that produces adenosine triphosphate (ATP), which the body uses as chemical energy.

More on what happens next – next, but by and large, that's it. Nothing much else in the body absorbs enough light, at least the colors of light that can get inside the body, strongly enough to do anything meaningful chemically. That makes things simpler to understand, actually. The other keywords you'll hear throughout the book, things that clearly have a positive healing effect on individual cells and bulk tissue and were triggered by light, must have gotten their power from some process that these four targets started when they absorbed the light. So, what are some of those things?

As a veterinarian, I would like to say that there are some cells and molecules that ARE susceptible to light that doesn't otherwise penetrate well into the *body. For example, we know that vitamin D synthesis depends on UV light incident on the skin. Some chemical compounds such as bilirubin can lead to photosensitization. And of course, the cells in our retina transform light into electrical impulses. But like he said, most of the effects in the cells come from these principal interactions.*

1.4   Absorption leads to ...

1.4.1   Heat

Heat is defined as the energy contained in a set of moving particles. So if anyone asks you how hot a single particle is, you yell at them. Heat is collective motion. Why would it be hard to believe, then, that the primary action of light (a wiggling electromagnetic wave) when it is absorbed by (i.e. transfers all of its energy to) a slab of matter (a bunch of really light particles attached by very "boingy" springs) is the generation of heat. Things that move (or in this case vibrate) cause – or in fact are defined as – heat. And I hate to ruin the surprise, but that's pretty much all infrared light does in the body: it creates little packets of heat where it gets absorbed.

I forgot to tell people who sell lasers to put their earmuffs on. Because they have been fighting against the notion that healing comes from heating the tissue for over a decade now. They fight against people who sell shock wave units or transcutaneous electrical stimulation (TENS) or the skeptics who cling to the "nothing more than a heat pad" argument. And now I'm saying it's all about heat? You should probably stop reading at this point if that's all laser therapy is about, right?

Not so fast. The key words here are "little" and "where." To give some perspective, let's talk about the scale of things. Take 1 joule of energy. That's about as much light as would hit your face in 12 seconds if you were 20 meters away from a 100 watt light bulb. In those 12 seconds you would be hit with about 16,000,000,000,000,000,000 pieces of light and not even notice a bit of warmth from it. So when each of those pieces of light gets absorbed, a very very small amount of heat is transferred. That said, cells are very small things. And molecules are even smaller.

It turns out, then, that a small piece of light has a pretty sizable effect on a small piece of matter like a water molecule. And as light shines, these little photons are getting absorbed at different rates at various depths in the body. So what though? What happens when they do get absorbed?

1.4.2   Changing shape

First, you have to understand that the main way chemistry works (i.e. the way that two molecules combine) is a very sensitive, physical lock-and-key mechanism. Things that fit together nicely (both spatially and electrically) tend to bond together. If they don't fit, they don't bond.

Second, you have to understand what heat does to an object, any object no matter how small: it causes that object to change shape. Remember, heat is just energy in movement. So whatever degrees of freedom

that matter has, the molecules will vibrate along those directions.

1.4.3   Physical chemistry

But changing shape, when it comes to molecules, means changing chemistry. Remember, if two molecules don't fit, they don't bond. And things that didn't fit naturally can fit after being heated. In general, by changing the shape of one part of a molecule, even slightly and even over a very short timescale, you can cause the molecule to shed parts of itself or grab onto new things. This is biochemistry at its very heart. Not a general rise in temperature across bulk tissue, but lots of microscopic heat sources that change what is and isn't bonded at a very small point in the body.

So when you have long chains of enzymes that have lots of parts in their synthesis or consumption processes, small changes can have very big impact, in good ways and bad.

1.4.4   Shapeshifting examples

For a water molecule, that means the O-H bonds will bend and twist and stretch and contract. Since water is in liquid form, and being that all the water molecules in a given area are vibrating to the same frequency of light, these minor absorptions lead to more and more resonance that propagates throughout its volume and cascades into micro-pressure waves.

For a hemoglobin molecule, the absorption in the iron core creates heat that propagates to its protein "claws," changing their folded shape. This is the same shape that naturally holds on tight to oxygen molecules. A slightly deformed shape holds on a little less tightly to that oxygen molecule. The claw doesn't naturally hold on very well to a nitric oxide (NO) molecule. Even though N-O is pretty similar in shape to O-O, the body is smarter than that and so NO–hemoglobin binding is usually very weak. But add a little heat and the claw's shape might be a little more likely to bond.

For cytochrome c oxidase, at one point in its cycle it "accepts" an oxygen molecule, then transports it, then releases it to another enzyme. Add a little heat – in the form of light absorption by that copper core – and the molecule may do this a little faster.

I've posed all this very hypothetically. After all, we can't see these individual molecules change shape in the femtoseconds (10^{-15} s) it takes for the absorption process to occur. We can see the results, though, and all of what I've mentioned here is very demonstrable.

Pressure waves in light-exposed water are very real and they change many properties of water including viscosity, pH, translucency, and permeability. Volumes have been written on the subject.[9–12] Supra-natural oxygenation of blood has been shown to be induced by light incident on hemoglobin.[13–15] We'll get into more of that when we talk about light in the blood. But I want to spend some time on what happens in the cells so we can better understand what the rest of this book is about.

1.5 Light's targets within the cell

In the mitochondria, where ATP (the cell's energy currency) is produced, and where a lot of the incident light is absorbed, some very productive things can be done with light.

First, some quick-and-dirty on how cells metabolize. Insert a full volume of textbooks on cellular biology. When you've spent years reading all of those, one of the only things you'll remember is a fundamental process called the electron transport chain (Fig. 1.2), which ends up with the production of ATP. On the membrane of a cell's mitochondria lives a complex that synthesizes ATP, quite conveniently called ATP synthase. The fuel for this complex is a cross-membrane proton potential. All this means is that when there are more

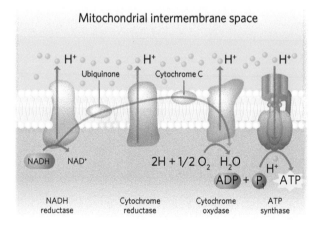

Figure 1.2 The electron transport chain. Once oxygen gets to the cell and migrates to the mitochondria, these membrane-based complexes act on it until ATP is produced by ATP synthase.

Illustrator: Elaine Leggett.

hydrogen ions (protons) outside the mitochondria than there are on the inside, this complex likes to produce ATP. Within this chain there are several processes that move electrons along and pump protons up and out of the mitochondria. The last and most powerful of these pumps happens inside the cytochrome oxidase complex. It involves an oxygen molecule (O_2) combining with four electrons and eight internal protons to create two water molecules (H_2O) and pumping four protons out.

So next time your kid (or grandkid) asks you why you need oxygen, you tell them it is the final electron acceptor in the electron transport system. Mr. Solomon, my ninth grade biology teacher, told me I'd use that once more in my life. Shout out!

1.5.1 Cytochrome C

This is the last "push" needed to turn the ATP synthase engine and produce a molecule of ATP. The mobile carrier that delivers the electrons to cytochrome oxidase is called cytochrome c, and so when they meet and cytochrome c delivers its electrons, it is called (again, quite fittingly) cytochrome c oxidase. But it only delivers electrons one at a time, and the oxygen molecule needs four of them for cytochrome oxidase to do its thing. So it has to go back and forth four times for each ATP molecule.

Enter, the light. Here is one of the most significant findings of laser research – ever – first discovered by Tiina Karu: "[laser irradiation] causes either a (transient) relative reduction of ... cytochrome c oxidase, or its (transient) relative oxidation, depending on the initial redox status."[16] In English? This means that if cytochrome c is in possession of an electron it is more likely to oxidate, i.e. give up its electron (thereby increasing its oxidation state) to cytochrome oxidase. And as if that wasn't cool enough, the converse is also true, that if cytochrome c is not in possession of an electron, it is more likely to reduce, i.e. accept an electron (thereby reducing its oxidation state) from its predecessor complex when it absorbs light.

This is the double whammy. Cytochrome needs to do both things in its natural process, called a "redox" cycle (see how they did that with the name: reduction plus oxidation equals redox). And light helps both, in whichever way the cell needs it to at that moment to produce more ATP. This can happen on very very short timescales, and so the more light incident on a cell in a given time period (say, as the hand-piece is being moved over the treatment area), the more ATP can be produced in cells. This phenomenon is what people call photobiomodulation, the increase in natural cellular function via the use of light.

1.5.2   Nitric oxide: a not-so-secondary effect

There is slightly more to the story inside the cell. Nitric oxide (NO) plays a very important role in cell signaling, both within the cell and between cells. An abundance of NO leads mostly to positive cellular function. There is, of course, a ceiling to this effect, where too much NO leads to nitrosative stress, but studies on several different cell lines show that light therapy enhances the production of NO, and within levels that lead to pre-dominantly positive results.[17] This is the "causal" effect that has been well documented: laser promotes the production of NO by somehow enhancing the conversion of nitrosyls (molecules containing the NO+ ion) to NO.[17, 18] But there is also a "resultant" theory. (NOTE: you can read more about NO in Chapter 3.)

N-O and O-O look very similar at the molecular level; the N is only slightly smaller than the O, and so the molecules tend to bind to similar things. This can be very bad, in the same way that C-O (carbon monoxide) binds to similar things as O-O, which will cause the cells to suffocate. If NO binds to things in the cells that need to (and normally do) bind to O_2, cells are inhibited. But the fact that light therapy increases the amount of NO available for the cell (all things being equal), means that it is making better use of the O_2, which is a VERY good thing for the body.

Remember that the cell needs O_2 as the final electron capture agent in the respiratory cycle. Well, NO competes with O_2 for this last electron capture. But again, amounts of extracellular NO have been shown to increase with laser, which means O_2 is being better utilized in more efficient ATP production.

While this is true, certain clinical situations can be particularly susceptible to NO production. For instance, ischemia-reperfusion injury. In a model in which blood flow from the cranial mesenteric artery was occluded for an hour, LT increased tissue damage, at least in the first few hours.[19]

Wow. That's three ways light inside the cell helps the cells function better. It enhances the redox cycle of cytochrome oxidase, which produces more ATP for cells to utilize in their natural functions. It helps produce NO within the cell, which facilitates cell signaling. And at the same time it forces the cells to use O_2 more efficiently, for things the body needs O_2 for (respiration), and makes available more NO for things the cells need NO for (cell signaling). Pretty cool.

So this is how light can enhance the usage of oxygen once it gets into the cell. But that is only the tail end of the circuit. This is akin to squeezing really hard on the nozzle of your garden hose in the hope of hosing down your burning trashcan without first opening the spigot past a slow drip. Without a plentiful supply of oxygen, the heightened efficiency of the cell will have little effect on the clinical outcome. There must be some way to increase local oxygenation with laser therapy …

Summary from a different perspective

Light can have a therapeutic effect if it penetrates the skin and gets absorbed by certain molecules. For light to penetrate the skin, wavelength is the first limiting factor. The therapeutic window is around 700–1000 nm. Melanin acts as a barrier by absorbing light in the visible to 750 nm range, but is more transparent to longer wavelengths. Light is absorbed by molecules such as H_2O, melanin, hemoglobin, and cytochrome c oxidase. The right type and amount of light can have the effect of increasing temperature, metabolic efficiency, and O_2 delivery.

CHAPTER 2

Blood and light

Don't be afraid of hard work. Nothing worthwhile comes easily. Don't let others discourage you or tell you that you can't do it. In my day I was told women didn't go into chemistry. I saw no reason why we couldn't.

— Gertrude Elion

2.1 Circulation basics

In a very simplified picture of things, the heart creates a massive pressure wave of blood, which like all fluids, will flow through the path of least resistance. This means flowing first through the widest vessels (arteries). In places close to the heart, it will also pass through the smaller vessels (capillaries) pretty forcefully, simply because there is a lot of pressure behind it. As you move farther from the heart, the pressure decreases, but so too does the number of available avenues for the blood, so it still gets to the capillaries. So, on the large scale, the circulatory system is a nothing more than a high-pressure pump with a series of tubes running to and from it.

In the capillaries, however, the flow is much more variable, depending on many smaller, local pressure sources. Whether these are caused by muscle contractions (how do you think blood gets up your leg against gravity on the way back to the heart?) or blockages in adjacent pathways, very small pressure changes can divert blood flow in a significant way.

2.2 Heat … again

It is fairly intuitive that pressure and temperature are related. We are taught this about gases in high school chemistry. But it's harder to make the assumption of constant volume inside a living, moving body made of less-than-rigid tissue. And so it's slightly less intuitive how these two are related when it comes to the circulation.

The first impulse may be to think that more heat equals more pressure. That's how a steam engine works, right? And if you have a sore back, putting a heat pad on it definitely loosens things up: the warmer the pad, the faster the relief. But do you put a heat pad on for 4 hours? No. Why not? First, because the body simply saturates. It's a very well-regulated machine that will soon start to counteract the external (foreign) heat source in order to regulate its own temperature.

But secondly, and perhaps more importantly, it is not the heat itself that causes the circulation of fresh blood into and waste-filled blood away from your aching back. Instead, it is the change in heat that promotes circulation.

What about cold? An ice pack is used for a sprained ankle, and it works very well to decrease the inflammation and get all the excess extracapillary blood away from the area. So low pressure (cold) leads to circulation too. Sort of. Can you leave an ice pack on that ankle for 4 hours? No, and for both the same reasons. The ice pack creates a temporary increase in local circulation not because it is cold, but because is it colder than the tissue around it. When the tissue around it becomes closer in temperature to the ice pack, the effect is quashed.

It is the creation of temperature differences (or gradients) that causes changes in pressure that lead to increased motion of fluid through vessels. Those differences can be temporal (in time) or spatial (in space): temporal being 20 minutes on, 20 minutes off with the ice pack, and spatial being hot here and cold there, right next to it. Both of these effects are present in the act of laser therapy.

As we've discussed, a beam of light is made up of lots and lots of tiny photons that are absorbed at various rates at various depths within the tissue. Microscopically, that means a lot of "hots" and "colds" throughout the tissue, which force blood through different pathways. And though we talk about arteries, veins, and capillaries as little tubes, the majority of the blood flow in the body is more akin to "seepage" through bulk tissue. This kind of fluid motion is even more susceptible to slight pressure differences, without the fixed boundaries that restrict blood flow in the vessels.

And temporally, you are consistently moving the path of light throughout a therapy session. In contrast to the slow results obtained using conduction, as seen with the ice pack, the energy of light is converted into heat in the tissue almost instantly. So you are continually producing lots of tiny "hots," whose heat very quickly dissipates on a microscopic scale. Moving the beam away from a site, however quickly, will cause a hot–cold pressure wave that gently guides blood to, through, and from the area.

This principle is demonstrated by an old anecdote from the early days of laser use in podiatry. Physicians were attempting to use laser to treat gout, which is basically an overabundance of uric acid in the foot. They began by simply treating the foot, but their patients complained of even more intense pain after treatment. Some doctors were discouraged; others were curious, as was I. Before long, we explored the actual mechanisms of treatment and realized that in order for laser to even have a chance of helping these patients, it would have to get the uric acid out of the foot and back through the lymphatic system to be excreted out of the body. Well, you wouldn't be able to do that by just treating the foot. You'd first have to open up some pathways for the uric acid to leave. So we began treating down the back of the knee during the first stages of therapy, then focusing on the foot, then finishing back up the leg, and voilà, no more pain. We first opened the lymphatic pathways, then pushed (against gravity) all that waste-filled blood back to the center of the body, where there was a much greater blood flow and where it could be scrubbed by the liver, kidneys, and lungs. Simply creating a series of temperature gradients along the path of the blood circulation lead to enough pressure differences to be clinically impactful.

While this is not usually necessary in practice, you really want to use it in cases of severe edema. Consider the lymphosomes or lymphatic territories involved.[20] For instance, if you have severe edema in a tarsus, treat the inguinal and popliteal areas first.

2.3 Push vs. pull

I use the word "push" for effect, but in fact this is only part of the truth (the lesser part). Once blood leaves the arteries and enters the capillaries, there are a combination of forces (beyond systolic blood pressure) that govern how well it perfuses into the tissue. Some of the forces push blood out of the capillaries: arterial pressure pushes outward and tissue oncotic pressure pulls blood into the tissues. Opposing these are forces keeping the blood in the capillaries: capillary oncotic pressure is holding the water inside while venal pressure is pulling the blood through the capillaries back toward the heart. These forces are in virtual equilibrium and so the perfusion rate of blood is relatively constant over time, even though it is highly skewed depending how far along a capillary you are: the closer to the artery, the greater the blood perfusion; the closer to the vein, the less perfusion, since most of the blood is being sucked back to the heart.

This is fairly intuitive, but what may not be is the fact that venal pressure plays a much bigger role in capillary pressure than does arterial pressure: five times bigger, in fact.[21] This means that even a fractional change in venal pressure can result in a significant change in the blood perfusion along a capillary. It is important to keep this in mind as you deliver therapy: it is more impactful to "pull" blood away from the area (or at least clear the way downstream) than it is to try to push blood through it.

2.4 Vasodilation: nitric oxide rearing its head again

We discussed earlier how light helps to produce nitric oxide (NO): by directly enhancing the nitrosyl reduction process to produce more NO, and by indirectly forcing the cell to make better use of its O_2, which often has to compete against NO for some local binding effect. In all cases, this means an increased abundance of NO available both inside and outside the cell. Besides its function in cell signaling, NO serves as a potent vasodilator when it is available outside the cell. After all, when the body senses a threat (whether an ischemic event or another local stimulus), it naturally secretes NO as the principle catalyst for vasodilation.

We'll cover the anti-inflammatory effect in more detail in Chapter 3, but microscopically (within the cell), this is a very important light-induced enhancement. Vasodilation not only increases local circulation, but also increases the permeability of the vessels, meaning more nutrients can pass from the blood to the damaged cells that need them. First and foremost of these nutrients is oxygen.

2.5 Oxygenation

The basis of oxygenation in the body revolves around hemoglobin. As mentioned earlier, this is a four-clawed molecule with an iron core that can bind to up to four oxygen molecules. The empty claws make their way to the lungs where they grab onto oxygen molecules,

since in that environment there is a very high "partial oxygen pressure" (i.e. a local surplus of oxygen). They hold on as they travel through the body in blood vessels until they find themselves in an environment with a low enough partial oxygen pressure (i.e. a local deficiency of oxygen), at which point they begin to dissociate and release their oxygen locally.

Part of hemoglobin's beauty is how efficient this process becomes. Figure 2.1 is a plot of the hemoglobin dissociation curve, where the percent oxygen saturation of hemoglobin is plotted against this partial pressure (sometimes called oxygen tension, since it refers to how strongly the oxygen is being pulled out of hemoglobin). This "slippery slope" is most easily understood like this: when the empty (0% saturated) hemoglobin is in the lungs (bottom left of the curve), capture of the first oxygen molecule is relatively difficult, but then after that first oxygen capture (the jump to 25% oxygen saturation, with one out of the four possible oxygen molecules bound), the slope becomes very steep, meaning capturing oxygen molecules two, three, and four is much easier.

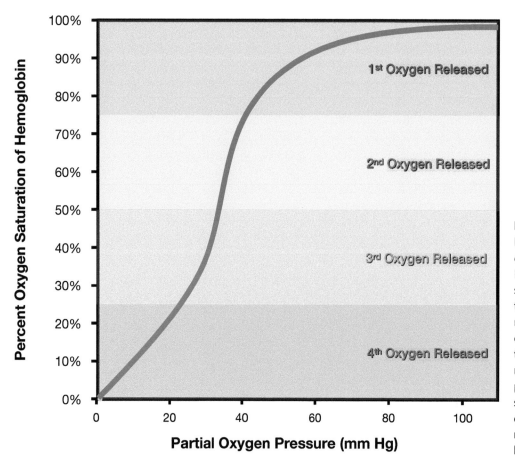

Figure 2.1 The hemoglobin dissociation curve. Notice the extra-steep slope in the middle of the curve. This is the reason for the cascade of oxygen binding (in the lungs) or oxygen release (in the distal parts of the circulatory system). Laser therapy can trigger this release mechanism in a localized way.

The exact same thing works in the opposite direction. To see how this works in the tissues, where hemoglobin has all four oxygen molecules bound, look again at the unique shape of the hemoglobin dissociation curve (Fig. 2.1). Fully oxygenated blood is on the top right of this curve (near 100% O_2 saturation). As you lose one oxygen molecule (equivalent to 25% of a single hemoglobin molecule's capacity), you move left and down on the curve toward 75% saturation. At that point, you can see that the curve is a much more slippery slope, and so the release of oxygen molecules two, three, and four (equivalent to moving to 50%, 25%, and 0% saturation) happens much more quickly.

Why, you ask? Well this is chemistry, remember, and chemistry is all about the shape of molecules. When one of hemoglobin's claws binds to an oxygen molecule (or releases it), the shape of the rest of the molecule changes in such a way that oxygen is more likely to be caught (or released) by the other claws. But what did we just finish discussing in Chapter 1 about how light interacts with these complexes? Light absorption in the iron core (heme group) of hemoglobin will cause a short-lived, tiny temperature change in the molecule. But that's all it takes. Not only does it take just a tiny bit of heat for a short time to trigger one of these claws to change form slightly, but if you do that just once (and force the first of the claws to release its oxygen), a cascade of oxygen release will follow. This is a four-for-one efficient process that can be triggered by just a little bit of light.

Summary from a different perspective

A quick summary is necessary here before we start talking about the wider effects of laser. The goal of laser therapy is to enhance the natural processes of the body and its cells. When we breathe in

air, oxygen from the air gets absorbed into the blood, and that blood travels through the vessels to a certain area. At this point, some of the blood releases its oxygen to the tissue. Oxygen then make its way from the outside to the inside of the cells and migrates to the mitochondria, where it is used as an electron acceptor in the respiratory chain of enzymes whose final product is adenosine triphosphate (ATP), the chemical currency the cells use to store and spend energy in their physiological reactions. Laser therapy can enhance this process in three ways.

- *Enhancement #1: light therapy can increase the local circulation, either by causing mini pressure gradients along the path, or promoting vasodilation via localized NO release (wherever the light is absorbed).*
- *Enhancement #2: light therapy can trigger hemoglobin dissociation, and therefore more efficient release of oxygen from the blood to the affected tissue.*
- *Enhancement #3: light therapy can stimulate the mitochondria in the cells to make better use of oxygen, producing more ATP and causing (either directly or indirectly) an increase of NO in the extracellular environment.*

The intervention of light does not fundamentally change the natural process. Instead it enhances the process at several steps along the way and in a variety of different ways. All roads lead to more chemical energy for the cells, given the same input of oxygen through the nose.

Now you'll read about all the wonderful secondary and tertiary effects that come when the cells of the body have a heightened ability to function.

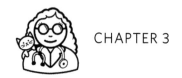

CHAPTER 3

Anti-inflammatory effect

Our own genomes carry the story of evolution, written in DNA, the language of molecular genetics, and the narrative is unmistakable.

— Kenneth R. Miller

The anti-inflammatory effect of laser therapy (LT) is probably the second most reported effect, after wound healing. It can be so significant that in several experimental studies it achieves results similar to well-known non-steroidal anti-inflammatory drugs (NSAIDs) such as indomethacin,[22] meloxicam,[23] or diclofenac.[24]

Let's review what exactly we mean by inflammation before we describe the effects of LT on this process. When we talk about inflammation, the first things that come to mind are probably the well-known signs of heat, tumefaction, redness, pain, and loss of functionality. These are consequences of the phenomena that take place in order to isolate, destroy, and prevent the propagation of noxious stimuli, because inflammation is actually part of the innate, natural, and non-specific defense mechanisms that enable an individual to fight and overcome an aggression.

The response can be triggered by internal (vascular and immune) or external (trauma, temperature, radiation, microorganisms and their toxins, etc.) factors. Different types of cells (e.g. platelets, leukocytes, and endothelial cells) are involved, as well as a broad spectrum of molecules called inflammatory mediators; an analogy can be made with the ingredients of a soup, so this mixture is sometimes referred to as the inflammatory soup. Among the inflammatory cells, which include neutrophils, macrophages, lymphocytes, and eosinophils, some are attracted to the injury site from nearby locations and some are already present, such

as the tissue's own macrophages. A certain degree of activation of the inflammatory cascade is necessary to achieve healing after trauma; the problem is that excessive or abnormal activation of the cascade, or its prolongation, can have serious consequences for the patient, from chronic pain to non-healing ulcers, autoimmune conditions, degenerative diseases, or even carcinogenesis (Fig. 3.1).

3.1 Changing the flavor of the inflammatory soup

It makes sense to try to explain how can LT be anti-inflammatory by breaking down inflammation into its cellular and molecular components. I am not saying it's fun – molecular biology is not as exciting as seeing a huge infected wound heal, of course, but it is what happens behind the scene.

Macrophages, leukocytes, platelets, endothelial cells, fibroblasts – all of these cells produce inflammatory mediators. These molecules are a substantial part of the language spoken by cells. The final clinical outcome depends on the right amount of the right inflammatory mediators at the right time, since their individual actions may vary according to their concentration and time of release – again, like words making sense in a language. There are different classifications of inflammatory mediators, and new ones may be investigated as research progresses. This is going to get a bit hard core and if you are not in the mood, just have a look at Table 3.1 and jump to section 3.2. What follows is a shortened description of the best known inflammatory mediators, with an explanation of how laser has been reported to modulate them. Remember, though,

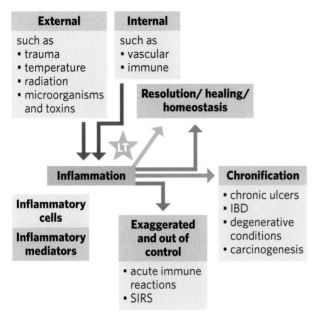

Figure 3.1 Laser does not abolish the inflammatory phase, but modulates the amounts of its components, and by doing so, it seems to help the body resolve the process faster and with better resulting tissue properties. Failure to modulate the inflammatory response is the common core of a very wide variety of clinical entities, and this is one of the reasons why LT is so versatile. In many of these conditions, the pathogenesis implies both an inflammatory component and a failure to properly regulate it. IBD, inflammatory bowel disease; SIRS, systemic inflammatory response syndrome. *Illustrator: Elaine Leggett.*

the global clinical picture is much more complex than each of these effects. Especially when a single mechanism is observed *in vitro*, it should be considered very valuable information but far from a full clinical effect: it would be like comparing a word or a few words with the meaning of a whole conversation.

3.1.1 Vasoactive amines

The most important of these are histamine and serotonin. Both induce an increase in vascular permeability. Histamine is released by mast cells, basophils, and platelets. It induces vasodilation of arterioles and vasoconstriction of larger arteries. Mast cells increase their histamine liberation when irradiated with infrared laser *in vitro*[25] and *in vivo*[26]; however, please remember this is far from being the whole picture and does not necessarily mean the clinical effect is going to be pro-inflammatory, since mast cells can influence not only the destructive events of inflammation but also analgesia and defense mechanisms.[27] Serotonin is also a neurotransmitter and can be found in the nervous system, as well as in platelets and enterochromaffin cells (a special type of neuroendocrine cell). It also plays a role in pain modulation, and **LT may influence its regulation: it increases serotonin levels, which in turn has an analgesic effect**[28, 29]; however, the inflammatory effect is species-dependent.

3.1.2 Acute phase proteins and plasmatic proteases

This category includes the coagulation cascade and the fibrinolytic, complement, and kinin systems. In experimental studies, LT was able to decrease fibrinogen plasma levels.[30] The end product of the kinin system is bradykinin, which attracts neutrophils and other inflammatory cells to the site. It also increases edema and generates pain in the inflamed area. **LT can modulate kinin receptors**[31] **as part of its anti-inflammatory effect.** Acute phase proteins such as C-reactive protein may also increase in response to exercise and muscle stress, and LT may be able to modulate this,[32] although the evidence is still scarce and does not

Table 3.1 Laser therapy has been reported to influence inflammatory mediators from every main group.

Group	Example	Influence of LT reported in literature (ref. nos)
Vasoactive amines	Histamine, serotonin	25–29
Acute phase proteins and plasmatic proteases	Bradykinin	30–32
Lipid mediators	PGE2	23, 33–37
Cytokines	TNF, IL-1, IL-6	38–48
Others	NO, CO, ROS	49–56

Note: some of these effects are described in *in vitro* studies, others *in vivo*, and some in both.

include other acute phase markers such as serum amyloid A or P.

3.1.3 Lipid mediators

These are the targets for most anti-inflammatory treatments, both with steroids and NSAIDs. This group includes platelet activating factor (PAF) and arachidonic acid (AA) derivatives or eicosanoids such as thromboxane A_2 (TXA$_2$), prostacyclin (PGI$_2$), and leukotriene B_4 (LTB$_4$). AA is part of the cell membrane, from where the enzyme phospholipase A_2 (PLA$_2$) detaches it. Once free, AA can be metabolized via prostaglandin-endoperoxide synthase, more commonly known as cyclooxygenase (COX), to form prostanoids (prostaglandins, prostacyclins, and thromboxanes) (Fig. 3.2). AA can also be transformed by the enzyme lipoxygenase (LOX) to form leukotrienes (LTX), which induce smooth muscle contraction, for example in asthma, and participate in chronic inflammation. COX-1 and COX-2 isoforms have been described; COX-1 is constitutive, but although COX-2 also has some physiological functions, it plays a central role in inflammation and hyperalgesia; if overexpression of COX-2 is prevented, so is tissue sensitization associated with inflammation. COX-2 also has a role in carcinogenesis. This was first investigated after observing a lower incidence of colonic cancer in regular NSAID consumers. Its expression is positively correlated with histological grade, infiltration, and staging of tumors. There is debate about COX-3: it has been suggested that this form is more commonly found in vascular and central nervous system (CNS) tissues and may be the target for paracetamol. But before you think about getting rid of all COX-2, remember it also has physiological functions. You may actually remember a famous drug that exclusively inhibited COX-2 and was sold as a super-aspirin, but had to be removed from the market due to cardiovascular risks. Now, how is all this related to LT? Several studies have reported a decrease in COX-2 activity and prostaglandin production at the inflammation site and in the blood and CNS after LT[23, 33–37]; this is probably one of the main anti-inflammatory effects that also influences analgesia. To date, no study has described a relationship between LT and leukotrienes.

3.1.4 Cytokines

Cytokines are a huge family of low molecular weight proteins that mediate intercellular communication and signaling. Almost every nucleated cell can produce cytokines if triggered by particular stimuli, and they play a part in acute and chronic inflammation and other immune processes. They activate other cells (macrophages, eosinophils, natural killer cells) and regulate

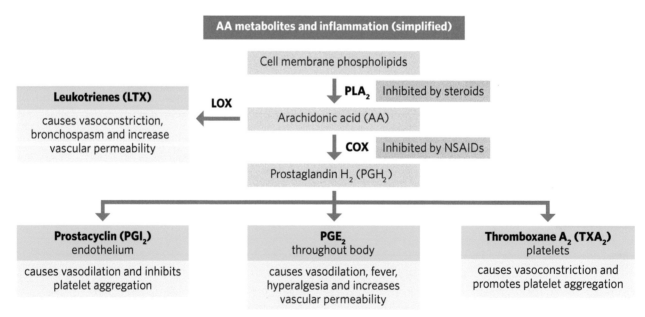

Figure 3.2 A simplified representation of arachidonic acid metabolites and inflammation.
Illustrator: Elaine Leggett.

cell survival, multiplication and apoptosis, tissue repair, and malignant transformation.

Regulation of cytokines is a fine piece of art, a really intricate net, since they may show properties such as antagonism, synergy, and pleiotropy – i.e. the same cytokine can have different effects on different cell lines (like a word can have different meanings depending on the context). They are also involved in downregulation mechanisms, in which the production of one cytokine stimulates the release of other cytokines with the opposite effect.

Some cytokines have kept their original names, for instance transforming growth factor (TGF) and tumor necrosis factor (TNF), while others are named interleukins (IL). Some of them promote inflammation (IL-1, IL-6, IL-8, TNF-α), while others are anti-inflammatory agents (IL-4, IL-10, IL-13, TGF-β). Many of the anti-inflammatory effects of LT are due to the shift in that balance, since it decreases the levels of pro-inflammatory cytokines, while promoting expression of the anti-inflammatory ones (Figs 3.3 and 3.4).

Pro-inflammatory cytokines increase vascular permeability, activate coagulation and lymphocytes, attract neutrophils, and stimulate the liver to release acute phase proteins such as amyloid A and C-reactive protein. The main pro-inflammatory cytokines are IL-1 and TNF-α, which may act synergistically. Regulation of IL-1 activity occurs naturally via the receptor antagonist (IL-1RA), which blocks the IL-1 receptor but does not generate IL-1 activity. IL-1 and TNF-α are released by macrophages and other cell types; they start the inflammatory response when they contact the endothelium, recruit leukocytes, and induce COX-2 synthesis, and are responsible for systemic inflammatory reactions. On the other hand, they promote fibroblast multiplication and collagen synthesis in the tissue repair phase, but with LT we can achieve this without the pro-inflammatory effect. IL-6 also increases during inflammation in proportion to the degree and duration of inflammation, and therefore acts as a diagnostic and prognostic indicator, but is also involved in the activation of anti-inflammatory mechanisms.

The decrease in IL-1, TNF, and IL-6 after LT has been described *in vitro* with different cell lines[38] and

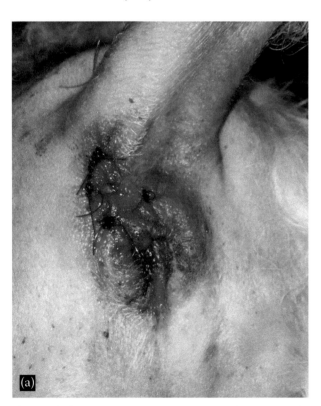
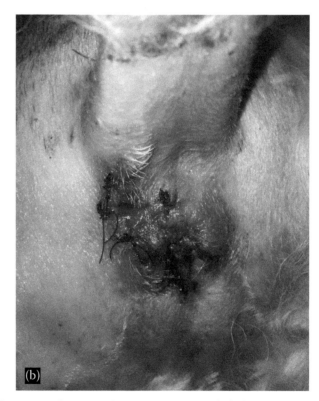

Figure 3.3 Sometimes one treatment is enough to impact the inflammation that is interfering with correct healing. (a) This patient underwent hepatoid adenoma excision and presented 5 days later with wound inflammation and initial dehiscence. His surgeon referred him for a laser treatment; (b) 48 h later the wound had improved enough to continue healing. Treatment dose was 3–4 J/cm², including base of the tail, with 0.2 W/cm².

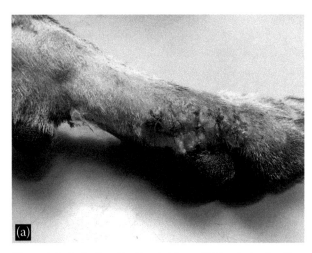
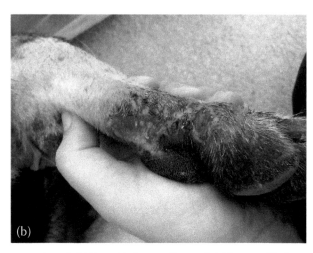

Figure 3.4 A similar situation to Figure 3.3 treated using the same parameters. (a) Wound inflammation and dehiscence 10 days after adenoma surgery. (b) Just one treatment was enough to reverse the situation. This picture was taken 72 h later.

also with *in vivo* experimental models of, for example, chronic nerve compression,[39] myocardial infarction,[40] acute joint inflammation,[41] acute muscle injury,[42] wound healing,[43] asthma and pleurisy[44, 45], among others. The deleterious and distant effects of these mediators, such as smooth airway muscle dysfunction,[46] can also be decreased with LT.

When the inflammatory cascade begins, the body also releases **anti-inflammatory cytokines**, such as IL-4 and IL-10, which inhibit the production of pro-inflammatory cytokines by macrophages and induce lymphocyte apoptosis, and TGF-β, which inhibits lymphoid cell proliferation but promotes multiplication of fibroblasts, osteoblasts, and smooth muscle cells. Other anti-inflammatory mechanisms include cytokine inhibitors, such as IL-1RA, which block the cascade, or at least attenuate the intensity or duration of the phenomena. Infrared light may also contribute to this shift from inflammation to repair, increasing the expression of anti-inflammatory cytokines in asthma models,[45] tendinitis,[47] wound healing,[48] and arthritis models.[41]

3.1.5 Molecule of the year and more

A final, heterogeneous group includes other molecules, like **reactive oxygen species (ROS), nitric oxide (NO), and carbon monoxide (CO).** These are some of the most intricately regulated molecules. For instance, an increase in ROS production can help neutrophils fight microbes better (actually, the respiratory burst they experience is oxygen-dependent; they need about 50 times more oxygen in those circumstances!), and LT

increases this response.[49–52] But an excessive amount of ROS production is damaging to the organs, even fatal, as seen in septic shock and systemic inflammatory response syndrome (SIRS).

With NO, regulation is also complicated and still raises some questions: NO is central to cardiovascular homeostasis, neurotransmission, and the immune response, but its oxidized metabolites are toxic and contribute to inflammation and oncogenesis. NO was named "molecule of the year" in 1992 by the journal *Science*, and more and more roles are still being discovered and investigated, for example in insulin-resistance and neurodegenerative diseases. NO can also react with O_2 to form reactive nitrogen species (RNS), which are produced by macrophages as part of the non-specific antimicrobial cytotoxic response, but these can turn into nitrates, nitrites, and eventually, carcinogenic nitrosamines. So the effect of NO at any given moment may vary in a sort of a bimodal way, depending on the amount and source, among other things. It sounds a bit crazy, but that is one of the wonders of how a living organism works.

NO is synthesized by nitric oxide synthase (NOS). NOS can be isolated in almost any tissue, but the neuronal (nNOS) and endothelial (eNOS) isoforms are expressed constitutively, while the inducible (iNOS) isoform is expressed by cells like leukocytes in response to bacterial lipopolysaccharides or pro-inflammatory cytokines. The cardiovascular effects of NO include endothelium-dependent vascular relaxation and inhibition of platelet aggregation, among others. The isoform iNOS can generate large amounts of NO for long periods of time. The body has several protective mechanisms, such as producing anti-inflammatory cytokines, which inhibit iNOS, or increasing glutathione, a radical scavenger that protects cells from toxicity caused by NO overproduction. But when NO escapes control, things like cytotoxicity and SIRS can happen. Yes, a bit of NO can be helpful on a wild Saturday night; it actually may save your life if you are having a heart attack or stroke, but too much of it can kill you. Sounds familiar, after all.

Since LT increases NO production,[53, 54] it could have a role in the treatment of myocardial infarction and ischemic stroke, and this is being investigated (see sections 5.3 and 9.8.3). LT delivered percutaneously *in vivo* was able to successfully reverse experimentally induced arterial spasm in atherosclerotic Yucatan microswine.[55] The reason for this is that LT induces relaxation of smooth muscle, as described in bronchoconstriction models,[56] but also the smooth muscle that is present in the vascular wall. What is more interesting is that this increase in NO would be coming from eNOS, and LT would actually be decreasing iNOS expression.[40] This would be great news, since we could benefit from the increased blood flow if needed, and still have an anti-inflammatory effect.

3.2   The anti-inflammatory effect of laser therapy on different cells, tissues, and conditions

Inflammation shows particularities depending on the tissue and condition; some inflammatory cells are more predominant in acute inflammation and others in chronification, and some specialized macrophages are exclusive to certain tissue types, such as the nervous system microglia. As a general process, damage to the endothelium, considered by many to be our largest organ, initiates the inflammatory cascade. The activation of certain molecules, such as integrins and vascular cell adhesion molecules (VCAMs), allows the adhesion (margination and rolling) of circulating neutrophils, the first cell type to be recruited, which then migrate (diapedesis) through the endothelial wall and into the inflammatory site. Neutrophils are the predominant cell type in the first 24–48 h of acute inflammation, and are replaced by macrophages later on.

Wounds are the most studied field of LT, including the inflammatory process (Figs 3.5 and 3.6). A few articles describe a stimulating effect on the chemotaxis of

leukocytes to burn wounds,[57] but most of them report a decrease in polymorphonuclear cell infiltration after LT and downregulation of lymphocytic proliferation during the healing process following experimental skin and mucosal wounds as well as burns. This correlates with the anti-inflammatory effect of laser.[5, 43, 58–60] The story with mast cells is a bit more complex; they are well known for their role in allergic reactions, and they are important in the early phenomena of burn healing, but a prolongation of their effects over time would perpetuate the inflammatory process and potentially the discomfort associated with the injury. LT modulates this; it increases the number of mast cells in the first 2 weeks after second-degree burns in rats, but then in the fourth week (remodeling phase) the number of mast cells decreases in laser-treated animals.[61] In rats with experimental linear incisions, mast cells were increased by day 4 but had decreased at day 10.[62] The different experimental models may explain why, although both studies indicate an early increase and later decrease in mast cells in the wound, the shift happens at different times – later in the burn than in the incision model. But after all, you would expect an incision to heal faster than a burn.

Laser can also benefit **mucosal** inflammation: interesting results have been published about its use in radiotherapy- and chemotherapy-induced oral mucositis. LT provided analgesia and better resolution of the oral lesions, both in an experimental model and in clinical studies with human patients, with associated functional improvement and a better ability to eat.[63–67]

In models of **pulmonary** inflammation, asthma, and edema, LT also decreases leukocyte infiltration. It has been proposed that this is because inhibition of inflammatory mediators decreases intercellular adhesion molecule-1 (ICAM-1) expression.[68] Also both *in vivo* and *in vitro* studies have shown that the hyper-responsiveness of **airway** smooth muscle cells, as seen in asthma and other respiratory disorders, can be significantly attenuated with LT.[56, 69] It also decreased the number of eosinophils in the bronchoalveolar lavage and the serum immunoglobulin E (IgE) levels in a model of asthma.[45] A similar result was described in a murine model of acute pleurisy,[44] in which inflammatory mediators and exudate volume were decreased after LT.

The **microglia**, which make up the immune system of the brain and spine, also seem to respond to LT. According to an *in vitro* study with neuronal cultures,

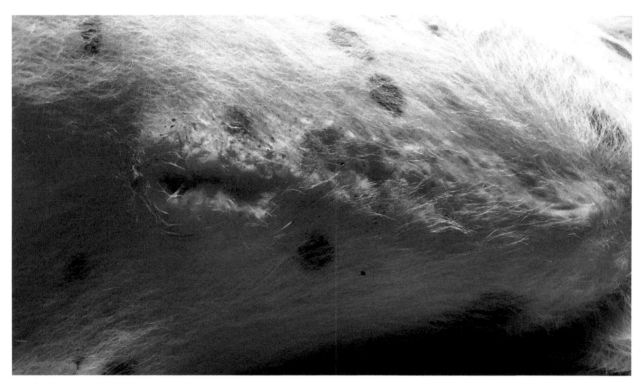

Figure 3.5 Sometimes a single treatment is enough to help wound healing take the right path. This dog showed progressive laparotomy wound inflammation 2 weeks after cholecystectomy.

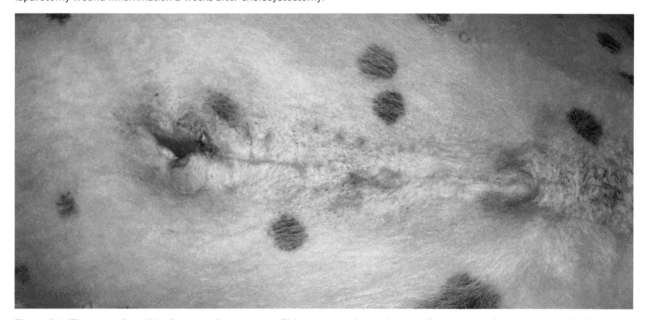

Figure 3.6 The same dog 48 h after a single treatment. This was enough to substantially improve inflammation and healing.

LT with different doses was able to modulate microglial transformation or polarization into different pro- or anti-inflammatory phenotypes,[70] which could affect how the CNS recovers after injury.

Several models have been used in **nephrology** showing the potential of LT in this field. In one of them, one of the ureters was occluded and then nine points distributed over the surface of the affected kidney received intraoperative laser.[71] When evaluated at 14 days, using immunohistochemistry, histomorphometric analysis, and polymerase chain reaction (PCR) for pro-inflammatory and pro-fibrotic molecules, LT-treated animals showed a decreased inflammatory and fibrotic response compared to controls. In a rat model of crescentic glomerulonephritis,[72] transcutaneous LT (daily for 14 days) decreased the expression of inflammatory mediators in the renal cortex, the infiltration of macrophages and lymphocytes, and the morphological damage to glomeruli.

In an experimental model of acute **muscle** injury, LT was more effective than topically applied diclofenac or cryotherapy in decreasing the release of pro-inflammatory cytokines. Higher doses did not seem to help. It decreased COX-2 expression while improving muscle injury healing, increasing collagen synthesis, and improving its organization to be more similar to the unharmed tissue.[37] In **osteoarthritis** models**,** LT decreased polymorphonuclear cell numbers in the synovial fluid and capsule.[41, 73] Tendinitis models also showed a decrease in inflammation with LT (together with better collagen repair and other effects).[47, 74] For most tissues you will find some scientific evidence of the anti-inflammatory effect of LT. For instance, **vascular** inflammation and abnormal metabolism are pathological components of several neurodegenerative and arterial diseases. LT was able to decrease abdominal aortic aneurysm progression in a mouse model.[75] Or in an experimental model of rat mastitis, LT decreased the number of neutrophils entering the mammary alveoli.[76]

Finally, let's consider two facts with potential clinical consequences.

- Steroids seem to play a role in the anti-inflammatory effect of LT. A study in rats found the anti-inflammatory effect was lost in adrenalectomized individuals.[24] Interestingly, in that study they compared doses of 1, 2.5, and 5 J/cm², and 5 J/cm² seemed not to work. But the same author, years later, described an anti-inflammatory effect with an even higher dose, 7.5 J/cm², using the same animal model.[77]
- In some reports, lower doses were found to be more

anti-inflammatory than those at the high end of the range. For instance, in a rat model of induced arthritis, 4.5 J/cm² applied with 0.4 W/cm² had a strong anti-inflammatory effect, decreasing the levels of inflammatory cells and mediators, but 72 J/cm² with the same power density lacked effect.[78] In a model of muscle injury (muscle damage induced by freezing), using 0.5 W/cm², 10 J/cm² was more effective than 50 J/cm² in decreasing COX-2 expression.[37] Remember this is a rat model and we are not transposing this figures straight into a dog; however, at some intuitive level it makes sense to think that strong stimulation is not the point when working with acutely inflamed tissue. But then think how little of the energy delivered to the surface can reach the tissues; the good news is that in the deep tissues, where less of the light penetrates, the effect is more likely to be anti-inflammatory.

Don't forget that a certain degree of inflammation is part of the healing process, even if we describe these effects separately. The other big effect of LT is analgesia. Of course, inflammation and pain are not independent either; after all, pain is one of the classical signs of inflammation.

Summary from a different perspective

Inflammation is part of the healing process, and the "soup" of mediators is a very complicated network of real-time balancing acts. Most of these molecules don't absorb light directly, but even minor changes in the soup, caused by the external stimulus of light, can initiate a cascade of events. Mysteriously enough, the vast majority of these types of cascade that have been studied lead to a positive effect. This supports a major theme in this book: laser doesn't determine the direction of the effect; the body (by and large) wants to heal itself, and laser simply enables it to do so.

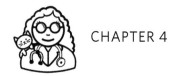

CHAPTER 4

Analgesic effect

The love for all living creatures is the most noble attribute of man.

— Charles Darwin

Pain is currently defined as "an unpleasant sensory and emotional experience associated with actual or potential tissue damage, or described in terms of such damage" (International Association for the Study of Pain). Note that pain is not just a physical stimulus or sensation, but it is also how it makes the patient feel about it. The psychological component is way more recognized, studied, and treated in humans, while often overlooked in veterinary science. This does not mean it does not exist: you are used to noticing how some patients seem to do just fine with conditions that you know are moderately painful, while others become paralyzed, highly vocal, or seem to panic with manipulations or conditions that you expect to elicit very little pain.

Pain should be treated both for ethical and clinical reasons. As veterinarians, we must work to prevent and treat pain in the most proactive way we can; it is a key component of our patients' quality of life. Under-treated pain leads to physiological changes such as increased glycemia and arterial pressure, immunological compromise, delayed wound healing, and increased risk of self-trauma to a surgical area. Pain increases not just morbidity, but mortality risk.

Let's review how the physical part happens. The origin of the noxious stimulus can be somatic, visceral, or neuropathic (central or peripheral), but pain can also be referred to distant sites. Once an injury or noxious stimulus activates nociceptors or free nerve endings of A-delta (mechanoreceptors and thin, fast-conduction myelinated fibers) and C fibers (polymodal receptors, slow conduction unmyelinated fibers), these get fired (they translate or transduce biochemical and physical signals into an electric impulse) and conduct the information to the dorsal horn of the spinal cord; from there, the spinothalamic tract carries the information into the brain. Different mechanisms can amplify or reduce the signal in the spinal cord. For instance, gamma-amino butyric acid (GABA) and serotonin act as signal inhibitors, but the inflammatory cascade that starts with the initial injury produces prostanoids and other mediators, which make fiber discharge persist and produce sensitization and primary hyperalgesia. Once the signal reaches the brain, pain is perceived and this triggers motor, endocrine, and biochemical responses.

Acute pain arises to minimize tissue damage after a specific disease or injury; it has a warning and protecting function and should disappear once healing is completed. An example is pain during surgery or in the postoperative period. The body has mechanisms to deal with pain and modulate it; serotonin, norepinephrine, and endogenous opioids are some of these neurotransmitters that inhibit nociceptive transmission. When the nociceptive information enters the brain, inhibitory descending pathways are activated. This may remind you of the anti-inflammatory mediators and mechanisms activated when the inflammatory cascade begins.

Chronic pain, on the other hand, persists after what would be considered the normal healing time for a particular injury, or remains because healing has not occurred; but it has no biological function and obviously affects quality of life. Think, for instance, about degenerative joint disease and the remodeling periosteum, oncological pain, or visceral pain in chronic enteropathies. It does not respond to an actual activation of peripheral nociceptors by trauma or temperature, and its intensity does not correlate with the stimulus. It often involves inflammatory pain, but it also changes the way the nervous system works, i.e. how the information is transmitted and processed. Briefly, persistent stimulation of receptors can lower their triggering threshold (peripheral sensitization) and repeated stimulation of afferent fibers can increase the excitability of neurons in the spinal cord and amplify signals (central sensitization). A decrease in the noxious inhibitory controls has also been described. These phenomena can lead to hyperalgesia and allodynia. Two of the main pro-inflammatory mediators described in Chapter 3, prostaglandin E_2 and IL-1, have a crucial role in this process.

Some cases could be classified as nociceptive pain, which occurs as a result of a disease or tissue damage, such as in inflammatory bowel disease, others as neuropathic pain, such as spinal cord injury or trigeminal neuralgia. But many patients fall into a mixed group: a neuropathic pain component is often found in chronic pain patients, which makes diagnosis and treatment more challenging. A study on spontaneous canine osteoarthritis (OA) demonstrated how OA was strongly associated with hyperalgesia: the nervous system of these dogs, compared with matching controls, overreacted to different types of sensory input in places that were distant but segmentally related to the arthritic joint.[79] A similar study described how inhibitory (analgesic) mechanisms were decreased in OA patients.[80]

Neuropathic pain is probably under-diagnosed in veterinary science; more than half of human patients with amputation stumps or spinal cord injuries report chronic pain and different forms of dysesthesia.[81] Traditional analgesic approaches using non-steroidal anti-inflammatory drugs (NSAIDs) or opioids are sometimes unsuccessful, and laser therapy (LT) has a place in the integrative multimodal approach that should be used in these animals.

4.1 How can laser therapy provide analgesia?

Different mechanisms have been reported to account for the analgesic effect of LT. Each of these may have a relatively greater importance depending on the type of pain (Fig. 4.1).

Mechanisms of pain modulation with LT

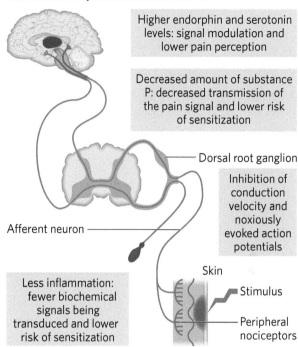

Higher endorphin and serotonin levels: signal modulation and lower pain perception

Decreased amount of substance P: decreased transmission of the pain signal and lower risk of sensitization

Dorsal root ganglion

Inhibition of conduction velocity and noxiously evoked action potentials

Afferent neuron

Skin

Stimulus

Peripheral nociceptors

Less inflammation: fewer biochemical signals being transduced and lower risk of sensitization

Figure 4.1 Proposed mechanisms for the analgesic effect of LT.
Illustrator: Elaine Leggett.

- LT decreases the inflammatory pain component by having an anti-inflammatory effect, as reviewed in Chapter 3. It **decreases pro-inflammatory mediators locally and centrally**, including IL-1 and TNF, PGE_2,[34, 36] COX-2,[33] and bradykinin,[35] as well as kinin receptor activity.[31]

- **Neural mechanisms,** i.e. changes in conduction and excitability. Initial experimental results suggested LT prevents depolarization of afferent type C fibers.[82] LT may slow down conduction velocity and inhibit noxiously evoked action potentials, decreasing their amplitude and increasing their latency for several hours.[83, 84] LT also decreases levels of substance P, which is a neurotransmitter involved in the modulation of pain signal transmission, as well as sensitization, hyperalgesia, and allodynia. LT inhibits the excitation of C fibers in the afferent sensory pathway by decreasing the amount of substance P in the spinal dorsal root ganglion[85, 86] and the spinal dorsal horn,[87] decreasing experimentally induced hyperalgesia and allodynia.

- Light may work differently for different types of pain; in an experimental model with rats, LT elevated the pressure threshold of treated animals, but had no effect in paw thermal threshold responses.[88] On the other hand, reduction of cold hyperalgesia after LT has also been described.[87] LT also improves nerve functionality and recovery in nerve entrapment neuropathy.[89]

• **Promoting inhibitory mechanisms**, such as serotonin[28, 29] and endogenous opioid production. LT increases beta-endorphin production in peripheral inflammatory models, and this mechanism is blocked by naloxone, an opioid antagonist.[86, 90, 91]

The scientific community does not have the same degree of agreement about all these mechanisms; for instance, there is a wide consensus on analgesia through anti-inflammatory mechanisms, but some studies don't agree on the modification of nerve conduction velocity or opioid release, or they find these effects in a narrow therapeutic window.[35] An increase in skin substance P after LT has also been described.[92]

Treatment of acute pain can even start before it happens, as in premedication for a surgical procedure. In chronic pain, treatment should start as soon as possible, both for ethical reasons and because this will decrease the likelihood of developing neuropathic pain. Treatment should be multimodal and LT can potentially help, in both acute and chronic pain management – it was already included in the WSAVA's 2014 Guidelines for recognition, assessment and treatment of pain,[93] both as one of the physical modalities used in rehabilitation and as a supplemental technique after ovariohysterectomy/ovariectomy for both dogs and cats. Nevertheless, these recommendations are made in the most part by transposing experimental results, clinical experience, and human studies, and more clinical studies should be carried out in small animals.

As a general rule, acute pain is treated with lower doses and power densities than chronic pain (Table 4.1). Pain related to superficial tissues is also treated with lower doses than conditions affecting deeper structures. For instance, an acute wound affecting skin and subcutaneous tissue would need 2–5 J/cm², while pain related to spondylosis may need 8–15 J/cm². In the first case, power density would be around 0.1–1 W/cm², with lower values if the subcutaneous tissue or muscle are exposed (Fig. 4.2). In the second case, we could go up to 2–3 W/cm² (Fig. 4.3). Remember LT can cause vasodilation, and higher parameters are similar to a stronger manual manipulation to some extent; so

if doses are too high for an acute case, this could cause discomfort, despite the anti-inflammatory or tissue healing effect. The potential scenarios are very varied, and so are your patients and their level of tolerance for discomfort and manipulation, so you will have to make adjustments within this framework.

I'll refer you back to the example in Chapter 2, section 2.2, of treating gout in humans, again to remind you of the importance of not just bringing fresh blood to an area, but also creating a drainage path for the toxin-filled fluid. Now, don't be silly and start treating the inguinal lymph node before treating an abdominal wound. These are very localized effects. But still, the point is that laser therapy is not a plug-and-chug modality where you have some "right" parameter-set preprogrammed into the machine. Clinical improvement is also dependent on the skill of the therapist (which you will have nurtured by reading this book).

4.2 Don't forget pain assessment

If we are going to treat patients in pain with LT and want to find out how effective our treatment is, we'd better assess it. To treat pain, we must first diagnose it and evaluate its intensity and progression. This evaluation can be based on certain physiological parameters (such as heart rate or blood pressure), changes in

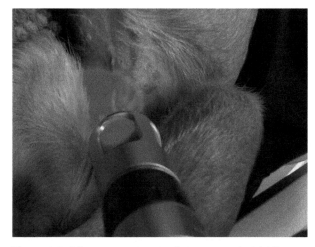

Figure 4.2 A laparotomy incision being treated with LT, using 2 J/cm².

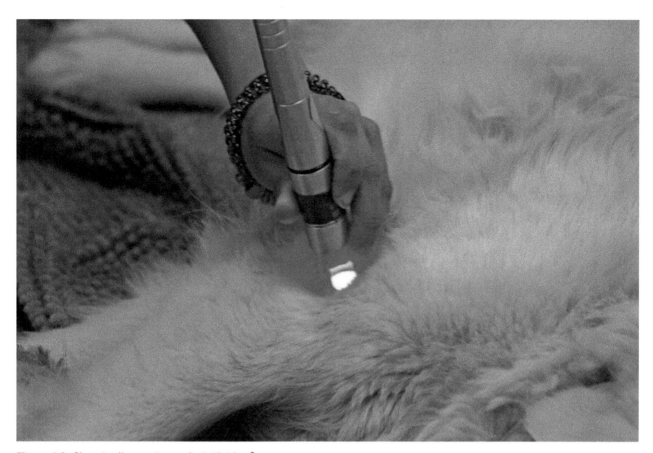

Figure 4.3 Chronic elbow pain needs 6–12 J/cm².

behavior (activities or postures), and subjective judgements such as visual scales. To achieve a proper and more systematic assessment of the potential pain and its associated behaviors, the species, breed, and individual are taken into account, as well as the clinical history and examination. Sometimes changes in gait, posture, or facial expression can be quite obvious, but a cat with chronic pain may only be hiding a bit more than usual or no longer being found on the kitchen counter.

Routine pain assessment is recommended. There are many available scales for this purpose and these are arguably a gold standard (Table 4.2). Some of them have been validated more than others, but it is always better to use a non-optimal pain scale than none at all, or many cases will go undiagnosed, especially in cats. By no means is this to underestimate the importance of validation, but rather to focus on integrating proactive pain assessment into your work routine.

Visual analogue scales (VAS) and numerical rating scales (NRS) represent the possible range of pain, from no pain at all to the worst imaginable kind or a very severe pain, in a way that depends on the particular

Table 4.1 Recommended parameters for pain management.

	Example	Dose (J/cm²)	Power (W)	Power density (W/cm²)
Acute superficial	Dog bite, acute tendinitis	2–5	1–4	0.2–1
Acute deep	Closed fracture	4–8	3–8	0.5–1.5
Chronic superficial	Non-healing ulcer, chronic tendinitis	4–15	2–5	0.5–1
Chronic deep	Spondylosis, hip dysplasia	8–20	6–15	1.5–3

Table 4.2 Overview of some of the available pain assessment scales and staging tools.

Condition	Scale or staging tool	Appendix
Acute pain, hospital setting	Glasgow – short form	A1, A2
Chronic pain	CBPI	A3
Lameness	Hudson VAS	A4
Feline musculoskeletal pain	FMPI	A5
Osteoarthritis	COAST, LOAD	

Notes: If none of these are possible, at least a simple NRS should be used. CBPI, Canine Brief Pain Inventory; COAST, Canine Osteoarthritis Staging Tool ; FMPI, Feline Musculoskeletal Pain Index; LOAD, Liverpool Osteoarthritis in Dogs; VAS, visual analog scale.

scale. VAS represents this range with a 10 cm line, where 0 represents absence of pain and 10 is extremely severe, or the worst imaginable kind. A mark is drawn on the line and the distance from 0 measured. NRS use numbers (e.g. from 0 to 10, or 0 to 4). Using descriptors of the ratings is useful to make pain assessment more consistent, especially when different evaluators are involved. For NRS, patients with a pain score of 3/10 or above should be treated.

It sounds simple and it is simple. So simple, that it is very often overlooked or not performed. Please choose one scale, either a basic VAS/NRS or one of the ones we will mention here, for acute and chronic situations, and start using it. You will shortly see how it becomes quicker and easier, and it is time well used for the sake of your patient.

Acute pain is easier to assess. The most common scenario is postoperative pain, and two of the most popular and more complete scales to assess it are the Botucatu and Glasgow Scales. The original Glasgow Composite Measure Pain Scale was developed in 2001,[94] and later a shorter form was also proposed for its speed and ease of use in a clinical setting[95] (see Appendix A1). A specific version of this scale has also been developed for cats[96] (see Appendix A2). The UNESP–Botucatu Multidimensional Composite Pain Scale, developed in Brazil,[97] was later validated in English,[98] and focuses on postoperative pain in cats. The function of such scales is not just to evaluate pain; they define an intervention level score above which measures should be taken to treat pain. They are very valuable tools for veterinarians and nurses, and quick and easy to use and implement in daily practice.

Chronic pain is more challenging to diagnose, but some scales and questionnaires have been developed. In this case, owner information is key to evaluating changes in dogs' behavior, which may be subtle. Some behaviors

may indicate the small animal patient is suffering neuropathic pain: frequent or constant licking, chewing, or scratching of an area where there is apparently no disease (to the point of self-mutilation in the worst cases), presence of hypersensitivity or allodynia, etc., but it is not always that obvious. You can read Chapter 9 for more information about chronic pain assessment.

In general, younger animals tend to be more vocal and expressive about pain; older animals in chronic pain can be more challenging to diagnose. It is important to understand how chronic pain can affect quality of life, and the most popular scales for chronic pain consider this as well as other descriptors (you can find them in section 9.6.1). To get a better, fuller picture and improve assessment, ask about the activities of the patient during the whole day; behavioral changes such as decreased exercise tolerance or difficulty with stairs, jumping, getting up, or lying down. Changes in the position or places they defecate or urinate. Cats in pain often decrease self-grooming. If necessary, get videos recorded for you of specific conducts. Quiet animals may just be a bit more withdrawn.

4.3 Analgesia in different conditions: clinical studies

Laser therapy has been used to treat different kinds of pain for quite some time now, and there is a good body of literature supporting different applications, most of them concerning musculoskeletal ailments in humans. There are inter-species differences, but a clinical study of musculoskeletal or chronic pain in people probably more closely resembles the dose and penetration needed in a dog than an experimental study in mice.

In human medicine, it has become evident in recent years that new tools to treat pain are necessary – not just to be able to treat cases that do not respond to conventional drug therapy, but as a safe alternative, to decrease the risk of drug abuse, especially opioid abuse, or drug toxicity, and LT is one of these options.[99]

In a systematic review of 16 randomized controlled trials including a total of 820 patients with neck pain treated with class III lasers, published in *Lancet* in 2009,[100] both acute and especially chronic cases improved, with an average improvement of 22 mm on a 100 mm VAS, and this improvement persisted in the medium term (up to 3–6 months). This means that if your pain score was 5 out of 10, and you had a typical response, your pain would decrease to almost half of its intensity. Functional ability was also improved. Overall, the evidence was categorized as moderate. Most of the included studies were performed by treating trigger points (average of 11 points per patient), delivering a wide range of doses, from less than 1 J/point to more than 54 J/point. The most statistically significant differences were observed with 2–6 J/point doses. Side effects were similar to those in the placebo groups, which points to another characteristic of LT that is very often reported: if properly performed, it is a very safe procedure.

The high safety of LT was also pointed out in another review of LT for lateral elbow tendinopathy (also known as tennis elbow),[101] which concluded that LT is helpful in pain and disability relief for this condition. Many of these patients initially had a poor prognosis, due to long-term disease and failure of other treatment modalities, such as steroid injections. In this compilation of trials, the average improvement on a VAS was 10.2–17.2 mm. A more intense analgesic effect was described in a review of LT for chronic joint disorders, including knee, temporomandibular, or zygapophyseal joints: an average of 29.8 mm on a VAS scale, provided the trial used a high enough dose and included the joint capsule in the treated area.[102]

More recently, a meta-analysis of LT and pain including 22 clinical studies in humans described the efficacy of class III LT for pain relief in different conditions, such as arthritis, carpal tunnel syndrome, low back pain, myofascial pain, or Raynaud's syndrome. The studies included varied treatment regimes, from 0.9 to 30 J/cm^2, wavelengths from 637 to 957 nm, and most patients received 10 to 20 sessions.[103]

Most studies concerning the use of LT in acute surgical pain refer to dental procedures, and the results are varied.[35, 104] There are few studies concerning LT and soft tissue analgesia: an early double-blind clinical trial of LT applied immediately after cholecystectomy laparotomy wound closure showed a significant difference in pain rating scores and analgesic demand.[105] Much more recently, a prospective, randomized, placebo-controlled clinical study reported an analgesic effect of LT in the postoperative period after bariatric surgery. Laser was applied to the laparotomy incision area, with a dose a bit higher than usual for wound healing, 10 J/cm^2 and 0.495 mW/cm^2, but with very good results.[106]

Laser therapy could be a coadjutant of regional intraoperative anesthesia; in a double-blinded, placebo-controlled, randomized clinical trial involving 48 patients undergoing radial fracture surgery, LT at the cervical nerve roots plus over the affected radius significantly improved VAS values during and after the surgical procedure.[107]

We have already mentioned that chronic pain is more challenging to treat, since a neuropathic component can often develop in these patients. In fact, traditional painkillers only work in about 30% of human patients with neuropathic pain. This field has also been researched in clinical trials with LT. One of them included amputated human patients with refractory neuropathic pain and showed a positive and lasting analgesic effect of LT over a 4 month follow-up period.[108] However, the paper only included three patients, and should encourage a larger scale trial, since persistent pain at the stump (due to spontaneous nerve activity, which sensitizes the nervous system and leads to hyperalgesia and allodynia) is described in a high percentage of cases in humans, and thousands of amputations take place every year in both the human and veterinary fields. In this trial, doses ranged from 8 to 15 J/cm^2 over the amputation scar and patients received nine sessions. Another typical example of neuropathic pain in people is trigeminal neuralgia, and a review on this topic concluded that LT should be considered for these patients. It also pointed out that the wider the dose and treatment regimens considered, the less consistent (yet still safe) the clinical effect becomes.[109] Eventually, in 2016, a systematic review[110] identified ten laboratory trials and five clinical trials regarding neuropathic pain and concluded that LT had a positive effect on neuropathic pain management, although again the wide variety of treatment regimens (e.g. doses from 0.9 to 42 J/point) made it impossible to perform a proper meta-analysis.

So, evidence supports the effectiveness of LT for pain treatment, but in some fields the body of evidence is still insufficient or lacks properly designed studies. This should encourage the performance of more clinical studies, especially now that class IV lasers are more easily available; treating pain with LT often requires higher doses than those used for wound healing or to achieve an anti-inflammatory effect. In his review, Bjordal[35] found 5 J to be the minimum energy needed to elicit effects, and 10–15 J/cm^2 is a very common dose. Higher power is also useful; in their review, de Andrade et al.[110] found the studies that compared lower and higher power reported that higher power was more effective in providing analgesia. Class IV lasers were approved for therapy by the Food and Drug Administration (FDA) in 2003, and of course they are less affordable than lower powered lasers. Therefore, it is plausible that when more clinical studies are performed with class IV devices, the evidence will become more consistent. Only a few have been published so far, regarding either analgesia or other fields. They include a randomized, controlled clinical study of patients with epicondylitis; a class IV (10 W) laser proved to be analgesic and improve arm functionality, using 3000 J/elbow (about 6.6 J/cm^2) and a total of ten sessions over 18 days. This regime is quite similar to the usual treatments we would perform for a large dog in small animal practice in terms of dose and frequency of treatment.[111] Of course, this does not mean we should always use super-high power for patients in pain. The pain itself can put them in a state in which they are especially sensitive to high power densities – keep that in mind – but higher power and higher dose is the first strategy when dealing with refractory pain.

Summary from a different perspective

Pain is the primary reason for a trip to the veterinary clinic. The causes and types of pain vary very widely, as do the mechanisms by which laser helps the pain to subside. All that said, the name of the game is consistency in measuring pain, over time for a given patient as well as across patients within your clinic. When you have an equation with this many parameters, you have to control the ones you can, and quality pain scoring is the best start.

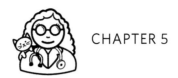

CHAPTER 5

Tissue healing

Healing is a matter of time, but it is sometimes also a matter of opportunity.

— Hippocrates

The most studied and reported effect of laser therapy (LT) is tissue healing; for almost every cell or tissue type you can think of, you will find related literature. There are clinical studies, *in vivo* experiments, and also *in vitro* experiments involving the particular cells that play a significant role in healing and their molecular mediators.

The common script for healing involves some kind of inflammatory response that triggers mechanisms to repair the damage, resulting in tissue that ideally resembles the original undamaged tissue as much as possible. Depending on the tissue type, the degree of this resemblance is variable with regard to structure, strength, and functionality. What LT achieves in tissue healing is to speed up this process and improve the final product, but it will not make cells do things they don't usually do; it increases their efficacy by a process similar to turning up the power of an engine and at the same time providing it with more fuel.

5.1 Wound healing

You can check Figure 5.1 for a summary of the wound healing process and some of the individual mechanisms that have been reported to be affected by LT. When the endothelium is damaged and its collagen exposed, the coagulation cascade begins. Every wound healing process starts with an attempt by the body to stop the bleeding.

Platelets adhere and aggregate to start with, and later the fibrin net holds the clot in place. When platelets are activated, they open up their granules, releasing (among other substances) the first factors that will start promoting cell multiplication and tissue growth. These growth factors are not exclusively produced by platelets, not even platelet-derived growth factor, but they do release a necessary initial burst, which is the basis of platelet-rich plasma therapy, a modality that is becoming very common.

A thorough explanation of their effects is beyond our scope, but their names are quite explicit and there is evidence that LT enhances the expression of the following growth factors, their receptors and the secondary pathways they activate:

Worth mentioning before María dives into the different tissue types and their individual responses to laser therapy, is the idea of enhancement of a process. What we mean to emphasize are two distinct, but related ways of measuring progress.

- *For a given time, an increased level of healing vs. conventional therapy.*
- *Getting to a given level of healing in less time vs. conventional therapy.*

I think you intuitively know the difference, but keep these in mind as you read the rest of this chapter (and book).

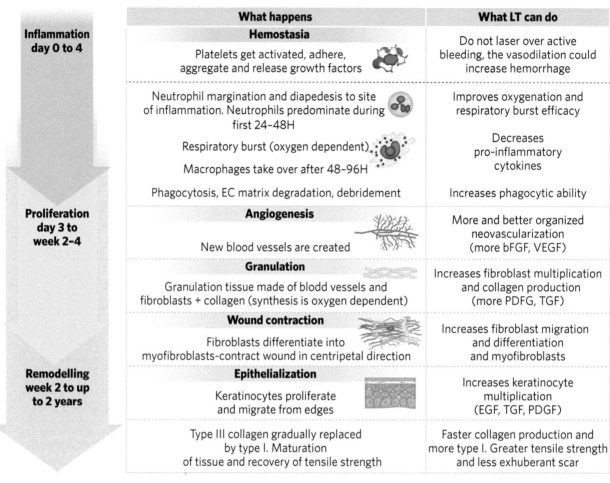

	What happens	What LT can do
Inflammation day 0 to 4	**Hemostasia** Platelets get activated, adhere, aggregate and release growth factors	Do not laser over active bleeding, the vasodilation could increase hemorrhage
	Neutrophil margination and diapedesis to site of inflammation. Neutrophils predominate during first 24–48H	Improves oxygenation and respiratory burst efficacy
	Respiratory burst (oxygen dependent) Macrophages take over after 48-96H	Decreases pro-inflammatory cytokines
	Phagocytosis, EC matrix degradation, debridement	Increases phagocytic ability
Proliferation day 3 to week 2–4	**Angiogenesis** New blood vessels are created	More and better organized neovascularization (more bFGF, VEGF)
	Granulation Granulation tissue made of blodd vessels and fibroblasts + collagen (synthesis is oxygen dependent)	Increases fibroblast multiplication and collagen production (more PDFG, TGF)
	Wound contraction Fibroblasts differentiate into myofibroblasts-contract wound in centripetal direction	Increases fibroblast migration and differentiation and myofibroblasts
Remodelling week 2 to up to 2 years	**Epithelialization** Keratinocytes proliferate and migrate from edges	Increases keratinocyte multiplication (EGF, TGF, PDGF)
	Type III collagen gradually replaced by type I. Maturation of tissue and recovery of tensile strength	Faster collagen production and more type I. Greater tensile strength and less exhuberant scar

Figure 5.1 A summary of how can LT enhance the different phenomena of wound healing. bFGF, basic fibroblast growth factor. *Illustrator: Elaine Leggett.*

- platelet-derived growth factor (PDGF)[43]
- vascular endothelial growth factor (VEGF)[6, 60, 112]
- transforming growth factor beta (TGF-β)[113]
- fibroblast growth factor (FGF)[114, 115]
- epidermal growth factor (EGF)[116]
- insulin-like growth factor (IGF).[114]

But wait ... before tissue growth starts to be significant, other things have to happen. Tissue growth does not predominate in this phase, but the seeds for it are already planted and these growth factors are fertilizing the soil.

Hemostasis could be considered the first step of the inflammatory phase, and neutrophils come in early to protect the organism from potential microorganism invasion. To achieve this task they use an oxidizing or respiratory burst, a mechanism that involves the production of free radicals of oxygen, among other

components. This is an important note: neutrophils need oxygen to do their job. And that is one of the reasons why ischemia facilitates infection: neutrophils can't get where they are needed, or not enough of them can, and if they can get there, they can't work properly. LT enhances blood flow, tissue oxygenation, and neutrophil activity,[51, 52] but at the same time it can decrease the number of these cells that infiltrate the inflammation site (you can review Chapter 3 for more on LT and inflammation). Could that mean less polymorphonuclear cells are needed because they are more effective?

Unless a purulent response persists, macrophages replace neutrophils after about 48 h. They remove neutrophils, debris, and dead tissue. Debriding can be more or less significant depending on the type of wound, and this phase is considered as either part of the inflammatory stage or separate from it, depending on the author. Macrophages also release proteolytic enzymes, which

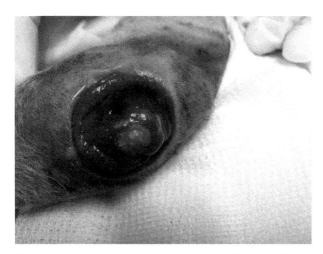

Figure 5.2 Deep wound over left olecranon. The formation of granulation tissue has started.

help degrade the extracellular matrix; this makes the matrix less dense and facilitates later migration of other cells. In a clean wound, the inflammatory stage persists until approximately day 4, but in wound chronification this catabolic state persists.

Around day 3, tissue proliferation should (assuming no infection or necrosis) start to predominate: fibroblasts, endothelial cells, and keratinocytes become the star players. Four processes take place: formation of granulation tissue, angiogenesis, wound contraction, and epithelialization. Granulation tissue (Figs 5.2 and 5.3) is made up of fibroblasts, blood vessels, and fibrin/collagen. LT increases fibroblast multiplication, migration, and collagen production,[4, 6, 112, 117–119] which is also an oxygen-dependent process. One study determined the hydroxyproline content of wounds as an indirect measure of the amount of collagen (since hydroxyproline makes up 10% of collagen) and found it to be three times higher in treated wounds compared to control ones.[120]

More and better organized blood vessels are created in response to LT.[121] Fibroblasts differentiate into myofibroblasts, which help contract the wound in a centripetal direction, and LT also enhances these phenomena.[48, 122] Once a healthy granulation bed has formed, keratinocytes will proliferate from the edges to cover the defect (Figs 5.3, 5.4, and 5.5), and their proliferation, maturation, and migration also increases with LT.[123–125] LT may also contribute to the enhanced wound repair by stimulating epidermal stem cells, which proliferate *in vitro* and migrate more after being irradiated.[126]

Proliferation may take 10 days to several weeks,

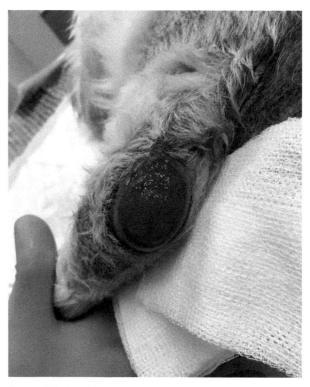

Figure 5.3 Granulation tissue now covers the wound bed and the margins start to epithelialize.

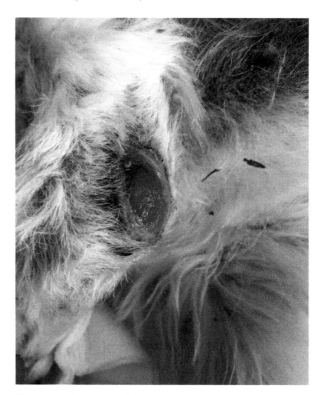

Figure 5.4 Both wound contraction and epithelialization have contributed to the decrease in wound size since the previous picture was taken.

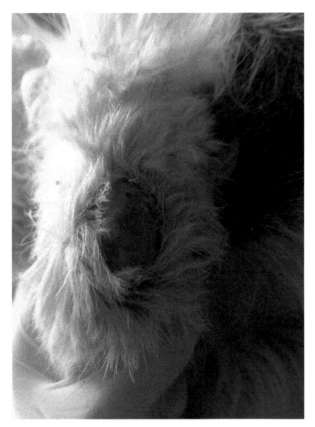

Figure 5.5 Epithelialization is almost complete. The area should be protected during the next few weeks to allow the tissue to regain more strength.

depending on the wound type and size, and by the second week the new tissue starts to reorganize, although it may still be proliferating. Type III collagen is gradually replaced by type I. Maturation of the tissue helps it to regain tensile strength, although this never recovers to its original values – only about 80% after 3 months! This process is also improved with LT, especially when it is applied in the proliferation phase. Stadler et al. performed an experiment in which they demonstrated that although tensile strength improved in all animals treated with laser, the effect on collagen was maximal if it was applied during the proliferation phase, rather than during the inflammatory phase. [127] This makes sense, although in a clinical setting you want to benefit from both anti-inflammatory and healing effects.

As you will have noticed, many studies of LT consistently report a benefit for wound healing, and systematic reviews conclude the same. [2, 128] Laser can promote wound healing even in adverse conditions, such as infected wounds, [129] diabetic individuals, [130–135] and

experimental burn wounds. [60, 119] Some have compared LT with other modalities: an *in vitro* experiment with fibroblasts found laser to be more stimulating than ultrasound in terms of fibroblast activity [136] and as good as electrical stimulation in experimental rat skin incisions – both electrical stimulation and LT decreased the duration of the inflammatory phase and increased the number of fibroblasts and the concentration of hydroxyproline compared with their control groups.

Steroid treatment may affect the efficacy of LT. One study concluded that LT was useless on open skin wounds in corticosteroid-treated diabetic rats (although it did accelerate epithelialization in the no-steroid group). [137] But using similar parameters, another research group [118] concluded that LT may help counteract the inhibitory effect of anti-inflammatory drugs on wound healing: while the groups treated with a non-steroidal anti-inflammatory drug (NSAID; celecoxib 22 mg/kg) or corticosteroid (dexamethasone 5 mg/kg) tended to have lower wound cellularity and more immature granulation, treating those animals with LT helped restore cellularity to the baseline level, increasing fibroblast migration, collagen synthesis, and re-epithelialization.

5.2 Healing of tendons and ligaments

Tendons are made up of dense connective tissue (a particular, well differentiated type of fibroblasts called tenocytes, and collagen), which is longitudinally oriented in line with the tension and traction forces. Ligaments are also made of connective tissue, although less cellular and not as dense and resistant. In both cases, the amount, quality, and arrangement of collagen plays a central role in the healing process and the result. Besides its effect on collagen, LT also increases blood flow and oxygenation, which are common concerns in tendons and ligaments.

Animal models have shown the potential of LT to enhance these aspects of the repair process. Some of these reports have remarkable results. For instance, in a rabbit model of calcaneal tendon injury, the proportion of collagen type I was increased up to four times in the LT group compared to controls. [138] A significant increase in the type I collagen proportion was also described in a rat model of Achilles tendinitis after mechanical trauma, as well as reduced infiltration of inflammatory cells. [139] Oliveira et al. performed an experiment in which laser treatment was found to restore collagen fiber alignment in damaged tendons to the point that no significant difference was found between the groups with standard treatment and 5 days of laser application.[140] Better collagen organization and functional recovery after LT has also been described in other experimental studies.[141] Animal models also show that LT can improve remodeling of the extracellular matrix during the healing process in tendons through simultaneous activation of matrix metalloproteinase 2 (MMP-2) and stimulation of collagen synthesis.[142, 143] An increase in tenocyte migration has also been described; the effect is mediated by a protein called dynamin 2.[144]

But having said great things about the *in vitro* and experimental results with tendons and ligaments, there really are few clinical studies. One of them evaluated the effect of LT on the recovery of digital flexor tendon injuries in humans and found a significant effect on edema reduction but no effect on analgesia or handgrip strength.[145] Again, a different treatment protocol might find different results, and more clinical trials should be performed to validate – or not – the good results obtained in animal models. We still need to find out the best way to get light into our bodies in the same way that we do in rats and rabbits!

5.3   Muscle healing

Three tissue types of muscle are recognized: skeletal, cardiac, and smooth muscle. The response of these three to LT has been documented, with different aims and fields of application. While the main applications of LT in skeletal muscle are related to injury recovery and sports medicine, recovery of ischemic infarct is the focus when treating cardiac muscle.

The precursors for skeletal muscle cells are called satellite cells, which become activated and differentiated when there is muscle damage. Laser can promote muscle repair by increasing the number of myofibers and satellite cell survival, proliferation, and differentiation, as reported both *in vitro* and *in vivo*[146, 147] and by having anti-inflammatory and pro-angiogenic effects.[148] It increases the biochemical activity of the muscle, which can be monitored with acetylcholine receptors, cytochrome c oxidase expression, and creatine kinase activity.[63, 149, 150] Also, transplantation of myogenic cells is being studied as part of the treatment of injuries with extensive muscle tissue loss, and their survival and functionality seems to improve after being treated with LT.[151]

In cardiac muscle, LT has the potential to reduce infarct size following induction of myocardial infarction in rats and dogs.[152] When mesenchymal stem

---

In a recent double-blinded study on standardized core lesions surgically created in the superficial digital flexor tendons of horses, some accelerated healing was noticed. Briefly, the recovery from this type of injury is broken down into two phases: inflammatory and remodeling. These typically manifest themselves firstly with the lesion getting bigger until about 5 weeks, then secondly turning a corner and starting to gradually decrease in size. In the study, this exact behavior was confirmed for the control group, as it had been in previous studies using this same surgical model, with the tipping point of transition from inflammatory to remodeling at week 5. For the laser group, there were several interesting points.

- *The initial slope was significantly greater in the laser group. This means that the inflammatory process was enhanced (by almost a factor of 2).*
- *In fact, the tipping point was achieved on average about 2 weeks early in the laser group than in the control group (again, statistically significant).*
- *Once the remodeling phase began (2 weeks earlier than in controls), the rate of healing was significantly better in the laser group than in the controls.*
- *After that tipping point, the average lesion size in the laser group was lower than in the control group AT EVERY measurement point EVEN THOUGH it was higher in the laser group at the tipping point.*

This represents a supra-natural response rate within the natural structure of tendon healing, which falls very nicely in line with the fundamental mechanisms of laser. Also worth noting is that this model is a condensed timetable for the real-world analog (and purposefully so, with almost full healing in 13 weeks, while these injuries usually take many more months to heal).

cells derived from bone marrow and adipose tissue were stimulated by irradiation and implanted into the experimentally infarcted rat heart, a 50% decrease in cardiac infarct size was achieved.[153] Laser increased survival of those stem cells, and the result was increased angiogenesis and reduced fibrosis. These experimental findings have started to have some clinical application: a clinical study in 58 patients (20 of whom made up the control group) showed that transthoracic LT decreased cardiac cellular damage and improved cardiac tissue healing markers following coronary artery bypass grafting operations for coronary vessel occlusion.[154]

The effect of LT on the third type of muscle tissue, smooth muscle, has also been tested: it stimulates smooth muscle cell proliferation and metabolism,[155] which is relevant to arterial diseases, among others, including aneurysm, where there is depletion of smooth muscle cells. This was later also proven in a rat model[75]: LT significantly decreases abdominal aortic aneurysm progression.

5.4   Bone healing

The first phases of bone healing after a fracture are quite similar to what happens in other tissues; there is hematoma formation and an inflammatory phase, with release of cytokines. Common growth factors such as VEGF or PDGF, which as you know can be enhanced by LT, start playing their roles, but also a set of particular proteins called bone morphogenic proteins. New blood vessels are created, and a few days after the fracture there is already an unstable net of early woven bone. Fracture repair usually involves a combination of intramembranous and endochondral ossification, with progenitor cells differentiating into chondroblasts and osteoblasts. The fibrocartilaginous callus is gradually (over a period of weeks) replaced by a more organized, calcified, and stable callus. This callus undergoes remodeling in the next few months, following stress forces, until its structure is similar to regular bone.

LT enhances osteogenesis: *in vitro* and *in vivo* studies report it increases osteoblast multiplication and survival, as well as osteoblast metabolism. It induces alkaline phosphatase (ALP) activity and also osteopontin, a protein involved in the attachment of osteoclasts to the mineralized bone matrix, among others.[156]

The clinical consequence is improved calcification and fracture recovery. For instance, an experimental study in rats using polymerase chain reaction (PCR) measured how LT can modify the expression of osteogenic genes during bone healing of tibial defects. Laser was applied every other day and induced upregulation of bone morphogenic proteins and ALP; histologically, treated individuals showed enhanced new bone formation.[157] Pulse frequency is important, and low frequency has consistently been reported to work better to enhance new bone formation.[158–161]

Some conditions make it more difficult for patients to form new bone, and LT has also been investigated in models of bisphosphonate treatment and osteoporosis. Bisphosphonates are used in humans for the treatment of bone metastasis and other skeletal conditions. They have resorptive and anti-angiogenic effects in the bone, and because of this some patients suffer a complication called bisphosphonate-related osteonecrosis of the jaws (BRONJ). *In vitro* models show different cell lines (including osteoblasts), proliferate more under laser treatment, even when they are incubated with bisphosphonates.[162] Primary osteoporosis is most commonly seen in elderly humans, but similar changes can be seen in small animals due to lack of use, poor nutrition, and endocrine and renal imbalances. Models of osteoporosis due to estrogen deprivation in ovariectomized rats show LT can enhance new bone formation, with and without metal implants.[163, 164]

5.5   Nerve healing and function

Animal models show peripheral nerves regenerate faster after transection and anastomosis when the animal receives LT.[165, 166] Laser also enhances autograft repair of peripheral nerves, and in models of nerve crushing injury, LT improves regeneration and accelerates functional recovery.[167–169]

In spinal cord injury models, the length of axonal regrowth can double in animals treated with laser, and those animals also achieve a better functional recovery.[170] The experimental effects of chronic nerve and ganglion compression can be alleviated with LT, which increases levels of nerve growth factor, accelerates functional recovery, and decreases the associated inflammation.[39, 89] Even in hemisection at T9, LT applied transcutaneously to adult rats increased axonal number and distance of regrowth and significantly suppressed immune cell activation and cytokine/chemokine expression.[171] For this study, they were using 0.53 W/cm^2 and about 450 J concentrated over a point at the hemisection site, irradiating for about 50 min/day with a 150 mW power device. They had calculated a 6% penetration of the power to the level of the spine for the wavelength used. So patients with intervertebral disk disease (IVDD) may also benefit from LT, shortening the post-recovery period and as part of conservative management if indicated, but of course we would need higher power to improve penetration to that level in our patients and to cover a broader area in a clinically reasonable time.

Laser has shown promising results in stroke, by improving cerebral blood flow and neurogenesis and decreasing apoptosis after experimental hypoxia of the central nervous system (CNS).[172] Another mechanism of action is the increase in cerebral adenosine triphosphate (ATP) stores induced by laser, especially by pulsed radiation, which seems to be more effective than continuous wave radiation to treat the CNS.[173] Transcranial infrared laser therapy improved clinical (behavioral) rating scores after experimental strokes in rabbit and rat models – only if laser treatment was initiated up to 6 h post-embolization in the rabbit model,[174] but at 24 h post-stroke in the rats.[175] You can read some more about studies of LT for neurological problems in Chapter 8.

So, in conclusion, there is quite some evidence that LT can improve nerve healing and survival in both central and peripheral nervous tissue, but it is no surprise that reviews of this effect on nerve healing and recovery again point out how "despite the potential benefit of the use of lasers on nerve repair, further double-blind controlled clinical trials should be conducted in order to standardize protocols for clinical application."[176]

5.6 Treating contaminated and infected tissues

The clinical outcome of a tissue infection depends on two types of factors: those that affect microbial survival/proliferation/toxin production and those that affect the host's immune response. We have already talked about how LT can improve immune functionality. *In vitro* and *in vivo*, LT increases polymorphonuclear cell activity, which is translated as an increase in phagocytic capacity, reactive oxygen species (ROS) production, and a better ability to kill microorganisms.[49–52] Bacterial challenge increases oxygen consumption by phagocytes over 50 times, and oxygen supplementation has been proven to decrease the risk of surgical site infection in humans.[177]

So LT can enhance the patient's own responses, increasing the ability to heal and fight infection by modulating the leukocyte response, but could it also affect microbial survival? And if the answer is yes, does LT promote microbial growth or inhibit it? Does it depend on the parameters of irradiation? Does it depend on the microbial species, since Gram-positive and Gram-negative bacteria have different morphology and bacterial wall structures?

Some reports describe a decrease in the number of pathogenic bacteria – but wait, this is not exactly the same as saying LT is antimicrobial, which by definition (American Society of Microbiology) would imply killing of at least three logs (99.9%) of a planktonic microbial population, and it does not mean it will sterilize a wound. However, decreasing bacterial burden is an important benefit when we are using LT to help in the healing/analgesia of a wound. We may think we

---

If you had asked a neurologist 20 years ago, "do injured nerves regenerate?" the answer would have been a resounding "no." But not anymore. Regardless of how you may have to redefine the word "regenerate," where there was no signal between two CNS cells, we can now repair the chain in such a way as to get that signal back. And not just on the periphery. There is some ground-breaking work being done on laser therapy of the brain that merits some serious attention. And though I will echo María's last quote here, cautioning against the jump to any major conclusions, I will also bring up the example of fire. If we had waited to use fire until we understood the ins and outs of combustion, we would literally still be in the Stone Age. As much as it pains me to say this, the world was pioneered not by physicists, but by engineers: people who care less about how/why it works, and more THAT it works. Once we convince ourselves that it is safe to treat a particular condition, we should push toward treating it. It is our responsibility to continually go back and understand the "why," but to wait for the detailed mechanisms to be uncovered is to deny potential benefit to your patients.

don't need to kill all the bacteria, just enough to help the patient deal with the rest. On the other hand, when an incomplete kill of bacteria happens with antibiotics, resistance can be a problem, but this has not been documented in laser therapy.

How does this happen? We certainly know it does not happen through genotoxicity: the photons of infrared and red light, by definition, just don't have enough energy. However, several mechanisms of action have been proposed for the antimicrobial effect.

- Light is absorbed by bacterial chromophores (porphyrins), producing an increase in intracellular ROS – the porphyrins act as endogenous photosensitizers – and a decrease in transmembrane potentials, which are related to cell energy generation and storage.[178] Because the types of porphyrin are not the same in all bacteria, their absorption peaks can also be different, thus making the optimal wavelength for a wound potentially variable if we are only talking about killing bacteria. Blue light seems to target porphyrins more than infrared.[179]
- Of course, you could consider a thermal effect if you are using a high-power laser, but thermal killing of bacteria in wounds is not what we do in LT; that sounds more like cauterization! The treatment always takes place while maintaining physiological temperature in the treated tissues.
- With a lower thermal effect, you could desiccate the surface of a wound, making it a less microbial-friendly environment.[180] But wound desiccation is not necessarily therapeutic; we try to make sure the wound has just the right amount of moisture to physiologically heal – a very dry wound does not heal better and does not encourage growth and maintenance of healthy granulation tissue.
- Last but not least: in living tissue, increased oxygenation in the area (which is part of what happens with LT) makes the microenvironment less friendly for bacteria (most pathogenic species grow less well in oxygen-rich environments) and more favorable for the aerobic metabolism of the host's cells, including leukocytes. When surgical site infections are studied, the most commonly retrieved bacteria are those susceptible to oxidative killing.

Again, the different technical parameters (wavelength, energy, power density, etc.) used in the published literature make it difficult to compare such studies and

their differing results. Some *in vitro* experiments seem to show decreased microbial growth after exposure to laser light, including common pathogenic and opportunistic species such as *Candida albicans*,[178] *Staphylococcus aureus*,[178, 181] *Escherichia coli*,[178, 181, 182] *Pseudomonas aeruginosa*,[183] *Trichophyton rubrum*,[178] and periodontopathic germs.[184] But others show no effect[185, 186] or even increased growth after laser exposure.[182, 183, 185] Some suggest pulsing frequency or pulse duration can have different effects at the same wavelength; for instance, Karu et al. found 950 nm could enhance *E. coli* growth at 26 Hz and decrease it at 5000 Hz.[182]

Results obviously depend on wavelength, dose, power density, and other factors, and few studies carry out a systematic parameter-by-parameter analysis. More recently, *in vitro* experiments have included biofilm models rather than just bacterial suspensions. These may be more appropriate and include more complex bacterial population dynamics, such as subpopulations of bacteria that are dormant, have a slower rate of growth, or are related to antibiotic resistance.[179]

In vivo studies have provided encouraging results in the treatment of infections with *E. coli*,[180] *S. aureus*,[187] MRSA,[178, 188–190] *P. aeruginosa*,[181, 187] and some other pathogenic species of bacteria[184] and fungal infections such as *T. rubrum*[178, 191] and *C. albicans*.[178, 181] One of these studies suggested that laser treatment could decrease/prevent pathogenic bacterial growth in burns, while increasing the number of non-pathogenic flora.[187] Decreased bacterial counts have also been described after irradiation of rats with an osteomyelitis model.[188] Again, not all *in vivo* experiments show such positive results: an experimental model of *S. aureus* septic arthritis in rats did not report a substantial benefit of LT, apart from a certain level of recovery in the articular cartilage and synovium. On the other hand, in this study the power, wavelength, and dose used were quite low and only one point was treated,[192] to be fair, so it would not have any similarity to what you do in practice.

These *in vivo* observations may assess the effect more globally and realistically, since a culture plate does not take into consideration the effect of laser irradiation on immune cells, cytokine release, and the complex interactions that occur in a living tissue. The increased vascularization and oxygenation of tissue also play a role in the fight against infection – a tissue with poor blood flow and oxygenation is more likely to get infected.

More research needs to be done, though, to try to clarify which parameters have more effect on particular

Table 5.1 *In vitro* research on the potential antibacterial effects of red and infrared LT.

Microbial spp.	Wavelength (nm)	Dose (J/cm² or total J)	Power (W)	Power density (W/cm²)	CW/Hz	Incubation time (h)	Results	Reference	Ref. number
Staphylococcus aureus	810	1–80	3	0.015 and 0.03	CW	20	1–80 J/cm² no effect	Nussbaum 2003	185
	940, 635	Total 60–360J	1–3		CW?	24	Decreased survival; more effect at 3 W and higher doses	Krespi 2009	181
	630, 660, 810, 905	1–50	1.1	15	CW	20	Non-significant decrease at 5 J/cm²; non-significant increase at 50 J/cm²	Nussbaum 2002	183
	870, 930	4074 and 3667	9–10	Around 5	CW	16–20	4074 J/cm² kills 98%	Bornstein 2009	178
	904	3	0.012 average, 30 peak		2000 Hz	24, 48	Daily x 7 d over a colony. No effect	Pereira 2014	186
MRSA	940 + shock waves	1400	3		CW?	72	Decreases growth in combination with shock waves	Krespi 2011	189
Streptococcus sanguis	632.8, 665, 830	3.2 and 6.4 (632.8 nm); 10.6 and 21 (665 and 830 nm)	0.003–0.1		CW?	48–96	Mild decrease with 632.8 nm; more marked with 665 and 830 nm	Chan 2003	184
Pseudomonas aeruginosa	940, 635	Total 60–360 J	1–3		CW?	24	Decreased survival; more effect at 3 W and higher doses	Krespi 2009	181
	810	1–80	3	0.015 and 0.03	CW	20	1–20 J/cm² with 0.03 W/cm² inhibits growth	Nussbaum 2003	185
	630, 660, 810, 905	1–50	1.1	15	CW	20	Decrease with 810 nm, 5 J/cm²	Nussbaum 2002	183
Escherichia coli	630, 660, 810, 905	1–50	1.1	0.015–0.03	CW	20	Increased growth with 20 J/cm² and 0.03 W/cm²	Nussbaum 2002	183
	810	1–80	3	0.015–0.03	CW	20	Increased growth, especially at 0.03 W/cm²	Nussbaum 2003	185
	940, 635	Total 60–360 J	1–3		CW?	24	Decreased survival; more effect at 3 W and higher doses	Krespi 2009	181
	870, 930	4074 and 3259	8–10	4.5 and 5.6	CW	16–20	4074 J/cm² (5.6 W/cm²) kills 98%	Bornstein 2009	178
	1300, 950	18–72	15	0.12	CW and 2,26,700, 1000 and 5000 Hz	1	1300 nm increases growth; 950 nm at 26 Hz increases but at 5000 Hz decreases growth	Karu 1990	182
Trichophyton rubrum	800		0.005–0.14		76 MHz		Decreased growth	Manevitch 2010	191
	870, 930	4074 and 4500	10–11	6.25 and 5.6	CW	16–20	100% killing	Bornstein 2009	178
Aspergillus fumigatus	940, 635	Total 60–360 J	1–3		CW?	24	Decreased survival; effect at 3 W and higher doses	Krespi 2009	181
Candida albicans	940, 635	Total 60–360 J	1–3		CW?	24	Decreased survival; effect at 3 W and higher doses	Krespi 2009	181
	870, 930	4074 and 4500	10–11	6.25 and 5.6	CW	16–20	100% killing	Bornstein 2009	178

Note: CW, continuous wave; MRSA, methicillin-resistant Staphylococcus aureus.

Table 5.2 *In vivo* research on the potential antibacterial effects of red and infrared LT.

Microbial spp.	Model	Wavelength (nm)	Dose (J/cm² or total J)	Power (W)	Power density (W/cm²)	CW/Hz	Tx regime	Tx technique	Results	Reference	Ref. number
Staphylococcus aureus	Third degree skin burns, rats	632.8	1.2 and 2.4	0.01		CW	Daily × 15 d	Grid pattern	Laser increases angiogenesis and with 2.4 J/cm² it prevents bacterial growth	Bayat 2006	187
	Rhinosinusitis, rabbits	940	90 J/rabbit						Decreases 2 log colony counts (99%)	Krespi 2009	181
	Septic arthritis, rats	660	2	0.03	0.47	CW?	Daily × 10 d	Only one point treated	No analgesia. Slight recovery of cartilage and synovia. None had positive bacterial cultures	Araujo 2013	192
	Osteomyelitis, rats	808	7.64–22.9	0.1	127	CW	Daily × 5 d	Single point of 0.7 cm² over wound	Decreases bacterial counts; 22 J more effect	Kaya 2011	188
MRSA	Infected, intact, and wounded skin, rats	658	5			CW	Daily × 3 d	Scanning technique	Laser reduces bacterial proliferation	Silva 2013	190
	Pilot study in humans, nasal	870, 930	83–110	10 each	1–2	CW	Days 0, 1, 3	10 cm² flat top diffuser to each anterior nostril	Reduces/clears bacteria	Bornstein 2009	178
	Humans with nasal MRSA but no sinusitis	870, 930, 904	200–600/nostril	3–4		CW	Days 1, 3, 5	Via a laser fiber diffuser, 3 cm, delivered inside each naris circumferentially.	Variable degrees of decolonization – 100% at 940 nm, 600 J	Krespi 2012	257
Streptococcus pneumoniae	Rhinosinusitis, rabbits	940	180 J/rabbit			CW			Decreases 2 log colony counts (99%)	Krespi 2009	181
Pseudomonas aeruginosa	Third degree skin burns, rats	632.8	1.2 and 2.4	0.01		CW	Daily × 15 d	Grid pattern	Laser increases angiogenesis and with 2.4 J/cm² it prevents bacterial growth	Bayat 2006	187
	Rhinosinusitis, rabbits	940	180 J/rabbit						Decreases 2 log colony counts (99%)	Krespi 2009	181
Escherichia coli	Infected skin wound, rats	810	130–260	10	6.5	CW?	Once	14 mm spot	Bactericidal at 260 J/cm²; may be related to desiccation? 45°C reached	Jawhara 2006	180
Trichophyton rubrum	Pilot study in humans, onychomycosis	870, 930	204–408	10 each		CW	Days 1, 7, 14, 60	1.5 cm spot	Eliminates nail fungus; clear nail grows	Bornstein 2009	178

Note: CW, continuous wave; MRSA, methicillin-resistant Staphylococcus aureus; Tx, treatment.

species, both in terms of dose, frequency, power density, etc., but also in terms of how often we irradiate. If you do some research, you can also find experiments with blue light, which seems to be more antibacterial, with light and photosensitizing agents, and with low-intensity visible light, which has been reported to increase the growth of some species.[193]

Check Tables 5.1 and 5.2 for a summary of what has been published regarding this direct antibacterial effect of infrared and red light, both *in vitro* and *in vivo*. In practice, an infected wound would be treated using around 1–4 J/cm^2 as a starting dose. Always consider bacterial culture for complicated, chronic, or infected wounds. If what you are treating is septic arthritis, be aware of how painful that is; you will have to use a lower power density than if you are treating osteoarthritis.

Summary from a different perspective

The take-home message is: use laser in your infected wounds, and also in the rest, of course. You will improve the clinical response and will probably end up using less antibiotics, which is always good news in terms of patient health and global resistance matters. Antibiotics are not always free from side effects, and the growth in antibiotic-resistant bacteria makes the development of new strategies to combat infection a must.

PART 2

Pointing the light into the patient

CHAPTER 6

Light's path to all these places in the body

We live in a society exquisitely dependent on science and technology, in which hardly anyone knows anything about science and technology.

— Carl Sagan

The goal of this chapter is to give you just enough understanding about light transport through tissue so that you can make good guesses about the clinical impact you can expect. So we will very broadly cover what light does when it runs into stuff, how its accumulation is quantified, the different ways to deliver it, and some clinically important implications of all of this.

Or if you prefer, we can go right into deriving and solving these equations …

$$(\omega \cdot \nabla)L(\mathbf{x}, \omega) = \varepsilon(\mathbf{x}) - \sigma_a(\mathbf{x})L(\mathbf{x}, \omega) - \sigma_s(\mathbf{x})L(\mathbf{x}, \omega) + \sigma_s(\mathbf{x}) \int_{4\pi} f_p(\mathbf{x}, \omega, \omega')L(\mathbf{x}, \omega')d\omega'$$

$$L(\mathbf{x}, \omega) = \tau(\mathbf{x}, \mathbf{y})L(\mathbf{y}, \omega) + \int_{\mathbf{y}}^{\mathbf{x}} \tau(\mathbf{x}', \mathbf{x})\varepsilon(\mathbf{x}')d\mathbf{x}' + \int_{\mathbf{y}}^{\mathbf{x}} \tau(\mathbf{x}', \mathbf{x})\sigma_s(\mathbf{x}') \int_{4\pi} f_p(\mathbf{x}', \omega, \omega')L(\mathbf{x}', \omega')d\omega'd\mathbf{x}$$

I didn't think so. You are much more interested in how to better predict the clinical outcomes of your therapy based on what flavors of light you are shining at the patient. To do so, you'll need to know some very fundamental pieces of the puzzle, and so my discussion will be guided throughout by its utility in helping you practice better medicine (and integrating partial differential equations is not gonna get you there). What follows, then, is a very high-level, albeit informal and qualitative discussion with quantitative analysis only when truly necessary. Keep in mind, as you will learn very quickly, that this is not a "skim through and find the 'right' value" kind of section, mostly because no individual subsection tells the whole story. Instead,

after reading this entire chapter, you will get familiar enough with everything that is going on to then go back and find which tidbit you find most useful toward whichever clinical effect you aim to target.

6.1 Attenuation via absorption and scatter

The amount of light present in the beam decays (or is attenuated) with depth inside your patient. This idea teeters between intuitive and counter-intuitive among different people. On one hand, you realize that the thicker the curtains you use to cover your windows, the less light gets through. On the other hand, especially with today's state-of-the-art digital radiography, you see right through your patients with ease and little-to-no technique manipulation on your X-ray machine, no matter the size of the patient.

But it's time to be publicly honest (more so than some laser manufacturers/distributors) about where laser therapy falls in that spectrum: infrared light is STRONGLY attenuated by the body.

I've always avoided (like the plague) the request to answer the question of, "So how deep does it penetrate?" because that is an ill-posed question. Light is not like a needle that will go to a certain depth and then not exist beyond that point. Instead, it is a decaying intensity that eventually dwindles down to being negligible at a certain depth … given a certain time. Wow … how vague, right? True, but that depth and that time very much depend on what you start with at the surface: how much power of which wavelength of light you shine for what amount of time.

I promise to shed more light than that, but not before I explain a little more about where the light goes.

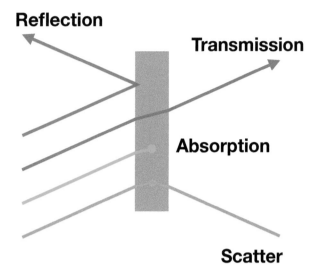

Figure 6.1 The four basic interactions of light.

We talked about absorption earlier. This is the way light "disappears" from the beam. Its energy gets transferred to the tissues and therefore, there is no more light. And this is the fate of virtually ALL of the light that enters the patient. That said, absorption is BY FAR the weaker of the interactions of laser light in your patients. The much more dominant interaction is scatter (Fig. 6.1).

6.2   Scatter: the primary interaction

Scatter is when light bounces off small particles within the tissue, changing the course of individual photons along its long and windy path to ultimate absorption. In the wavelength ranges relevant to therapy and given the body as the incident material, the type of scatter that occurs is termed "elastic," which means the light retains all of its energy as it bounces around. This is an important concept that merits being repeated in slightly different terms: light does not lose pieces of its energy along its path, so there is no slowing down during the pinball game. It remains in full effect until it gets absorbed, and when it does, it is completely absorbed – all the energy gone. So the only thing that changes is the direction of the photon as it gets pinged around the body.

To give some scope to the relative difference between these interactions, a single photon is likely to bounce around almost a THOUSAND times before it gets absorbed. Now granted, we don't talk about scatter (or absorption) in terms of the paths of individual photons;

we would lose count for a single photon very quickly, not to mention the billion billion photons delivered every second. Instead, we talk about probabilities and the average distances traveled, with terms like attenuation coefficients and mean free paths.

6.3   How much and in which direction?

I know I promised to spill the beans and give you an answer, but not quite yet. There are two very distinct and equally important concepts here: amplitude and direction. So you are not allowed to jump to any conclusions before I explain both.

For amplitude, I have to talk a VERY little about math and the idea of exponential decay. I won't bore you with the differential equations that govern light transport, but the amount of light that remains unattenuated (i.e. not absorbed or scattered) from a beam over distance is an exponentially decaying proportion that looks something like $I(x) = I0 \, e^{-\mu x}$, where I is intensity at distance x, and $I0$ is the starting intensity (at distance 0), e is the natural logarithm, and μ is the attenuation coefficient. OK, that's all the math you need. In English, this says that intensity will decrease by 36.8% for every section of distance equal to $1/\mu$. This distance ($1/\mu$) is called the mean free path, which is basically the average distance between attenuating interactions.

NOTE: Notice I've used only percentages here in my description. This is exactly how these values are defined, as the ratio of the quantity you are left with over the quantity you started with. Flexibility like this is very useful to understand how we SHOULD be talking about penetration.

Now, as we've covered, attenuation is a combination of absorption and scattering, so the attenuation coefficient μ is made up of two components, the absorption coefficient μ_a and the scattering coefficient μ_s. The inverse of these numbers is then the mean free path (or the average distance) between absorption and scattering events, respectively.

Remember how I said that scatter dominates over absorption when infrared light enters the body? Well, Table 6.1 shows exactly that. You can see that the average 800 nm photon scatters once about every millimeter in soft tissue, but is only absorbed about once every 33 centimeters.

This is awesome. Laser therapy penetrates SO far into tissue. WRONG. Those equations hold for interactions ALONG THE PATH of a photon. And so yes,

Table 6.1 Values for the mean free path between scattering and absorption events (calculated as the inverse of μ_s' the reduced scattering coefficient and μ_a the absorption coefficient, respectively) for 800 nm infrared light in some common tissues.[193] The last column shows how dominant scattering is over absorption.

Tissue	Mean free path between scatter events (cm)	Mean free path between absorption events (cm)	Average # scattering events before absorption
Skin	0.04	40.00	944
Brain	0.09	32.73	378
Breast	0.10	47.62	487
Bone	0.06	42.21	654
Soft tissues	0.10	33.48	344
Fibrous tissues	0.08	35.32	420
Fatty tissue	0.07	50.43	671

if a photon moved in a straight line through the tissue, it would go a long way before disappearing into tissue. But … it doesn't.

So while the values in Table 6.1 start to answer the "how much" question, the bigger part of the story describes the "where."

But first we need to understand a little about the importance of angles when it comes to light. An example from everyday life is very useful here. Why is it hotter in the summer than it is in the winter? I used to ask this question on the first day of my physics lectures to the pre-meds and engineering majors and sadly 80% of these brilliant minds that hold the future of our health and technology in their hands got it wrong – well, half wrong. Most people understood that it had to do with the angle of the earth's rotational axis relative to the plane of the orbit around the sun, so that the northern/southern hemisphere is pointed toward/away from the sun and therefore experiences summer/winter. During spring and fall the axis is pointed perpendicular to the sun and so they are about the same.

But the earth gets warmer NOT because the distance from the sun to a hemisphere is shorter. In fact, because of the earth's elliptical orbit around the sun (that's right, it's not a perfect circle), the earth is about 3,000,000 miles FARTHER from the sun on July 5th than it is on January 4th. But that's only about a 3% difference, which is why it has virtually no impact.

Instead, the reason for our seasons is the incident angle of the sun's light on each hemisphere during the summer/winter. Earth's axis is tilted 23.5° and this angle makes all the difference. Scatter is very VERY angle-dependent. At right angles (when the beam is perpendicular to the surface), scatter is very much forward-pointing, meaning the deflections to the angle of incidence are very small and most of the light continues in the same general direction – inside the patient. As the incident angle changes, the amount and angle of the scatter increases dramatically. This is called anisotropy, and again, we don't deal with individual photon paths, so we use a characteristic called the *anisotropy factor* to describe things. Technically, this is defined as the average cosine of the deflected angle. Or in English, if this value is 1, the average deflection is straight ahead; if the value is 0, the average deflection is at a right angle to the original beam (lateral deflection); and if the value is –1, then the average deflection is reflection (straight back at you). Figure 6.2 helps to illustrate this idea.

Anisotropy is an important concept since as we saw earlier, scattering events happen very often (multiple times per millimeter in some instances), making it virtually impossible to keep track of individual trajectories. Instead, we deal with averages, and so the scattering coefficient gets weighted by the anisotropy factor to give us a *reduced scattering coefficient* μ_s', calculated as $\mu_s' = \mu_s(1-g)$. The mean free paths in Table 6.1 used this reduced scattering coefficient in their evaluation ($mfp_s = 1/\mu_s'$).

You can see from Figure 6.3 that most anisotropy factors are in the range 0.75–0.90, meaning the average deflection (again assuming you started the beam perpendicular to the surface of the patient) is inside the patient, but at a 25–45° angle.

So now you're supposed to say, "Final answer: how far does light get inside the patient?" Then I say, "A few

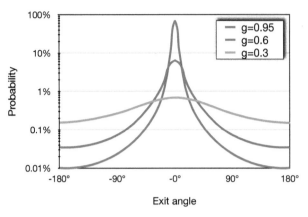

Figure 6.2 Probability of scattering at a given angle for several values of the anisotropy "g" factor. The way to read this figure is to pick a g factor (say 0.95 for example), and follow that line (red, in this case). What this tells you is the probability that a photon is scattered at a given angle, measured from the incident angle. So you can see that for g = 0.95, about 70% of the scatter is directly forward (angle θ = 0°) and at least 99% is scattered "mostly forward" or between 45° and −45°.

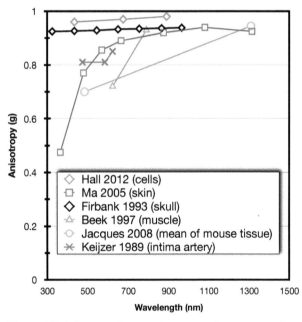

Figure 6.3 Anisotropy factors of common tissues at a variety of infrared wavelengths. Based on a range of published data. [194-199]

centimeters." Then you say, "Really? All this complicated analysis and that's all you come up with?"

Yup. With all this pinball action of scattering photons bouncing in all directions and incrementally being absorbed along their winding paths, that's about as precise as we can be. I can show you Monte Carlo

simulation data on a perfect slab of tissue with a perfectly cylindrical, homogeneous beam of photons incident perfectly perpendicular to the surface. And even in that case you'd see some serious spreading of the beam and decaying intensity over the first few centimeters of depth. In fact, Figure 6.4 is based on some of this data.[200]

But does that description of perfect geometry and homogeneous tissue sound like your Beagle's hip? Not even close. Also, do you plan to keep the hand-piece in exactly the same spot for the entire treatment? If you're not too discouraged after this let-down of an answer to your main question and decide to keep reading, you'll learn that treatment technique is not realistic either.

There are several pieces of good news though.

- Most of the light gets inside the patient (with good technique).
- Virtually all of that light gets absorbed somewhere in the body (you don't see massive exit beams of light coming out the opposite side of the body).
- Dose accumulates from various treatment paths (the intersection of two treatment beams, even if from opposite sides of the elbow for example, provides more dose at that intersection than along the two individual paths).
- Dose accumulates at depth over treatment time (more detail to follow in section 6.6 on Power).

So what does this mean to you as the clinician? Well, two things: first, that WHENEVER you are treating, it is CRITICALLY important to keep the treatment head PERPENDICULAR to the patient at all times. If not, much if not most of the beam will be deflected laterally or back at you, rendering your therapy fairly useless.

 He used a lot of capitals here because this is really important. In practice, what this means is illustrated in Figure 6.5.

Second, the beam profile inside the patient is not AT ALL what it looks like outside the patient. It doesn't matter if you have a shower-head-like treatment head or a very narrow "pencil" beam. If you are treating in one spot, you are getting light inside the body across an area that is much wider (in all directions) than the spot size you see on the surface of the patient.

This is a big deal. When you use a scalpel, you are cutting where you see the blade. Even when you apply

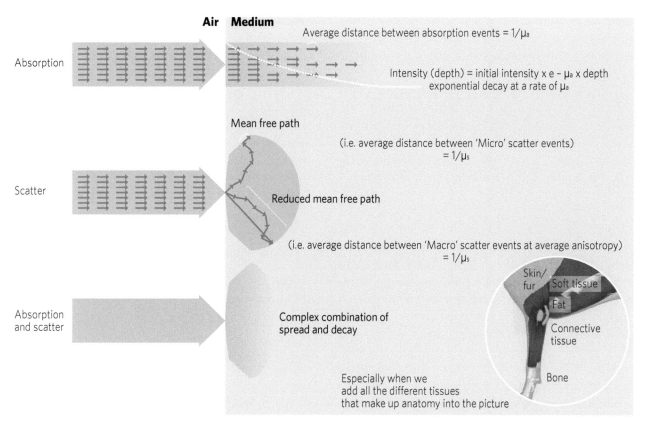

Figure 6.4 Pictorial representation of absorption, scatter, and the "real-life" combination of both. *Illustrator: Elaine Leggett.*

an ice pack, only the tissue underneath (or very close to) the ice pack is getting cold. But with laser, you will be administering therapy well outside of where you see the light.

This is a good thing, but also leads to some confusion.

There are two critical values: energy and power. Energy is the total energy of the beam INCIDENT at a given spot and is measured in joules. Power is the total energy of the beam incident on a given spot PER UNIT OF TIME and is measured in watts, with 1 watt = 1 joule per second.

I emphasize the word "incident" because we do not talk (in this industry) about the absorbed energy. In fields that deal with X-rays, we do talk about absorbed dose (in units of energy per volume or energy per mass of tissue) because, for X-rays, absorption is the primary

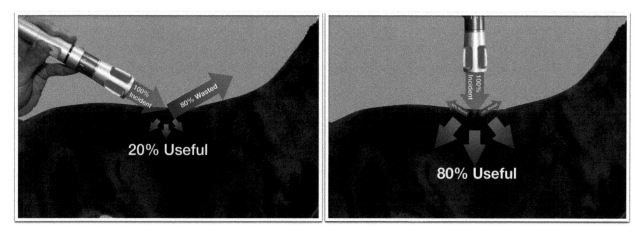

Figure 6.5 (a, b) The effect of the angle of the incident beam on light dispersion.

interaction. With infrared light, since scatter is the primary interaction, it is more appropriate to talk about the energy that passes through a given cross-sectional area, rather than a given volume.

So now we have to revisit those two critical values and add some spatial dimensionality to them in order to be useful. We started with energy and power. Now we move to energy density, better known as dose (J/cm^2) and irradiance (W/cm^2), or what is more commonly referred to (especially in this book) as power density.

6.4   How this adds up to dose

Talking about the number of joules of energy you delivered in a therapy session is a little like talking about how much water came out of the hose as you water your garden. Is 20 liters a lot of water? If you poured it all into a single flower pot, then yes. If you watered your whole lawn, then absolutely not. The same goes with light.

If you deliver 100 J of energy to an entire hip, you're not going to get much of a therapeutic effect. The hip of a medium-sized dog spans something like 500 cm^2 and so this 100 J divided by 500 cm^2 yields an average dose of 0.2 J/cm^2. If you gave that same 100 J to an affected paw that spans only 50 cm^2, then you would have given an average dose of 2 J/cm^2. Now we're talking.

However, there is still the lateral spread of light, even if you are diligent enough to keep the treatment head

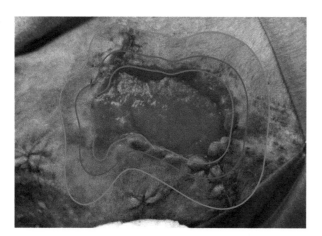

Figure 6.6 Treatment boundaries for an example wound. The blue area represents the boundaries of the actual wound. The purple encompasses the recommended treatment area (the amount to cover when aiming your beam). The red approximates the area through which you actually deliver a subdermal treatment dose.

exactly perpendicular to the surface at all times. So if you were to treat an exact area of 500 cm^2 – i.e. the very edge of the visible light you see on the surface of the patient is exactly 500 cm^2 – you are actually treating an additional 20% around the edges of your treatment area (Fig. 6.6). BUT that extra 20% is virtually all subdermal treatment. So when treating the fringes of a wound, make sure you cover (with your visible aiming beam) an extra 2–5 cm along the periphery, and then you will get the benefit of this additional 20% beyond that.

That extra 20% is welcome, since there is no disadvantage from treating healthy tissue (except for the usual contraindications). Having said this, 20% of a 1-5 cm^2 spot is a small area, so don't think that treating a few points in an area is the same as spreading a full dose over every square centimeter of it. Unless you are treating trigger points or acupuncture points, your aim is to cover the whole area.

The following chapters will give you specific recommendations for a variety of treatable pathologies and anatomies, but these basics of measurement set the stage. Almost.

6.5   Interpreting dose *in vitro* vs. *in vivo*

The simple calculation above is just that: simplified. It gives the average dose delivered to the SURFACE of the patient. We've just spent many pages talking about how complex the light transport and penetration situation is. And if you are talking about treating wounds, the simplified calculation in the last section is pretty much the whole story. But the majority of what you'll be treating won't be superficial; it will live within the soft tissue and bones and joints of animals ranging from 2 to over 50 kg.

This is important to keep in mind as you continue to read through the rest of this book, especially as we cite dose values from publications.

Virtually all of the empirical investigations that attempt to narrow the optimal treatment parameters have been performed *in vitro*. These studies have the advantage that the majority of the parameters can be easily measured and well controlled, and many of the results of these experiments have indeed shown an optimal dose region for biostimulation above which very little clinical benefit results. There are, however, inherent limitations in extrapolating these results to conclusions on the effects in bulk tissue, as well as some fundamental shortcomings in the breadth of their investigations.

The first is the fact that the amount of light incident on a monolayer of cells in a Petri dish is quite different than the amount of light that penetrates the skin/fur, through some fat and soft tissue, to an affected bone, for example. What you CAN take from an *in vitro* study on bone cell repair initiated by laser therapy is the amount of light it takes to stimulate those cells. From there you need the rest of this discussion to better understand what proportion of the light you start with at the surface actually gets to the bone, then work your way backward to understand how much you need to start with in the first place.

The second point of hesitation is the range of doses used and the *a priori* assumption that there is only one peak in the biostimulatory spectrum (i.e. one sweet spot of dose that gives the only hope for healing). Tiina Karu, among others, has shown this to be an invalid assumption, and that for a given cell line, there may be several peaks with similar biostimulatory effect separated by several orders of magnitude of dose.[194] There will clearly be a lower limit, below which no effect is possible. But I'll warn you that if some paper claims an upper limit – some maximum dose above which there is no effect, or some inhibition – they simply may not have measured enough of the dose domain to see the next peak.

With this there also has to be an admission concerning the opposite end of the dose spectrum. Most people who preach on the use of higher powers (as we do) quickly dismiss anecdotal reports on the clinical efficacy of much lower-powered lasers. And there is certainly a threshold below which no effect will be observed. But that threshold, as mentioned here, can be orders of magnitude different.

So things treated with a lower dose – or structures much deeper into the body treated with a higher dose – can still be getting the light they need to respond and repair. However, keep reading for the method to our madness when it comes to using the higher end of the dose domain.

6.6 Power

Dose is the accumulation of energy over a given area. How quickly that energy accumulates is dictated by the average output power of the laser. Average power is simply the total energy per unit time, where that unit of time is virtually always measured in seconds, and so the units of power are watts (1 watt = 1 joule per second). This is important to stress: a higher-power laser beam is simply producing more of the same light than a lower-powered laser (when all else is equal). Maybe it is better to say that a higher power setting on the same laser produces more of the same light as its lower power setting. But each photon still packs the same punch; remember that energy per photon is determined by its wavelength.

So the difference is about how many photons are delivered by each laser in a given time. Or from a time perspective, how long it will take with each differently powered laser to deliver a given amount of energy.

6.6.1 Average vs. peak power

A word to the wise: for the purpose of therapy lasers, always always always make any decision (purchasing or protocol selection) based on average power. Again, this is the total joules of energy emitted in a second, and given in watts. If you move your focus to surgical or body contouring or tattoo removal or even equine regenerative lasers, then you'll need to bring peak power into the conversation.

Photo-acoustics

There are some very cool things you can do when you have a very bright laser that emits its light in very short bursts: those short, but powerful pulses will force absorption events within the tissue that happen faster than the thermal relaxation time of the tissue, which causes the creation of a shock wave. These photo-acoustic waves (so named because they are caused by light – photo – but end up as shock – acoustic – waves) can permeate farther through tissue than the original light and can mechanically shake the tissue in their path. Sometimes this is good for imaging (photo-acoustic imaging), sometimes for bursting trapped ink packets (tattoo removal), sometimes for ablating the water in tissue (surgical), and sometimes even to force the release of growth factors from the extracellular matrix near dormant/hypoxic/necrotic tissues so as to stimulate healing where the body otherwise wouldn't (regenerative laser therapy).

Power vs. penetration

After I gave my annoying, imprecise "a few centimeters" answer on how far light penetrates, I made a comment on accumulation of dose at depth over time and promised you more detail. I come back to it here, as it relates to power.

The penetration profile of a beam is determined by the tissue being treated and the wavelength(s) of light used. Light that interacts (via either scatter or

Figure 6.7

absorption) with tissue in a stronger way leads to a steeper decay in intensity with depth. But no matter what the shape of that attenuation, if you start with more light, then you are left with more light at each

depth. In fact, any percentage increase in power will lead to that same percentage decrease in treatment time to deliver the same dose to the same depth. So it should be obvious that if you use twice the power, then you'll get the same dose to the same depth in half the time. But that doesn't say anything about penetration. Or does it?

The flip side of that same coin is what happens if you fix the treatment time. Let's consider the example of treating for a fixed amount of time and calculate the depth to which each laser will deliver the same dose. In Figure 6.7, you have two identical lasers treating at different power settings, with an exponential decay in intensity as you go deeper into the patient. Treating for 20 seconds with a 2 watt laser will deliver 20 joules of energy to depth A (50% intensity of 2 joules per second times 20 seconds). Now, even though the transmission percentage is four times lower at depth B (where the beam has decayed to 12.5% of its intensity), because you start off with four times more photons with the higher-powered laser, the same 20 joules of energy can be delivered to this deeper target (B vs. A) in the same treatment time.

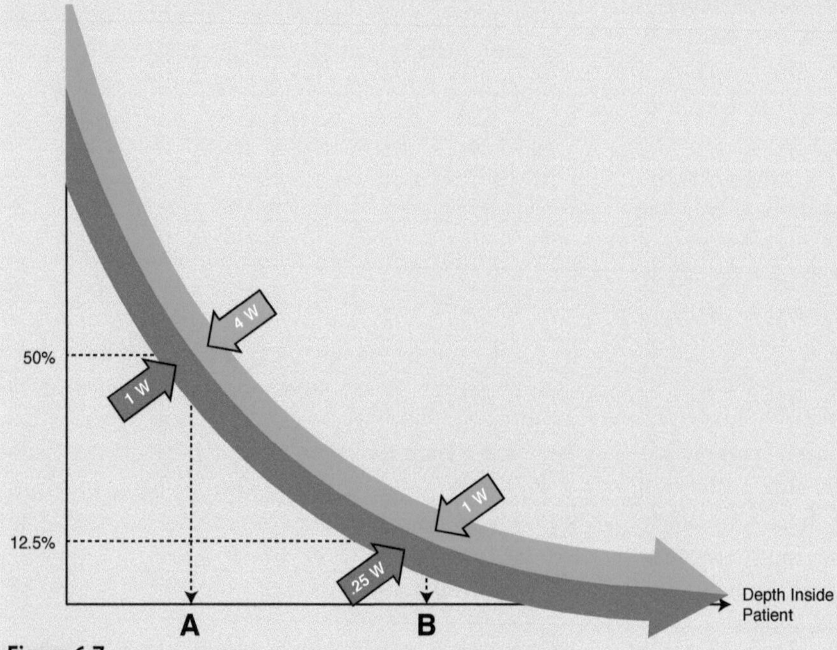

But for the scope of this book, average power tells the story. With continuous wave (light) where the light is always on, peak and average power are one and the same. But when you pulse the light, they diverge ... importantly. Chapter 8 dives into the importance of pulsing and the variety of effects it has on different tissues in the body. But here we will limit our discussion to what the light is doing and how it is structured.

Pulse frequency simply describes the number of pulses per second. If you try to reconcile which realm of thermal or biochemical effects discussed above is relevant to a laser pulsing at 20 Hz, good luck to you.

A simple picture may help here (Fig. 6.8). Our variables are pulse width t_{on}, dark period t_{off}, duty cycle DC, pulse frequency f_p, peak power P_p, average power P_a, and energy per pulse E_p.

You need t_{on} to tell you if the light absorbed during the pulse is going to cause an acoustic wave (i.e. if t_{on} is in the low microsecond range) or if it can be dissipated away during the pulse. You need t_{off} to tell you if the time between pulses is going to coincide with whichever thermal or biochemical process you aim to take advantage of. But you can get either from the other if you have the frequency or the duty cycle, so you need one of those (you could also have t_{on} and t_{off} or f_p and

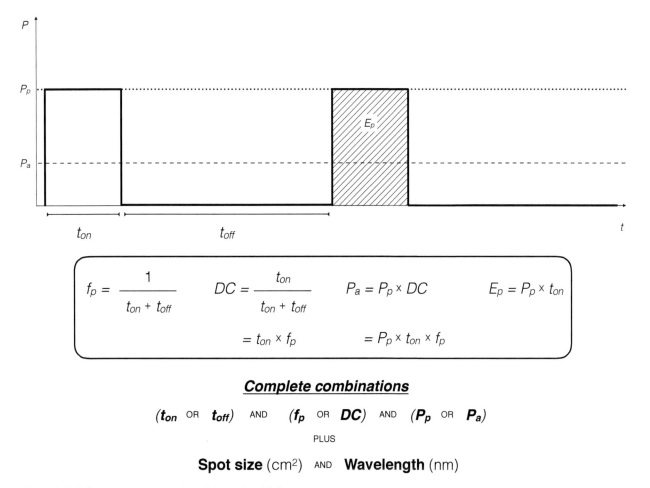

$$f_p = \frac{1}{t_{on} + t_{off}} \qquad DC = \frac{t_{on}}{t_{on} + t_{off}} \qquad P_a = P_p \times DC \qquad E_p = P_p \times t_{on}$$

$$= t_{on} \times f_p \qquad\qquad = P_p \times t_{on} \times f_p$$

Complete combinations

(t_{on}   OR   **t_{off})**   AND   **(f_p**   OR   **DC)**   AND   **(P_p**   OR   **P_a)**

PLUS

Spot size (cm²)   AND   **Wavelength** (nm)

Figure 6.8 Relevant parameters describing pulsed light.

DC to get what you need). Then you need one of the power values to determine the energy per pulse.

Obviously the wavelength and spot size round out the story, wavelength giving you information as to the absorption/scatter/penetration/target chromophore of the light, and spot size giving you the values of energy density (dose) and power density.

All that said, the average power P_a is what matters when it comes to understanding how much time is required to deliver your clinical effect. You will hear the term "superpulsed" thrown around a lot in this industry. That word in itself can be good or bad. In the good form, there are superpulsed lasers that deliver high average power, but with enough time between pulses to allow for thermal relaxation of the tissue. In the bad form, there are superpulsed lasers that have substantially high peak power, but their pulses are so short and so few that the total energy delivered per second (average power, by definition) is only about as much

as a laser pointer (in the low milliwatt range), which would take hours or days to deliver the necessary clinical dose.

But how long is too long?

6.7   Treatment time and reciprocity

In general, a serious question is whether the accumulation of dose is a sufficient predictor of clinical effect. With respect to pulsing, it is clear that the rule of reciprocity (i.e. that total exposure or dose determines clinical effect) does not hold across the board. The whole beneficial nature of pulsing relies on a specific timing of pulses (either in the time they are on or in the time the light is off between them) and so it is clear to see that if you modified the pulse structure (e.g. by decreasing the peak power but increasing the pulse width proportionally) you could expect a very different intra-tissue effect, even though the total energy per pulse and therefore the delivered dose was identical. Your new pulse may not be short enough to produce an acoustic wave, or there may not be sufficient dark time before the next pulse to allow the redox reaction to reset. That said, it may coincide with some different reaction rate or resonant effect. Or your changes might have been too subtle to make a difference. The point is, the pulse structure has at least some impact on the biological effect; if not, why are we pulsing at all? Chapter 8 will answer that in much more detail.

But an equally important question is the timescale of treatment, both within and between treatments. Should a treatment that aims to deliver 2 J/cm^2 of light take 2 minutes or 20 minutes or 2 hours? Should those treatments be repeated every hour or every day or every week? Or does it matter at all; i.e. will all of these situations produce the same clinical effect as long as they deliver the same total dose? These are ultimately clinical questions that I have no business answering, but there are some useful limits governed by concepts in my realm that we can cover before turning the question over to the clinician in the next few chapters.

The first limit is on the short side. Remember, there is a maximum power density that can be delivered to the skin before inflicting pain. This number depends somewhat on wavelength, since melanin absorption in the skin is the primary tissue heating mechanism and since melanin's absorption falls sharply from its peak in the ultraviolet (UV) and visible ranges (an evolutionary advantage that protects us from the sun's ionizing radiation) to virtually zero in the mid-infrared. But for reference, about 1–2 W/cm^2 of 800 nm, continuous wave light will begin to hurt after a few seconds, and about 2–5 W/cm^2 will inflict immediate pain. So you can't deliver too much energy at a time before heat comes into play. Then, there is the issue of area coverage. Whatever your dose prescription, odds are you'll want to deliver that dose uniformly to every part of the treatment area. And you can only move your hand so fast when trying to be predictable and repeatable, so you can't deliver 2 J/cm^2 to an entire hip in 10 seconds, even if your laser is capable of delivering that much output light.

On the high side, a clean example is to look at the sun. Figure 6.9 shows the solar irradiance data recorded by the National Renewable Energy Laboratory.[195] Surprising to some is the fact that the majority of the radiation we experience from the sun is not in the UV or visible spectrum, but rather in the infrared range.

How much though? Table 6.2 shows the integrated power densities (a quantity we will cover soon) for some relevant wavelength ranges as well as the resultant accumulated doses of each that we are exposed to per hour of sunshine. You can see that you are exposed to 33 mW/cm^2 of light in the "therapeutic window" (the region in the near infrared between the peaks of melanin and water where the greatest penetration into the body occurs) from the sun (Fig. 6.9). Some dose prescriptions you'll find in the coming chapters are attainable by sitting in the sun for an hour or two at this exposure rate. Does that mean that the clinical effects would be the same if you received all that light in a few seconds or minutes? Again, who knows, but this element of time (i.e. determining the minimum threshold of light per time that can stimulate a clinical effect) plays a crucial role and should influence your decision-making process when it comes to selecting a light source, as well as choosing a protocol once you have done so. In any case, if you are delivering light therapy at even close to that low a power density (and therefore over the lengthy treatment sessions you'd need at that power to deliver a therapeutic dose), then you'd probably be better off prescribing walks in the park rather than laser therapy.

Then there is the idea of energy storage in cells. One idea behind the "lasting" effect of a laser therapy session is that the cells produce enough energy during treatment to be used later. Leaving aside the biological processes in between, as well as fats in adipose tissue, excess cellular energy can be stored in the form of glycogen, which is synthesized when blood glucose and insulin levels are high, and which can be useful to the cells as energy for up to 12 hours. So if we indeed stimulate cellular metabolism and enhanced production of adenosine triphosphate (ATP), and if we think this leads to the storing of energy, then the timescale for effectiveness is about daily, or half that. Keep in mind though, that many laser treatments of acute injuries aim to actually "fix" what is "broken" and so the effects can last far longer than this.

So while reciprocity does not seem to hold across the board, there are certain windows within the broad treatment spectrum where you can be reasonably confident that slight tweaks (because a pet owner couldn't get to the clinic that morning or because you have the chance to deliver a second treatment since the animal is boarded overnight) will not severely impact your standard expectation of therapeutic outcome.

Spectrum of solar irradiance
(Power density at each wavelength)

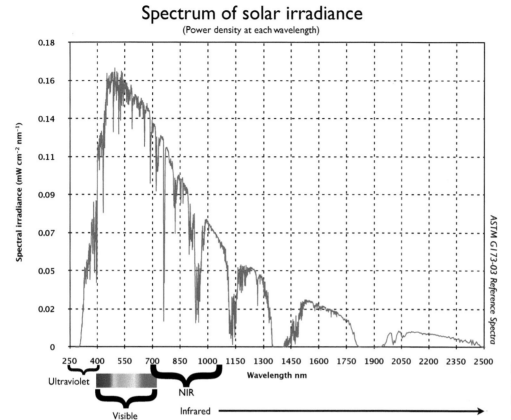

Figure 6.9 Solar irradiance data recorded by National Renewable Energy Laboratory.[195]

We may not speed up more tissue growth by treating every 12 hours instead of every 24 hours, but if you have an acute inflammation and the animal is staying overnight at the hospital, why not benefit from the extra anti-inflammatory effect? I do think you are likely to see a difference in short-term inflammation at least, but the truth is that there are no clinical studies comparing these two treatment regimes.

6.8   Power density and patient comfort

On the high limit of the dose range, another limitation presents itself: one of thermal accumulation. Whatever energy of radiation is absorbed in the monolayer of cells and the serum environment is converted to heat, and in a Petri dish, thermal diffusivity is extremely low. Dose is defined as energy density and so the higher the dose, the more energy is absorbed, and thus the higher the thermal accumulation. To get a real idea of what contribution this has to the cellular environment, let's

do a very first-order thermodynamic calculation to see if higher doses even have a chance at biostimulation before creating thermal damage.

Imagine we are testing the viability of 100 J/cm^2 of 980 nm radiation on a monolayer of cells in a Petri dish with (as standard radiobiology protocols suggest) irradiation in nutrient-rich growth medium to simulate *in vivo* pH and temperature. I won't go into the back-of-the-envelope calculations,[196] but suffice it to say that this amount of energy deposited in the serum would inevitably raise the temperature of the cellular environment well above the viability threshold.

It is well known that bulk tissue can undergo irreversible tissue damage when raised above 40°C, never mind in a monolayer of cells with only two degrees of freedom to dissipate heat. In fact, this thermal accumulation is often taken advantage of, and clinical hyperthermia is an increasingly popular technique in oncology. It turns out, using 980 nm light, that the threshold of thermal damage to cell culture would be around 30 J/cm^2, even though we know that light can have a beneficial effect on the body at these doses.

Remember, this effect is simply an artifact of *in vitro*

Table 6.2 Solar irradiance data from National Renewable Energy Laboratory.[195]

Wavelength range	Irradiance (power density) (mW/cm²)	Hourly dosage (J/cm²/h)
Total (280–4000 nm)	100	360
UV (280–400 nm)	6.4	23
Visible (400–700 nm)	46	160
Infrared (700–4000 nm)	48	170
635 ± 20 nm	5.8	21
800 ± 20 nm*	4.3	16
"Therapeutic window" (700–1100 nm)	33	120

Note: * Very few people would argue convincingly that 780 or 820 nm radiation has a significantly different therapeutic effect from 800 nm, hence the bandwidth listed here.

experimentation, where there is (intentionally) a lack of thermal diffusivity to maintain cell viability. The body, on the other hand, is very well suited to deal with both internal and external heat or cooling sources. After all, we live in an environment that ranges from much cooler to marginally warmer than our internal temperature; we also have the ability to drink hot coffee or hold an ice cube in our mouths without experiencing hyper- or hypothermia. To properly simulate this effect *in vitro*, some microfluidics designed to measure real-time temperature and simultaneously carry away heat would have to be employed.

In any case, it is clear that while *in vitro* experimentation is absolutely necessary to isolate individual chromophore absorption characteristics and cellular mechanisms of action, the Petri dish environment is quite different from our bodies. This idea resonates throughout the entire biological community: the reaction of a macroscopic matrix of cells that form tissue is NOT the sum of the reactions of each of the individual cells. One of the great mysteries of biology involves the complexity of cell–cell signaling and the ubiquity of bystander effects. A prime example of this intrinsic communication is in radiation oncology, where researchers have used X-ray needles (microscopically narrow beams of X-rays) to irradiate individual cells growing in a monolayer. Amazingly, cells far away from the irradiated region received information from the irradiated cells and underwent apoptosis (programmed

cell death) in a way that is characteristic of cells that absorb ionizing radiation (even though they didn't).

Accordingly, we have to narrow the scope of individual cell and single cell monolayer studies to the search for absorption sites and the cellular functions affected by these sites, and stay away from making broader tissue-scale generalizations.

I think by now you'll have had enough of "if you point light into the tissue," and you're ready for the more hands-on chapters that discuss what happens clinically when you do.

Summary from a different perspective

Keep in mind the type of absorption we talk about in laser therapy (Fig. 6.4), but also how much this is influenced by wavelength, and the type and color of the tissue. Remember to keep the beam perpendicular! (See Fig. 6.5.) Pulses have some advantages, but don't just focus on their peak power. Average power is always what defines how much energy a laser will deliver in a given time. We need enough power density to have a therapeutic impact, but not so much as to cause any thermal damage to cells or make the patient feel any discomfort. Laser therapy should always feel pleasant to neutral for the patient.

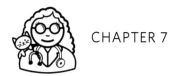

CHAPTER 7

Pointing light at soft tissue: clinical applications

The wound is the place where the light enters you.

— Rumi

Previous chapters have included a lot of references about what has been published in different fields; you will also find some here, but the focus is more on practical clinical tips and experience-based advice, which I hope will help you in daily practice.

Some particular soft tissue conditions will be discussed in this chapter; since the list of applications is so extensive and still growing, it is unlikely that all of them will be included, but you will get the foundations and examples to help you infer the appropriate treatment regime to apply when faced with a potential new case. Muscles and ligaments are soft tissue but will be covered in Chapter 9, together with bone problems, in the sections on musculoskeletal conditions (see 9.3 and 9.4).

7.1 General treatment considerations and parameters

After all that's been said in Chapter 6, some of the following information may seem redundant. Nevertheless, becoming completely familiar with laser therapy (LT) and its parameters requires repetition, so many basic calculations are detailed again.

7.1.1 Dose

Soft tissue treatments may include superficial areas, such as skin wounds, but also deeper targets, such as intrathoracic structures. The dose range can be as broad as 1 to 30 J/cm²: you will find suggestions under each condition described. In general, both dose and power will have to vary according to the following factors.

- **The depth of the condition:** treating a superficial wound is different than treating a deep fistula or otitis in the external ear canal. The deeper the target, the higher the dose you need on the surface of the patient, since most of it will be lost in the tissues in between. But of course, trying to deliver a high dose with a high power may excessively heat the surface – a surface that can be sensitive enough already, with a wound or inflammation – so the power used in wounds is lower than in musculoskeletal conditions. Some wounds will require higher doses than some musculoskeletal cases, though, but always delivered using a lower power, which means a longer delivery time.
- **The chronicity of the process:** after acute damage to the body, its repair mechanisms are activated; what we try to do with LT is push those mechanisms in the right direction and in the shortest time possible, and a lower dose is usually enough. But very often in chronic wounds, the body's resources seem insufficient or altered, and we need to "wake up" those mechanisms with a higher dose, and also a slightly higher power.

7.1.2 Power

The **power** (W) used in soft tissue conditions usually ranges from 1 to 6 W. There are several related parameters and treatment techniques this decision will influence (and be influenced by).

- **How long it takes to treat an area:** the higher the power, the shorter the time a treatment will take (W = J/s). You will first decide the dose you want, calculate the treatment area, and then decide the power you want to work with; this will determine the time spent on the session. Remember the power used for this calculation is the AVERAGE power, not the peak power.

  Many devices will have preprogrammed treatments. In some of them, preset parameters will coincide with what you want. But manufacturers' guides are not always clear. For instance, the laser device may have a program that just indicates treatment for a 10 cm² wound takes 1 minute. That information is NOT enough to go on: if the device is working at 1 W of average power, and we deliver the treatment just over the wound, having it on for a minute (60 s) will deliver 60 J in total, or 6 J/cm² over the wound area. Will that be enough? Many times it will. But if 1 W is the peak power because you are working with modulated frequency (Hz), you could actually be using 0.02 W, for instance, and the amount of energy used would be 1.2 J in total, or 0.24 J/cm², which will be an insufficient dose for most conditions.

- **What density of photons penetrates the surface:** higher power means more photons are delivered per second, and we need a certain amount of photons to elicit a clinical response. So, in order to reach deeper with a higher photon density, we need higher power.

- **How warm the surface gets:** this does not only depend on power itself, but on **power density.** Using 4 W of power with a 1 cm² spot hand-piece feels very different to the patient than using the same power over a 10 cm² spot. In the first case, power density would be 4 W/cm², and in the second, 0.4 W/cm². Of course, power and its density are not the only factors affecting how warm it gets: if we move the hand-piece instead of having it over a fixed spot, the tissue will have time to cool off. And the faster we move, the less warm it will get.

> Most patients will feel uncomfortable over 2–3 W/cm² and some even over 0.5 W/cm², especially if there is an open wound. If the patient's skin/hair is dark, the melanin will absorb more radiation and the hair/skin will become warm faster than in a light-haired patient (especially with lower wavelengths).

- LT treatments should both be safe and comfortable; of course we have to avoid thermal injuries, but we don't even want to get to the point where the patient starts feeling uncomfortable. So this comfort threshold can change according to the patient, its own skin temperature, its darkness of coat, and the condition. For instance, a hot spot or a first-degree skin burn will tolerate less power density than a chronic ulcer.

Calculating your treatment in four steps

1. Decide the dose (J/cm²) you will deliver, based on reference values and clinical progression of that particular case.
2. Estimate or measure the treatment area (cm²).
3. Multiply those two values to calculate how many J you want to deliver in that session, in that area (J/cm² × cm² = J).
4. The average power you work with (W) will then determine how long it takes to deliver those J (time in s = J/W).

DO NOT select a treatment time and just deliver a preset protocol, as some devices prompt you to do.

Example

1. You have decided to apply 2 J/cm² to a large wound over the lumbar area.
2. The wound and its 5 cm margins cover a surface of 24 × 20 cm (480 cm²).
3. Therefore, you want to deliver a total amount of energy of about 960 J in that session.
4. If you work with an average power of 2 W, it will take you 480 s to deliver that energy, which is a bit less than 7 min.

If you are treating a patient that seems somehow uncomfortable with the LT, check and try the following.

- **What are the power output and the power density?** You can decrease power density by decreasing power output but also by increasing the spot size of the beam. Depending on the manufacturer, this can be accomplished by adjusting an integrated "zoom" dial (which moves an internal lens closer to/farther from the fiber termination), increasing/decreasing the collimation of the treatment beam or selecting a treatment head with a wider diameter, or defocusing by increasing the distance to the surface of the patient. In most cases, this will suffice to improve comfort. Note that if you decrease power, you will decrease the final amount of energy applied, unless you compensate for this by increasing the treatment time.

Compensating for decreased power

Imagine you wanted to deliver 300 J over a certain area, using 4 W, which would take you 75 seconds. The patient seems uncomfortable, and one of the things you can do is treat with a lower power, such as 2 W. But then, if you were to treat for the same 75 seconds, the delivered amount of energy would drop to 150 J. If you still want to deliver 300 J, you should be treating for 150 s. In other words, if you use half the power, you need to double the treatment time.

- **What is your hand speed?** You can't move faster than the speed of light, but you can move faster than the speed of heat. So if you find that the surface temperature trailing the treatment area is getting warmer, increase the speed of treatment. But make sure you are getting uniform coverage of the area.
- **What are the wavelengths used?** Darker coats will absorb more energy, especially with lower wavelengths.
- **What is the temperature of the patient?** A cold skin has a lower threshold for thermal discomfort and pain than a warm one.
- **What area are you treating?** Areas with a thinner skin can be more sensitive.
- Try decreasing or eliminating the time you work with continuous wave (CW) (as opposed to pulsed mode), since CW has a more warming effect.

7.1.3 Pulsing frequencies

You can deliver your desired dose either with the light always "on" (CW), or by pulsing it with different **frequencies**. CW is the fastest way to deliver your treatment compared to modulated frequency (Hz; light is on/off and the energy is only delivered when it is on) but will also give the patient a warmer sensation. It will also increase blood flow more, which is something that can be worth considering (think for instance about a distal wound with compromised vascularization in that limb). Pulsing the light has shown biological benefits for wounds. The range of effective pulses described is very broad, though, from 2.5 Hz to 20,000 Hz.[48, 201] You can read a detailed discussion about pulsing in Chapter 8.

7.1.4 How often?

Generally speaking, acute conditions need a more fractioned treatment (lower doses but more often) and chronic conditions often need higher doses to "wake up" the metabolism again, but once some improvement is noted they can be treated less often.

These are examples of general treatment regimes, but there is some flexibility. The frequency of treatment should be discussed with the owner, since it generally implies several appointments (although maybe not long visits). Particularly for wounds, treatments should be coordinated with bandage changes as much as possible. More treatment regimes are described under each condition.

- **Acute conditions:** treat daily for 2–3 days, then every 48 h for 2–3 more treatments, and then twice a week if needed until resolution.
- **Chronic conditions:** treat every 48 h until you see a clinical response, then decide if twice a week will be enough. In some cases, such as otitis, a weekly dose or another maintenance regime is needed for some time to prevent relapse.

7.2 Wounds and burns

Wound healing is the most documented benefit of LT, and since it is such a safe therapy, it should be considered in almost every case in which you want to stimulate healing, decrease inflammation, and treat pain. (NOTE: remember, of course, the contraindications such as malignancies.) The analgesic effect on wounds can often be noted within minutes; if you don't believe it, just try it on yourself next time you get bitten or scratched. Wounds are a great way to start in the LT world, since more than 90% of them will show a positive change with just 1–2 sessions. This does not mean they will be closed with one treatment, of course, but the following effects are generally seen.

• Acute wounds that are becoming more instead of less inflamed after the first 48 h, which would be the physiological process, will evolve from this inflammatory/catabolic state to an anabolic/proliferative one, and produce new tissue and less inflammation (Fig. 7.1).
• Chronic wounds that are stuck in an underactive metabolic state will change to a more reactive phase, where new tissue can be created.

Since the required penetration is less than for musculoskeletal tissue, for example, and there are hygiene and patient comfort considerations, treatment is usually performed in non-contact mode. The exception could be when we treat the periphery of the wound and the patient is comfortable enough; in this case, we could also combine a non-contact treatment directly over the wound with a soft contact treatment over the periphery.

It is highly recommended to take pictures of the wounds and measure them at different stages (or at every visit) to help evaluate progression objectively. Always include a distance reference (ruler or index card) when taking pictures of wounds, and whenever possible, take the picture from the same angle in similar lighting conditions. Pain assessment should also be performed.

Dose (J/cm²): the range of appropriate doses or energy densities can range from 1 to 30 J/cm², and if you try to find literature to support the choice of a lower or higher value, please note factors such as how a monolayer of *in vitro* cells behaves differently from a real, full thickness wound, or how an acute experimental wound over the back of a mouse can be different from a chronic ulcer on a dog's footpad.

Some *in vitro* studies have suggested that high doses can be damaging, but where is the point where energy density becomes "high" or "too much"? An *in vitro* model with a keratinocyte culture found that doses of 0.1–1.2 J/cm² increased cell proliferation and migration, while 10 J/cm² was inhibitory[125]; however, the

experimental groups differed both in the dose and the power density. In another *in vitro* study, fibroblasts proliferated more under 3 J/cm² but not under 5 J/cm².[4] In her experiment with wounded fibroblasts, Houreld found that 5 J/cm² stimulated proliferation while 16 J/cm² was damaging.[115, 202] A similar result was described by Hawkins and Abrahamse,[117] who found 0.5 to 5 J/cm² to be stimulating for the *in vitro* growth of fibroblasts, while 10 and 15 J/cm² were inhibitory.

But the same doses (10–30 J/cm²) that seem to be too much for *in vitro* cultures have been found to be stimulating *in vivo*,[106, 123] and in fact, several peaks of stimulation have been obtained *in vitro* with both low and higher doses[203]; **dose may not necessarily be proportional to effect.** Even higher doses may be beneficial: a murine model of healing by secondary intention found even more collagen and glycosaminoglycan synthesis, cellularity, vascular density, and faster wound closure with 30 J/cm² than with 3 J/cm² doses[121] and 36 J/cm² improved random skin flap survival in a rat model.[204]

Again, the different parameters used in each study make it difficult to compare results. Most *in vitro* studies use a dose of 0.5 to 4.0 J/cm², but of course *in vivo* treatments may require and tolerate higher doses. A review including 47 studies with mice and rats concluded that there was a consistent benefit for wound healing.[128] The average dose in those studies was 4.2 J/cm².

To summarize, the usual starting dose for wounds is 1–4 J/cm². But we have also learned from clinical experience that high doses (10–30 J/cm²) may be beneficial to treat some chronic wounds, and remember dose is just a part of a bigger picture that includes other important factors, such as power density and time: taking 1 hour to deliver 4 J/cm² may not be as efficient (or practical) as doing it in 3 minutes.

Table 7.1 has suggestions about dose, power, and power density when treating soft tissue. Rather than considering these figures as something rigid you have to abide by, take them as a general framework, but always be aware of the values you are using.

When treating wounds, you need to include not just the wound bed, but a margin of healthy tissue. And of course, **that area needs to be included in your calculations.** Let's imagine an example: if you had a wound with an area of 150 cm², and you wanted to use 4 J/cm², applying 600 J is NOT what you need. If you were to include a 2 cm margin, your area of treatment would be 266 cm², and if you wanted a margin of 5 cm around

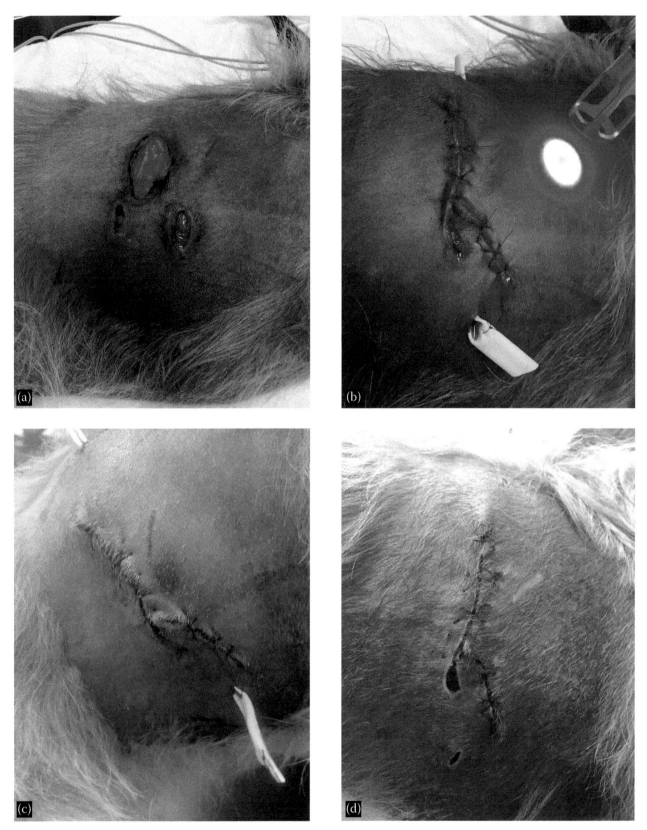

Figure 7.1 (a–d) A 48 h bite wound. All compromised tissue was removed, the remaining skin was closed with a Penrose drain and a laser treatment performed. Image (c) shows the wound 24 h later.

Table 7.1 Recommended parameters for management of mucocutaneous conditions.

	Example	Dose (J/cm²)	Power (W)	Power density (W/cm²)
Acute superficial	Skin incision, hot spot	2–5	1–3	0.1–0.5
Acute deep	Acute sacculitis, penetrating wound	4–6	3–6	0.3–1
Chronic superficial	Non-healing ulcer	4–25	2–4	0.3–0.6
Chronic deep	Deep fistula	5–20	3–6	0.5–1.2

the wound bed, this would mean a total treatment area of 500 cm². So if you really want to apply those 4 J/cm², you would need between 1000 and 2000 J, roughly 2–3 times the original value! I am not saying treating a chronic wound with 2 J/cm² will have no effect; but you need to be aware of the applied J/cm², so if the wound does not progress the way you expected, you know what parameters you started with.

Together with the wound margin, another strategy you can consider is to first treat the proximal blood supply area, and then the wound. This is often done in human medicine when treating distal diabetic ulcers.

> **NOTE:** Include at least the metacarpal/metatarsal area when treating wound in the foot pads

Regarding **frequency of treatment**, these are the guidelines for an uncomplicated surgical/acute wound.

- You may do the first treatment on the operating room table or in the immediate postoperative period (unless there is active bleeding or oncological concern), or at the time of initial wound management.
- If the patient is hospitalized, you may treat twice a day for the first 24–48 h, or daily until it can leave the hospital and then at the rechecks: since most surgical and uncomplicated wounds are expected to heal uneventfully, you may treat during the first recheck at 24–48 h and the second recheck at 5–7 days. Some of these wounds will need no further treatment, but you may add a last treatment at the time of suture removal.
  - If you feel the wound deserves closer follow-up, treat on 2–3 consecutive days and then treat every 48 h until suture removal.

Note that in acute surgical wounds, the first effect you will notice is a decrease in the expected degree of inflammation. But the effects on the tensile strength of the wound require more time to allow collagen and fibroblasts to be produced, so resist the impulse to remove sutures at day 5, even if the wound looks really pretty.

In chronic wounds, treatment is usually performed initially every 48–72 h and can be even less frequent later, but if possible, recheck no longer than 48 h after the first treatment and decide whether you want to continue with the same parameters or change them. I prefer not to spread treatments further apart until I see a change in the wound.

Frequency of visits should be considered together with the type and amount of discharge, since this will also determine the type and frequency of wound care. If the wound requires daily bandage changes in the clinic, then perform LT at that time. If it's every 2–4 days, adapt to that once the wound has started progressing; it is not difficult to schedule both events together. This way, we will avoid unnecessary bandage changes that would increase the risk of wound infection and affect tissue regeneration, patient comfort, and cost of care.

7.2.1 Acute wounds

Acute wounds (both traumatic and surgical) can be treated initially with 1–4 J/cm². What's more, we can take advantage of LT before the procedure starts, as in the example shown in Figure 7.2.

The first treatment of a surgical wound can be on the surgery table (Fig. 7.3), unless it is an oncological surgery and we want to wait for the pathology report to confirm surgical margins are clean enough.

If there is active bleeding, we do not want to laser the area of course, since the increased blood flow would worsen the hemorrhage. Just wait a bit and start the treatment a few hours later. If cryotherapy is going to be used over the wound area after the surgical procedure is completed, which can be very useful to decrease

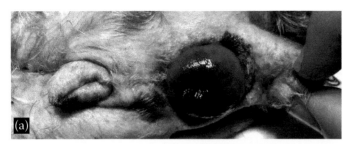

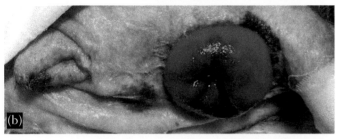

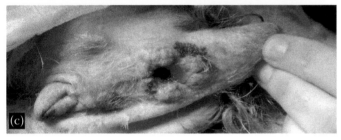

Figure 7.2 A 4-year-old Yorkshire Terrier about to undergo surgery for rectal prolapse. Even if we're going to remove this portion, it is preferable to operate on better vascularized tissue. The images show the prolapse (a) before LT, (b) immediately after LT, and (c) after surgery. Two consecutive treatments were performed, each using 2 J/cm^2 and 0.15 W/cm^2, and with 2 min time off between them. Another dose was delivered after surgery and 2 days later at the recheck. Healing was satisfactory and uneventful.

incision bleeding and inflammation, do it before LT and not after, since that would inhibit some of the effects of LT.

It is OK to use the laser with surgical staples and osteosynthesis implants, as any absorption by them will lead to negligible heat in the tissue. Colored substances like antiseptics should be washed out because they could potentially cause a photosensitivity reaction or an increase in local temperature, although a bit of a residual stain of dilute chlorhexidine is not a problem.

Surgical wounds treated with laser have the following properties.

- Less edema and erythema. LT also helps to deal with postoperative complications if they appear (Fig. 7.4).
- Less risk of complications, such as seroma formation or infection (see Case no. 12).
- They heal faster and better[106]: the tensile strength of the wound is increased.

Scar malleability can also be improved with laser[205]; this may significantly affect patient comfort (thick and poorly malleable scarring is a well-known source

of chronic pain in humans) and range of motion. So a thinner scar, a more resistant tissue … it is all advantageous.

By the way, clipped hair regrows faster as well, which will be appreciated by some of your clients. LT has also been used to successfully treat canine non-inflammatory alopecia.[206]

In fact, the reason we've had the honor of writing this book is due to this effect. The beneficial effects of laser were actually discovered via hair regrowth … accidentally. In 1967, Endre Mester was attempting to determine if laser light was carcinogenic to mice. The study results were negative (thank goodness), but interestingly enough, the hair on the back of the mice in the laser group grew back quicker than in the control group. And photobiomodulation was born.

LT can also benefit flap and graft survival, and it has been studied in experimental models of skin grafts[207] and axial pattern,[208] musculocutaneous,[209] and

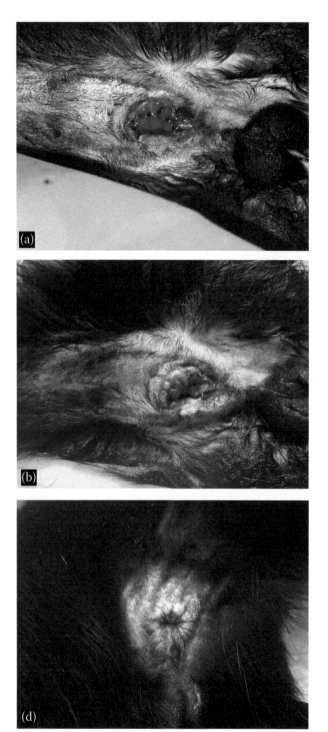

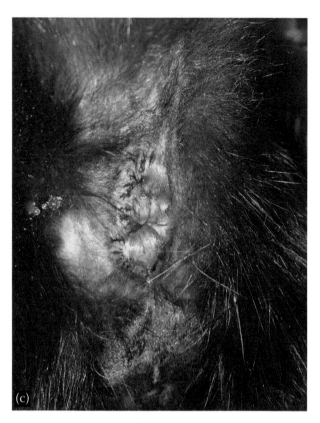

Figure 7.3 Another example of perioperative use of LT in anal surgery. (a) A chronic (1 years) rectal prolapse was resected. (b) After the procedure, LT was applied over the anal and perianal area, with 2 J/cm^2 and 0.2 W/cm^2. Immediately after the treatment, an improvement in tissue inflammation can be noted. Two more treatments were applied, (c) 24 h, and (d) 72 h after surgery, respectively. The patient started to defecate comfortably during the second day. Recovery was uneventful and complete.

random skin flaps.[204] If you were to work with a low power laser, and had to choose a point-type technique over uniform scanning, the most effective site to apply the light would be the base of the flap, where blood flow is going to come from initially. In an experimental model of abdominal muscle flap in rats, both single point irradiation over the vascular pedicle at the base of the flap (3 × 5 cm) and multi-point irradiation over its surface achieved a significant improvement in flap survival and angiogenesis.[210] It can also help accelerate wound healing at the donor site, of course: treat both areas in these patients. If you enjoy flaps and grafts,

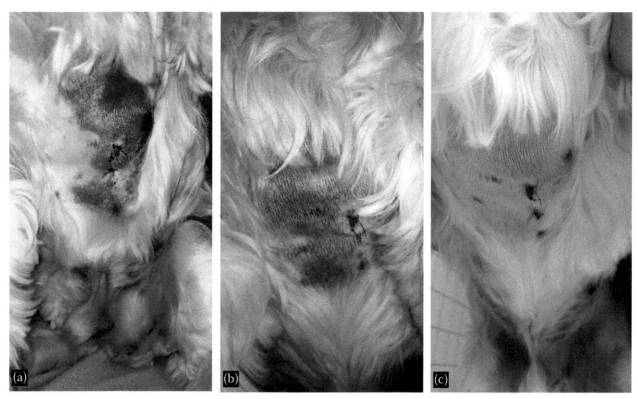

Figure 7.4 (a) Hematoma and swelling 24 h after surgery for lipoma in the sternal area. Laser treatment was used with a low dose of 2 J/cm² but over a 200 cm² area. (b) 48 h later tumefaction and hematoma have improved and a second treatment is performed. (c) The last picture was taken another 48 h later.

the "bad" news is that with laser therapy available, you will need to perform less reconstructive surgical procedures, since some cases will resolve with LT. But of course this is beneficial for the patient.

7.2.2 Chronic wounds

First of all, what really is a chronic wound? The Wound Healing Society defines a chronic wound as "one that has failed to proceed through an orderly and timely reparative process to produce anatomic and functional integrity or has proceeded through the repair process without establishing a sustained anatomic and functional result." So it may be taking too long to close, not progressing at all, reopening after an initial closure, etc., but LT can help in most cases.

The reasons behind chronicity can be multiple, but bacterial infection and hypoxia are common problems in chronic wounds, and both can benefit from laser therapy (see Chapter 2 and Chapter 5, section 5.6, for more on LT and blood flow as well as treating infected tissues). The conclusion is that although *in vitro* results are sometimes contradictory about the effect of LT on bacteria, *in vivo* studies show bacterial counts decrease with LT, whether this is the result of a direct antimicrobial effect, a consequence of the immune modulation, or a combination of both. This is interesting in all infected tissues, but especially when there is a multi-resistant infection or when antibiotics are not well tolerated.

The usual starting dose for chronic wounds is 4–5 J/cm², but some chronic cases will require gradual increases up to 20–30 J/cm². In a clinical case series, doses ranging from 6 to 21 J/cm² were used.[211]

We have three basic scenarios when we recheck a chronic wound.

- **The tissue looks the same:** in this case, you may either repeat the treatment and wait another 24–48 h, or consider increasing the dose and/or power density. You may be dealing with a weak reactor, a patient that shows a weak biological response to a standard dose or treatment regime. You can see an example in clinical Case no. 2 at the end of this chapter. Consider treating blood supply area.
- **The tissue looks metabolically healthier:** you can repeat the same treatment parameters, as in Case no. 7.
- **The tissue looks more active, but a bit too exuberant:** this is actually a good sign for a wound; it means you are dealing with a strong reactor, but use half the dose and half the power that you used the first day (see case study no. 6). In many devices this means switching from "chronic wound" settings to "acute wound" settings. Also give the patient some time before the next appointment (e.g. 2–3 days instead of 24 h). In all cases, I am talking exclusively about dogs and cats: other species may have a different type of tissue response, and the exuberant granulation may require a different approach.

7.2.3   Burns

As with any other type of wound, the benefits of helping **burns** heal with LT will include faster healing, decreased pain, and decreased risk of infection.[187] Experimentally, LT can increase the number of intact mast cells in the tissue during the early phases of burn healing, but decrease them in the remodeling phase.[61] The qualitative improvement in the new tissue formed can have a great impact on the quality of life of these animals, both because the new tissue will have more organized collagen and greater tensile strength, and because the increased malleability and decreased inflammation will make chronic pain and central sensitization less likely.

Nevertheless, this is probably the type of patient in which you will have to take measures to decrease power density and thermal accumulation, since hyperalgesia and allodynia are common (Fig. 7.5) – see section 7.1, "General treatment considerations and parameters."

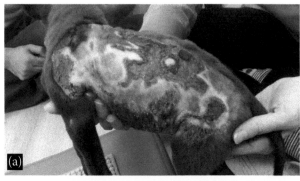
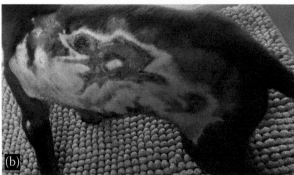
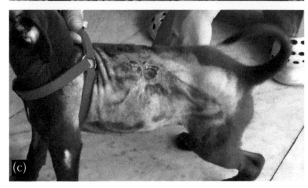

Figure 7.5 (a) Second-degree burns in a puppy. This is a typical example in which power density should be decreased due to hyperalgesia and decreased tolerance by the patient – only 0.2 W/cm² was used in this case, with 2 J/cm². (b) A week later, the same patient could now tolerate 1 W/cm² of power density. (c) Ten more days and the threshold is now normal, with no signs of discomfort at 2-3 W/cm².

This means decreasing power density, increasing hand speed, etc.

7.2.4   Wound care, dressings, and laser therapy

If you wonder what LT has to do with wound dressings, let me ask you a couple of questions.

- Do you think that once you have a laser, wound care will actually matter? After all, with such an amazing

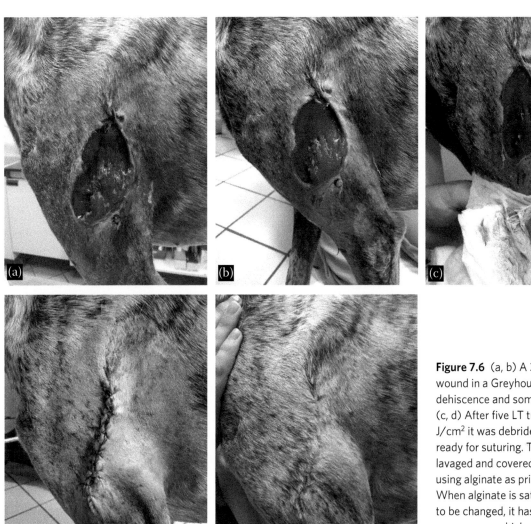

Figure 7.6 (a, b) A 3-week-old bite wound in a Greyhound presented with dehiscence and some necrotic tissue. (c, d) After five LT treatments with 5 J/cm² it was debrided and granulated, ready for suturing. The wound was also lavaged and covered with a bandage, using alginate as primary dressing. When alginate is saturated and ready to be changed, it has this jelly-like appearance, which should not be mistaken for infection. (e) The sutures were removed 12 days later.

tool, tissue healing is going to be enhanced. Well, of course wound care is at least as important as LT.

- If you do moist wound care and you do not want to remove the primary dressing, would the light be absorbed in the same way through alginate, a hydrogel, or a transparent film? The answer is no: some material will transmit much more light to the underlying tissue and we will discuss this here.

Appropriate dressings and bandages prevent trauma (including self-trauma) and contamination. When properly used, they contribute to patient comfort and can help remove exudates and create an optimal environment for wound healing. The selected type of dressing depends on the amount of exudate you expect and the phase of healing the wound is at, but as a general rule, wounds are better if covered; moist wound care has been proven better for a long time in humans, and is gaining ground in veterinary medicine, as opposed to the old paradigm of "let it dry and breathe."

For highly exudative wounds, especially if some debridement is needed, one of the best contact layers to choose is an alginate dressing, either with plain calcium alginate or silver-impregnated. It is also hemostatic; but remember you do not want to laser an active hemorrhage though. This is more often used whenever there is still some debridement to do and a higher amount of exudate to evacuate. Bandage changes are performed every 24–72 h, depending on how fast the dressing saturates. When it is ready to be changed, it looks like jelly and comes off very easily, making the change comfortable for the patient (Fig. 7.6). If the alginate dressing looks dry, you should either space changes further apart in time, or switch to a less absorbent type of dressing.

> A study of burn wounds showed LT was sufficient to stimulate myofibroblastic differentiation, but when it was combined with cellulose films or sodium alginate/chitosan-based dressings it improved epithelialization, angiogenesis, and collagen synthesis with a higher proportion of organized type I collagen.[212]

Once granulation tissue starts to appear or the amount of exudate is moderate, polyurethane foams and hydrocolloids are a good choice. In this stage, bandage changes usually take place every 2–4 days. Check the dressing to make sure it is not too saturated and if so, consider more frequent changes or a more absorbent material such as alginate. If there is little exudate, bandage changes are often postponed to every 3–5 days; hydrocolloids will maintain optimal moisture, and when there is extra desiccation risk, a hydrogel is added. Manuka honey is also useful and can be added in all phases – it sounds more sticky and messy than it is; it is worth trying if you haven't already done so. Much more novel than honey, a new type of dressing based on a galactomannan matrix made from locust bean gum and an antioxidant hydration solution containing curcumin and N-acetyl-L-cysteine (HR006) has been marketed, which forms a hydrogel matrix that is able to absorb exudates while promoting an optimal microenvironment that enhances healing.[213, 214] With this type of product, the primary dressings are usually changed every 5–7 days, which can be a great advantage.

Some membrane-type wound dressings and gels may transmit more than 50% of the laser light.[215] Quite an extensive study was performed with different kinds of occlusive wound dressings and wavelengths,[216] showing that, depending on the material of the dressing and the wavelength, the amount of power transmitted could range from 96% to 0% of the incident power. Hydrocolloids and thin, translucent dressings all allow transmission of more than 40%. Others, such as opaque tape and bands, activated charcoal, and other absorbent dressings, allow very little to no power transmission. Opacity and thickness, rather than density or the presence of any adhesive, were the most relevant factors. The 904 nm beam had the highest transmissivity. So you may consider keeping the gel/translucent membrane dressing and increasing exposure time; but

opaque dressings should be removed to perform LT over a wound. If you want to maintain that primary layer intact, you could still remove the tertiary and secondary bandage layers and laser the periphery of the wound.

Having the best materials available is ideal, to make sure you need fewer bandage changes, improve patient comfort, and promote healing. Nevertheless, if these types of dressings are not available or affordable, you can still do decent wound management with cotton-based gauzes and paddings. Remember to avoid loose cotton that could leave some threads in the wound, use a sterile contact layer (with some hydrocolloid ointment if possible), and if there is thick exudate, to remove it using a wet-to-dry technique.

So when a bandaged wound comes in, the overall plan is as follows. First, remove bandages and coverings. If they are stuck to the wound surface, which is avoided in moist wound care technique, moisten with saline to facilitate separation. Inspect and smell these materials. Lavage the wound with lactated Ringer solution or, as a second option, with sterile saline, to remove debris and reduce biofilm and inflammatory mediators. Perform the LT. If the wound has signs of infection, you may lavage with antiseptics after this, preferably with chlorhexidine at 0.05% concentration: a higher concentration can inhibit healing, and a lower concentration is not enough to be antiseptic. After a few minutes of contact, wash the antiseptic off with more lactated Ringer solution and cover again with a new dressing and bandage. Consider sedation if necessary, depending on the amount of manipulation, discomfort, pain, or stress expected with the procedure and the patient's clinical situation.

7.2.5 How to improve results

- **A+ Wound care:** LT helps create a better local environment to promote wound healing, because perfusion increases, oxygen delivery improves, white blood cells work more efficiently, there is less necrosis and an overall better metabolism. But you still need to lavage, debride, cover, and manage the wound properly. Good wound care acts synergistically with your LT, but poor wound management will decrease or eliminate the positive effects of LT. It is not a magic wand – you cannot do LT and forget about the rest.
- **Don't be afraid to increase stimulation:** as we

have said, if you treat a chronic wound with 4–5 J/cm^2 and after 1–2 treatments (in 24–72 h) it looks the same, stimulate it more. You can use a higher dose (more J/cm^2), a higher power density (more W/cm^2) or both. I tend to maintain power density around 0.2–0.5 W/cm^2 but increase dose (by 30–100%) by increasing treatment time when I want to stimulate a wound more. Underdosing is much more common in LT than overdosing; just don't try to give that extra energy too fast (too much power) or over too small a spot (too much power density).

- **Consider other factors that may interfere with the healing process:** I suggest you read the "Guidelines to aid healing of acute wounds by decreasing impediments of healing"[217] for a more extensive review of local and systemic factors affecting wound healing and the level of evidence behind them. The Wound Healing Society categorizes local factors into wound perfusion, tissue viability, hematoma and/or seroma, infection, and mechanical factors. LT improves blood supply, oxygenation, and metabolism, which affects both perfusion and viability. LT should not be used if there is active bleeding, since we would increase hematoma, but after bleeding is controlled it can help resolve the hematoma faster, decrease the risk of seroma formation, and decrease bacterial counts in infected wound and burns. Mechanical factors such as licking or other forms of self-trauma to the wound are very common in small animal practice, much more than in human medicine. Many owners report their that animals pay less attention to the wound after LT, but we still need to find the best way to protect the wound while keeping the patient comfortable.

If local factors seem to be under control but the wound is not properly progressing, consider systemic factors that may be contributing to this delay – these are just a few.

- **Steroid treatment** affects wound healing, whether you laser the wound or not. But LT will help counteract those inhibitory effects of steroids.[118] One paper described no effect of LT in steroid-treated rats,[137] but they were using 1–15 mW/cm^2, whereas you will be using around 200–600 mW/cm^2 most of the time while working with class IV devices and wounds. You need a certain power density to achieve a biological effect, and steroid treatment may also change that threshold.

- **Endocrine disorders:** diabetes, Cushing's, hypothyroidism, and Addison's can be quite a challenge, especially Addison's.

- **Paraneoplastic syndromes** can dramatically alter wound healing – usually other symptoms are present.

- **Nutritional deficits:** an insufficient caloric and/or protein intake will affect wound healing. Some situations, such as burns, post-ops, and severe infections, require a higher protein intake. Vitamins A and E, zinc, copper, magnesium, and omega-3 fatty acids are especially relevant to proper wound healing.

- **Immune and/or infectious diseases**, such as leishmaniasis (which is unfortunately very common in Southern Europe) will have an effect. This does not mean you will not achieve wound closure in an immune-suppressed patient, but it may take longer. In an experimental study with hydrocortisone-induced immunosuppressed rats, LT improved wound closure and decreased inflammation.[48] Interestingly, 10 Hz seemed to work better than 100 Hz in these rats. Leishmaniasis patients may experience more challenges when it comes to wound healing, but in my experience LT is very likely to help them too when it comes to wounds and pododermatitis.

7.3 Lick granuloma

This is one of the conditions in which you often have to significantly increase the dose, and it is not uncommon to end up using 20–30 J/cm^2, especially in the more chronic and hyperplastic lesions. Nevertheless, some patients respond to 4–5 J/cm^2, which is a usual dose for chronic wounds. You can use 2–4 W. Do not hesitate to broaden the treatment area and treat a 5 cm margin (Table 7.2).

The etiology of lick granulomas is multifactorial, and often not even diagnosed. Behavior disorders, atopy, folliculitis, and other causes are considered, but some animals enter this cycle because a painful condition is present, in the granuloma area or at a distant site, and this should be ruled out and treated if diagnosed. Neuropathic pruritus and dysesthesia may also occur, for example in intervertebral disk disease and nerve root irritation. Investigate these as potential causes; if you think there is such a component, you need to

Table 7.2 Recommended parameters for lick granuloma.

Dose (J/cm²)	Power (W)	Power density (W/cm²)
4–30	2–4	0.5–0.8

address it, whether it is with LT, manual therapy, or however indicated.

Make sure the animal cannot lick the area, but consider the stress that Elizabethan collars (E-collars) represent for some cases and think of alternatives if necessary. Treat 2–3 times per week and if the area is bandaged, schedule its change for the same day. My advice is that you continue with a twice a week schedule until the lick granuloma is resolved, and then keep treating the area once a week for 2–4 more weeks. If after the first 2 weeks there is no substantial improvement or if the granuloma is too old and hyperplastic, you may consider granuloma ablation (by conventional surgery or CO_2 laser) and laser treatment for the postsurgical healing (Fig. 7.7).

7.4 Dermatitis

7.4.1 Acute and chronic dermatitis

Acute moist dermatitis, commonly known as hot spots, can be the result of self-trauma or acute focal

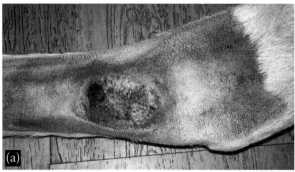
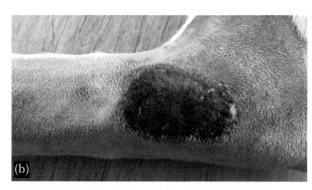
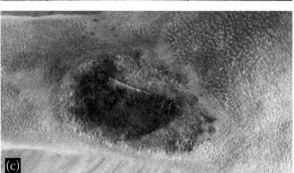
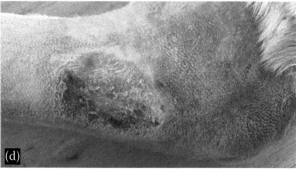
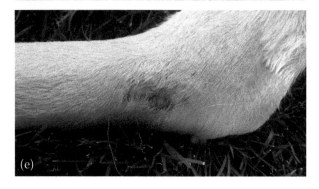

Figure 7.7 (a–e) Some granulomas require surgical treatment. In this case, ablation with CO_2 laser. Ten treatments of LT with 5 J/cm² were used postoperatively to help with healing.

Table 7.3 Recommended parameters for dermatitis.

	Example	Dose (J/cm^2)	Power (W)	Power density (W/cm^2)
Acute superficial	Hot spot	2–5	1–4	0.1–0.5
Chronic superficial	Chronic dermatitis	4–15	2–4	0.3–0.6

pyoderma (and usually both). Traditional treatment includes clipping the area, using topical antiseptics and a variety of topical and/or systemic corticosteroids and antimicrobials. The systemic use of these medications can (and should) be avoided in most cases, and LT is a very useful adjunct that quickly decreases inflammation and discomfort and helps with the skin infection and regeneration.

Rinse off topical treatments before LT. Use 1–3W and 3–5 J/cm^2, but keep a low power density in the most acute phase and inflamed cases. Treat daily for 2–4 days, then gradually decrease frequency of treatment (Table 7.3).

Chronic dermatitis can be more challenging to treat due to the permanent tissue changes we encounter. Nevertheless, LT can be a very useful adjunct – and sometimes substitute – to traditional pharmacological treatment. Consider increasing dose and power compared to what you use in acute cases, i.e. use 4–8 J/cm^2 and 2–4 W. Start with the lower settings but consider increasing values if after 2–3 sessions you don't see a significant change. Chronic steroid therapy can delay the response, but in most cases you will notice improvement in both lesions and patient comfort (Fig. 7.8).

7.4.2   Pododermatitis

This is a general term that comprises a number of presentations of local, dermatological, and systemic conditions leading to inflammation of the skin in the paws, with or without concurrent infection (Fig. 7.9). You will probably have been faced with frustrating cases, and LT does help, but before you run to get your laser, please work a diagnosis: fungal, bacterial, and parasitic infections are on the list,

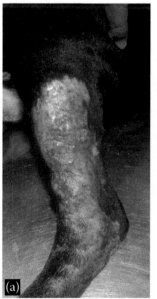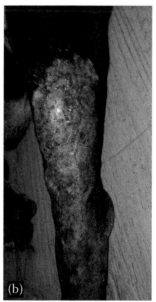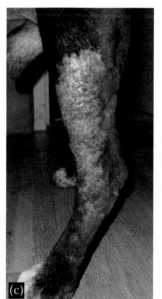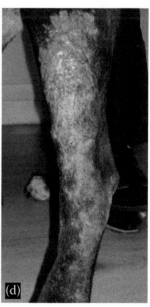

Figure 7.8 (a–d) This 11-year-old male castrated (MC) Pit Bull had been on different courses of steroids and antibiotics for over 9 years. He had a deep pyoderma and was referred for LT due to gastrointestinal side effects of the medication. The pictures show the progression over 5 weeks and 14 treatments. All medications were discontinued when LT started (progressively in the case of steroids). By the middle of the treatment, dose was increased from the initial 4 J/cm^2 to 17 J/cm^2. Average power was initially 3 W, and later increased to 4 W. Power density was kept around 0.5 W/cm^2. The whole circumference of the hindlimb was treated, from the proximal tibia to the foot.

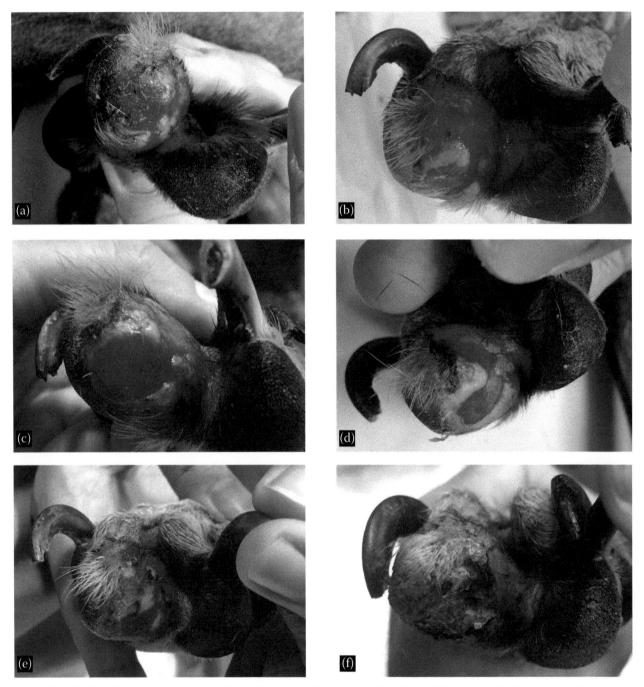

Figure 7.9 Healing of a chronic wound and dermatitis in the left forelimb pad and interdigital space of a 10-year-old MC Greyhound. The dog suffered from leishmaniasis. The nail was lost. He had been adopted 4 years before and the wound and dermatitis were already present by that time. The treatment dose was 5 J/cm², which was increased to 10 J/cm² later on. One to two treatments per week were performed. A grade 3/5 lameness in the same limb disappeared as the wound healed. (a, b) Before initial treatment; (c) 48 h later; (d) after 10 days; (e) day 20, fifth treatment; (f) day 45, ninth treatment.

with endocrine disorders, atopic dermatitis, sterile interdigital pyogranulomatous pododermatitis, just to name a few, and often several factors will be contributing – plus the self-trauma perpetuates the problem. The success of LT depends on the etiology and full management of the condition, but in most cases it will at least be a valuable adjunct, with the following effects.

♦ Lesions will likely heal with less scarring; scars contribute to susceptibility to future infections.

♦ Self-trauma will decrease with the relief of pain, inflammation, and pruritus.

♦ The enhanced perfusion you can achieve with LT is actually well sought after in some deeply seated bacterial infections, where even pentoxifylline is considered.

A couple of clinical papers have been published addressing LT in canine pododermatitis. One of them describes how LT with daily treatments for five consecutive days was effective in treating sterile pyogranulomatous pododermatitis in a case–control study in five dogs.[218] Some cases will not respond so dramatically, but in my experience LT will allow you to decrease the use of glucocorticoids in such cases.

Another paper reports how a regime of three treatments per week for 2 weeks plus two treatments per week for the next 2 weeks, using 4 J/cm², was not effective in decreasing two scores in atopic dermatitis dogs: localized canine atopic dermatitis severity score (LCADSS) and owner localized pruritic visual analog score (LPVAS).[219] Interestingly, in this study one paw was treated with LT and another paw in the same patient was used as a control. The study had to conclude LT was not effective because there was no difference between the paws ... but both treated and control paws did improve.

If tissues are very inflamed, start treating with 2–4 J/cm² and low power density, even if it takes longer, on at least 3 consecutive days. If the inflammation is less severe, you can start with 4–8 J/cm² and more focused energy every 48 h – gradually increase if you don't get a response, though. Treat both the dorsal (Fig. 7.9)

and palmar/plantar surfaces, and if the patient allows you, separate the digits to improve interdigital skin exposure to laser. Remember to try to keep the beam perpendicular to the skin surface. Your treatment area has to be calculated for both the dorsal and the palmar/plantar surfaces, and it is usually a good idea to include all the area up to the carpus/tarsus.

We always need to be aware of the patient's eye safety, and treating the front paws can put the beam and the head in positions where eye exposure is relatively easy, especially when the palmar surface is treated or in very nervous animals.

7.5 Ear disease

7.5.1 Otitis

LT can help acute and chronic cases of external otitis. It is not uncommon to find patients respond to LT after a challenging and frustrating series of other more conventional treatments. Nevertheless, proliferative otitis is more refractory (depending on the case you will have to consider surgery and LT postoperatively), and some cases need a maintenance treatment regime to prevent relapse, or a new course of treatment with seasonal worsening, most commonly in the spring time.

Other segments of the ear can potentially benefit from LT; an experimental animal model showed LT could help the tympanic membrane heal faster, while decreasing inflammation and preventing excessive fibrosis.[220] LT may also be useful in the recovery of hearing and cochlear hair cells after different types of damage, such as gentamicin-induced ototoxicity[221] and noise-induced hearing loss.[222] *Ex-vivo* dosimetry measures show how penetration into the cochlea is

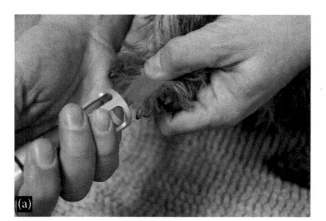
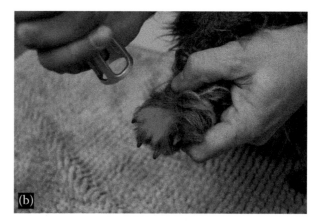

Figure 7.10 (a, b) Interdigital treatment from the dorsal and cranial directions, opening the interdigital spaces.

about 100 times better through the tympanic membrane than through the mastoid portion of the temporal bone.[223]

The first benefit you will notice from adding LT is a faster resolution of inflammation and pain. Some mild cases will not need any treatment other than LT, but others will definitely require topical medications, and sometimes also oral. A severe, purulent, and ulcerative otitis does need other treatments. Plus LT is never a substitute for a local ear cleaner. My advice is that when you first start to work with LT, you do not change your usual treatment protocol; just add the laser. Once you become more used to it, you will feel more confident in predicting its clinical effects. Please, remember the importance of antibiograms.

Before you start treating, eliminate debris and secretion to a reasonable extent and remove topical products to a reasonable extent – full removal is usually not possible in this location. The **pinna** can be treated as if it was an acute/chronic wound, in non-contact mode, with quite similar considerations for dose and power – usually acute wound settings are enough (Table 7.4).

- Use 2–6 J/cm²: start with the lower dose, but consider increasing it if by the third treatment you don't see a response, especially if it is a chronic case.
- Use 1.5–3 W of average power.
- This area can be more sensitive than a wound in some dogs and keeping a low power density is important. Depending on the patient's tolerance, use 0.2–0.6 W/cm². In an acute flare-up, with very inflamed skin, choose a lower power density; for chronic refractory cases with not so much reactivity, you may choose the higher end of the range. Nevertheless, the patient will tell you if it is too much, for example by flinching the ear.

With proper positioning of the ear, light can be focused inside the vertical **ear canal** in non-contact mode (remember to keep moving your hand-piece),

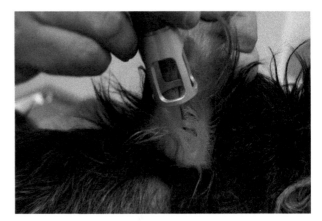

Figure 7.11 Direct exposure of the vertical ear canal.

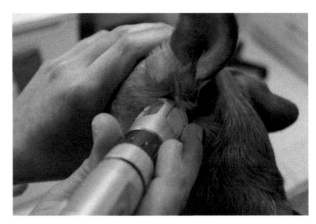

Figure 7.12 Contact treatment of the ear canal through the skin.

from a caudolateral position, aiming down the canal as you do when you move the ear to explore it with an otoscope (Fig. 7.11). To reach within the ear canal from the lateral, cranial, and caudal aspects, more power, dose, and power density are used (about double for each) to penetrate skin and cartilage, and contact, if tolerated, improves penetration (Fig. 7.12). It is advisable to combine both direct exposure and treatment from outside, and to include the projection area of the bulla in the outer treatment.

Table 7.4 Recommended parameters for otitis.

	Dose (J/cm²)	Power (W)	Power density (W/cm²)
Acute, pinna	2–4	1–3	0.2–0.6
Acute, canal	4–6	3–4	0.6–1
Chronic, pinna	4–6	2–3	0.2–0.6
Chronic, canal	6–12	4–8	0.8–1.2

Table 7.5 Recommended parameters for otohematoma.

Dose (J/cm²)	Power (W)	Power density (W/cm²)
4–6	1–3	0.2–0.5

For acute otitis and severe flare-ups, consider treating daily for 2–3 days, then spread out treatments to every 48 h, then 72 h, according to progression. For chronic cases you can start treating three times a week and then decrease to twice a week once there is an improvement; do not decrease the frequency of treatment until you notice a clinical response. You should notice an improvement in 1–2 weeks, otherwise reconsider treatment and/or diagnosis.

7.5.2 Aural hematomas

Most aural hematomas have a concurrent otitis that explains the ear shaking, scratching, and trauma that break the blood vessels in the pinna's cartilage. A few cases will report trauma without otitis, and a few others will have an underlying condition that interferes with blood coagulation (e.g. ehrlichiosis) – you may want to check this if there is absolutely no otitis or history of trauma.

There are almost as many approaches for aural hematomas as for cruciate ligaments. If drainage and bandaging is your preferred approach and works for you, I will not try to convince you to change and do more surgeries. If the punch technique is your thing, keep doing it. My preferred treatment is surgery with transfixation mattress sutures (always monofilament), with or without an otohematoma pad – the pad helps to keep the ear straight but makes it more difficult to use the laser and clean the wound. Whatever you do, LT will help to:

- absorb the hematoma faster
- produce less exuberant fibrosis, with a better cosmetic result
- decrease the inflammation associated with the otitis and/or surgical procedure
- make the patient more comfortable, which will also decrease trauma to the ear.

Use 4–6 J/cm², with 1–3 W and a power density of 0.2–0.5 W/cm², very similar and with the same frequency as you would do with a wound or otitis

(Table 7.5). If you have placed an otohematoma pad, you obviously have to treat from the external/convex surface of the pinna, so you can use about double the dose and power/power density. If you want to apply cold packs, do it before you laser the area. If you have placed sutures, it is probably a good idea to leave them for 14–21 days, even if the skin wound healing is accelerated, since sutures here are holding the cartilage and not just the skin.

7.6 Sacculitis and perianal fistulas

Most acute cases of anal sac impaction do not require systemic therapy, although some patients will feel more comfortable with a short-term course of non-steroidal anti-inflammatory drugs (NSAIDs). The very mild cases just require sac expression; moderate ones benefit from flushing (using a small gauge IV Teflon catheter, for instance) and packing with antimicrobial and anti-inflammatory topicals. In both cases, LT can provide fast and side-effect-free relief of the local pain and inflammation. In severe cases with fistulous tracts and cellulitis, systemic medication should be added, but LT will accelerate fistula healing (Figs 7.13 and 7.14).

If the patient tolerates it, and there is no open wound or fistula, treat in contact mode to improve penetration. If the hand-piece can't be properly cleaned afterwards due to its design, cover it with a disposable or disinfectable cap (Fig. 7.15). Improving penetration can be more important in German Shepherds than in other breeds, since their sacs are located more deeply, lying against the rectal wall.

If you choose to use a disposable/disinfectable cap, make sure it has been approved by the laser manufacturer. Some of these plastics can absorb/attenuate the light. And virtually all of them will do so if there are any scratches or debris in the light's path, so be sure to keep these clean and dry when in use.

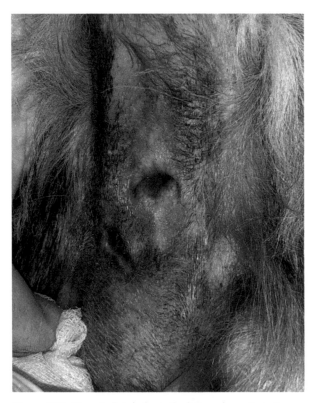

Figure 7.13 Chronic fistula from the left anal sac, 5 cm in depth, undergoing treatment with antibiotic.

Immune-mediated perianal fistulae, typical of but not exclusive to German Shepherds, always require systemic treatment; their etiology is not anal sac impaction and abscessation, and current standard care involves a variety of systemic immunomodulating drugs and topical tacrolimus. Complete healing of the fistulae is not always achieved, and this disease and the pain that it involves can heavily impact the quality of life of the patients – and their owners.

While LT will not cure the disease, it will significantly help with the inflammation, pain, and lack of healing. A clinical study with 20 German Shepherds that were unresponsive to oral cyclosporin and topical tacrolimus reported a reduction in pain and dyschezia in all 20 patients (complete resolution in 18 cases), and a decrease in lesions in more than half of them when LT was added to the treatment. Animals were treated every 48 h for the first 3 weeks and then twice a week for 2 more months. A maintenance regime of LT was able to perpetuate the remission in 15/20 cases.[224] A potential enhancement of the therapeutic effect of tacrolimus (oral form, in this case) had previously been described in an experimental mouse model of atopic dermatitis, using phototherapy with 850 nm light at 25 J/cm2.[225]

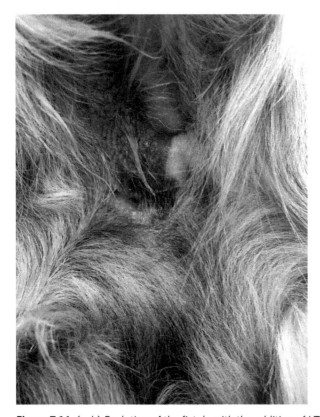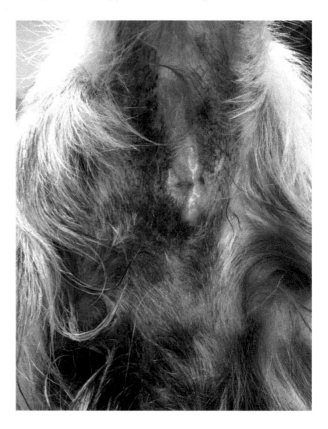

Figure 7.14 (a, b) Evolution of the fistula with the addition of LT.

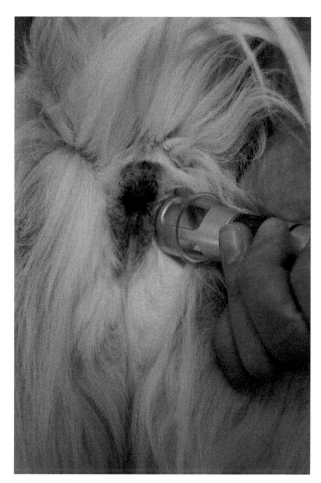

Figure 7.15 This type of cap allows comfortable treatment of the perineal area and it is easy to disinfect.

LT has also been investigated in humans for the treatment of anal fissure with some clinical results.[226] Patients in the laser group significantly improved after 5–10 sessions: pain, spasm, bleeding, and constipation decreased, by as much as in the group that received botulinum toxin injections for chemical sphincterotomy, with no side effects.

Treat fistulae like deep chronic wounds, in non-contact mode, with 2–4 W and 4–20 J/cm² (Table 7.6). Include all the perineal area (tuber ischiadicum to base of tail). The patient may be reluctant to have its tail raised initially, but this will soon improve. In severe cases, start treating on 2–3 consecutive days; milder cases can be treated every other day for 2–3 weeks.

Once the patient improves, decrease the frequency of treatment. For chronic cases, once apparently healed, it is recommended to recheck and treat every 2–4 weeks, depending on the case. Use these visits to palpate and empty the anal sacs if necessary.

7.7 Hygroma (false bursitis)

This is a false bursa that can develop over bony prominences and pressure points. If a lot of fluid is present, drainage may be necessary, and of course bandaging and proper padding of surfaces. It is not uncommon to need 6–15 treatments. The most common location is the elbow, where it can be mistaken for true bursitis, since there is a true bursa situated under the tendon of the triceps brachii, where it crosses the proximal part of the olecranon (bursa subtendinea olecrani). Be aware that these are different clinical entities; a true bursa is an anatomical structure that cushions moving parts, such as tendons, ligaments, and muscles. True bursitis is associated with pathological changes in the associated structures (tendon straining, fracture, etc.), for example in shoulder bursitis/tenosynovitis, and treatment has to consider this.

Surgery is usually the last option for elbow hygromas, due to the risk of wound breakdown and chronic ulceration, and damage to the triceps tendon and true bursa. Chronic ulcers of the elbow can heal with LT and proper wound care; or you can choose to improve tissues locally, get a partial closure, and then perform surgery over healthy tissue – but as previously mentioned, LT can avoid many flaps.

A callus usually develops over the false bursitis, but a chronic cavity may persist below the surface, with alternating chronic fistulae – again, LT would be your best option here. Treat hygromas and callus (Fig. 7.16) as chronic wounds in terms of parameters, although very often you will be able to treat in contact and improve penetration.

7.8 Gingivitis and stomatitis

The main benefits of LT (tissue healing, decreased pain and inflammation) can also be applied to the oral

Table 7.6 Recommended parameters for perineal treatments.

Dose (J/cm²)	Power (W)	Power density (W/cm²)
4–20	2–4	0.5–1

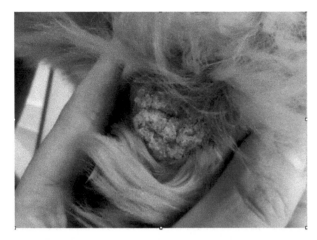

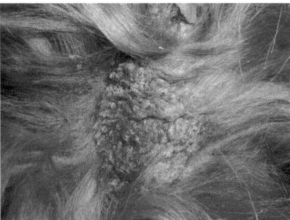

Figure 7.16 (a) This 15-year-old hypothyroid dog shows hyperkeratosis and chronic inflammation of the lateral elbow skin. (b) The change after two treatments, once a week, with 4 J/cm² and average power 3 W, was notable.

tissues, whether we are talking about stomatitis, periodontal disease, or wounds in the oral cavity, all very frequent conditions presented in canine and feline practice. Of course, gingivitis and/or stomatitis is very varied in its causes and usually multifactorial: from dental plaque or tooth malposition, to feline viruses and overreaction of the immune system, among others.

LT as an adjunctive treatment sometimes leads to a decrease in the need for medication, especially in cats with chronic stomatitis, and helps provide better pain management. Very often you may notice a reduction in pain, which translates as a better ability to eat, even without an improvement in the macroscopic lesions. Animal clinical studies are missing in this field, but let's have a look at what has been published in human medicine.

LT has been used in clinical studies with human patients to reduce gingival inflammation, decrease dentin hypersensitivity,[227] and improve mucosal healing after oral surgery. The majority of studies have been performed with low power devices, though, in a variety of protocols (most of them using 2–10 J/cm²), and sometimes some of the parameters are not specified. Laser improved clinical and biometrical parameters of mucosal healing after gingivectomy in human patients with bilateral procedures in which one side served as control and the other received treatment at 4 J/cm².[228] In a double-blind clinical study in which, again, one side served as a control, the addition of LT to scaling and root planing reduced probing pocket depth, plaque, and gingival indices.[229] In cases with conservative treatment, LT also improved plaque index, gingival index, and bleeding on probing index in a case–control study.[230] Cytomorphometric analysis of gingivitis in children improves after LT.[231] Recent systematic reviews conclude that LT improves management of chronic periodontitis,[232] mucosal healing, and dental pain.[233] Sometimes higher doses (not necessarily power, especially if there is high sensitivity) are used for immediate postoperative pain and inflammation treatment than for tissue proliferation.[234]

LT has also been used in human implantology to improve implant integration. *In vitro* studies show laser can enhance the attachment to the titanium implants and proliferation of human gingival fibroblasts in a dose-dependent manner.[235] *In vivo* models demonstrate laser increases osteocyte count and viability and accelerates osteogenesis and integration of titanium dental implants,[236] while reducing the inflammation.[237]

Radiotherapy- and chemotherapy-induced oral mucositis is a common problem in patients undergoing oncological treatment. There are several clinical trials in humans reporting both the efficacy[64] of LT and the lack of it[238] in preventing the development of mucositis, but once the mucositis appears, LT seems to significantly decrease its duration.[65] This has many consequences, including patient comfort among others, and the possibility of eating better and maintaining a better nutritional status.[66, 67]

The treatment plan will change according to the affected area, the clinical status, and the handling of our particular patient. The gingiva can often be quite well exposed in cooperative patients by manipulating the lips and slightly opening the mouth (Figs 7.17 and

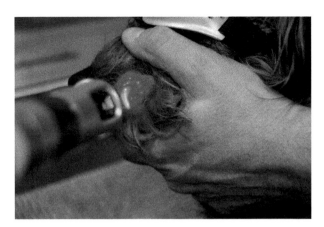

Figure 7.17 Lip retraction to expose the gingiva.

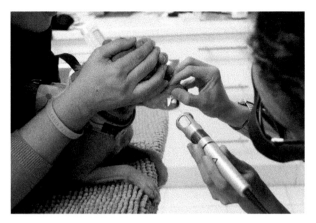

Figure 7.18 If the patient does not tolerate doggles, the assistant can help protect the eyes and the therapist will retract the lips.

7.18), but caudal stomatitis may benefit from sedating the patient to better reach those surfaces. Of course this is not always an option, especially if the patient is in a very poor clinical condition, as often happens in cats with severe oral pain, unable to properly eat for quite some time and with concomitant systemic disease. For these cases, though, LT with a closed or partially open mouth can help provide analgesia and improve oral feeding, with an awake patient and no side effects, until the general condition allows sedation if necessary for better exposure.

The dose and power used depend on whether the treatment is directly over the mucosa, with the mouth open, or with the mouth closed, from the outside. For a direct treatment, the starting dose is 2–4 J/cm², with 1–3 W of power and a low power density, 0.2–0.8 W/cm². If our aim is to treat from the outside, then these parameters increase 2–3 times: 6–10 J/cm² and 4–6 W, and we also need a higher power density, about 1 W/cm², unless we are dealing with a very sensitive patient (Table 7.7). For your treatment area calculations, include the intermandibular space. I tend to treat at least half the mouth, even for localized problems, rather than using the laser for a few seconds over a small spot.

In cases of severe pain, start treating on several consecutive days until you achieve good analgesia

– of course, you may combine LT with other medical approaches. Once the condition improves, treat every other day for a week and then try to decrease to twice a week, and so on. Chronic cases will, of course, require maintenance treatment, for which the frequency is very dependent on the case.

The best technique for cats is to place them with the head over the edge of a table, and have an assistant/owner holding them from the back, protecting the eyes. Most cats like being surrounded or embraced even if they don't enjoy other manipulations. The person holding the laser can then access the mouth from both sides and from under the cat, to reach into the intermandibular space. Very often, you will notice that after 1–2 minutes the cat seems more relaxed and moves the tongue a bit, feeling more comfortable.

7.9 Abdominal organs

Abdominal organs also suffer from inflammatory and painful conditions, and therefore they may also be a target for LT. As with any treatment, how we treat intra-abdominal organs depends on how we reach them and what amount of energy and delivery mode we want to use. They can be reached during a laparotomy

Table 7.7 Recommended parameters for oral treatments.

	Dose (J/cm²)	Power (W)	Power density (W/cm²)
Direct treatment	2–4	1–3	0.2–0.8
Through skin	6–10	4–6	0.6–1

or with a transabdominal approach. Wait, wait, I'm not suggesting you cut your patient open to perform LT!!

7.9.1   Transabdominal treatments

The list of potential applications includes conditions such as inflammatory bowel disease (IBD), cystitis, and pancreatitis. But the evidence to encourage this does not come from clinical studies; it is based on experimental models, clinical cases, and clinicians' experiences.

Reaching the middle of the abdominal cavity is probably not mandatory; some organs, such as the urinary bladder, are just "behind" the muscle wall, and even closer lies the peritoneum, which plays a central role in paracrine abdominal inflammation regulation – you have probably noticed how different degrees of peritonitis can be seen when an intra-abdominal organ is inflamed. An experiment in mice with lipopolysaccharide-induced peritonitis described how LT at a point "over the peritoneum" was able to reduce the inflammatory infiltrate.[239] If the patient tolerates being treated in contact, a gentle massage can really improve penetration. The coat is usually less dense here, and clipping is also better accepted than on the thorax, for instance.

Reports of the effect of LT on **pancreatic** tissue come from experimental studies, but represent examples of potential uses that could be developed in the future. An *in vitro* study with pancreatic islets treated showed laser light significantly increased cell function before transplantation (higher insulin secretion after a glucose challenge test).[240] A promoting effect of laser on pancreatic β-cell replication and cell cycle progression has also been reported,[241] as well as exocrine function of this organ in cases of chronic pancreatitis.[242] In experimental models of induced diabetes, laser enhanced antioxidant defense capabilities in the kidney[243] and the liver[244] of those animals, and improved renal function too.

Some cases of **intestinal** inflammation can show improvement with less common modalities of LT. An experimental model of acute colitis in mice, in which 850 nm light was applied endoscopically, reported an improvement of colonoscopic scoring at different doses.[245] A clinical study in human patients with gastroduodenal ulcer described shorter times for ulcer healing in patients treated with LT than for those in the control group.[246]

The **liver** could be another potential target for LT,

if what has been achieved in experimental models can be reproduced in patients, but clinical studies are necessary.

- The ability of LT to enhance liver regeneration after partial hepatectomy: in a rat model, after removing 70% of the liver, the group that received LT showed a 2.6-fold increase in the number of proliferating cells and a 3.3-fold increase in the number of newly formed vessels.[247] Mitochondrial activity and serum alanine aminotransferase were also increased in another study.[248] In contrast, in a similar hepatectomy model carried out in elderly rats, LT was not able to improve liver regeneration.[249]
- The protective effect of LT in models of ischemia-reperfusion injury of the liver, applied transcutaneously: LT seems to decrease both histopathological changes and serum levels of biochemical markers such as aminotransferase, TNF-α, malondialdehyde, and glutathione.[250]
- Transcutaneous LT over several points of the liver ameliorated induced cirrhosis in a rat model: it improved liver function, decreased formation of cirrhotic areas and inflammation, inhibited the induction of hepatic stellate and Kupffer cell accumulation, and restored liver protein synthesis.[251]
- The protective effect of LT against oxidative stress in a rat model of acute and chronic diabetes: it did help for acute cases, but not for the chronic ones. LT restored normal glutathione reductase and superoxide dismutase activities and increased glutathione peroxidase and glutathione S-transferase activities.[244]

The **urinary tract** is another candidate for LT. As discussed in Chapter 3, several experimental models have reported effects such as decreased inflammatory and fibrotic response in kidneys and decreased morphological damage in the glomeruli after different types of renal insult.[71, 72] Secondary kidney damage due to metabolic syndrome has been investigated; in a randomized, placebo-controlled study in rats with progressive renal failure induced by a metabolic and hypertensive disorder (nephropathy, hypertension, hyperlipidemia, and type II diabetes), LT, especially in the higher dose group, which received 12 J/cm^2 for 5 days a week during 8 consecutive weeks, showed better preserved glomerular filtration rate (despite no differences in plasma creatinine between groups), reduced interstitial fibrosis, and better blood pressure control. [252] If these were to be transposed to small animal medicine, the results would be considered promising but the same treatment regime would be quite challenging in terms of frequency.

LT can be used as an adjunctive therapy for cystitis, especially for idiopathic cases, due to the anti-inflammatory effect. In my experience, some neurological bladders may also benefit from transabdominal LT. In the extra-abdominal portion, urethritis is also a good candidate for LT in cats with feline lower urinary tract disease (FLUTD), especially acute cases.

For transabdominal treatments, your parameters would be as follows (Table 7.8).

- Starting dose of 4–6 J/cm^2 for a bladder, peritonitis, or IBD (cat), but if after a couple of treatments there is no improvement, you may increase to 6–10 J/cm^2; 6–10 J/cm^2 would be the initial dose for kidneys, or treatment of pain related to pancreatitis.
- Normally 4–8 W of power are used, up to 10 W in larger dogs.
- Use 1–2 W/cm^2.

Your treatment area will be focused over the projection area of that organ, but will probably include about a half of the abdomen at least; for instance, consider how the size and projection of the bladder can change depending on how full it is, and you want to aim at its surface from different angles. The bladder projection area in the cat is proportionally larger than in the dog.

7.9.2 Laser therapy during laparotomy

Really? Yes, it can be done. You don't need to touch the surface of the organs, of course, and you will use much less dose, power, and power density: 1–3 J/cm^2 with 0.5–2 W and around 0.1–0.2 W/cm^2. You can use LT to improve blood flow to areas or organs, but as a surgeon, you know reperfusion injury can be fatal and some organs or parts of organs with ischemic damage should not be reperfused, but removed. If you think

the tissue has a chance, you may use LT; the effect will be obvious in few minutes: tissue color and motility (if working over the intestine) will improve.

In a model of renal ischemia (30 minutes) and reperfusion injury, LT decreased tissue damage when applied over the kidney area shortly after reperfusion and 1 and 2 hours later. The protective effect included decreased nitric oxide production and myeloperoxidase activity, and maintenance of renal tissue glutathione, superoxide dismutase, and catalase levels. Blood urea nitrogen and creatinine levels were also lower in the LT group. [253] The same research group found LT could protect skeletal muscle from reperfusion injury.[254] But if there has been severe sustained hypoxia in the intestines, once the metabolic balance has shifted to cell death for good, laser would not be such a good idea (could it increase peroxynitrites?); an intestinal ischemia-reperfusion injury model in rats described such deleterious effects: the cranial mesenteric artery was occluded for 60 minutes, and LT applied before or immediately after reperfusion, using 0.5 J/cm^2 in CW over the serosal surface of the jejunum, in a point-to-point technique, with a low dose of 0.5 J/cm^2 and very low power density (0.035 W/cm^2).[19] The histopathology of the treated animals initially showed more advanced infarction and damage, although 6 h after reperfusion there were no differences between the treated and control group and the animals were not studied further in time (could there be a difference after those initial 6 h or by using different irradiation parameters?). Interestingly, despite the more severe local damage shown in the treated group, LT had a protective effect against secondary damage to the lung. The protective effect on lung damage in gut and limb reperfusion injury has been reported by several studies, when LT was applied over the bronchus.[255, 256]

Other examples of the use of LT would be after cystotomy or intestinal suture (your oncological contraindications apply here too, though). Once the laparotomy is closed, use LT to improve its healing, and consider transabdominal therapy benefits, such as those described in the liver and kidney injury models.

Table 7.8 Recommended parameters for transabdominal treatments.

	Dose (J/cm^2)	Power (W)	Power density (W/cm^2)
Cat/small dog	4–10	3–6	1–2
Large dog	6–12	4–10	1–2

For open abdominal treatments, your parameters would be as follows.

- Dose: 1–4 J/cm². If you are unsure, use 1 J/cm², wait for a couple of minutes for a tissue response, and decide whether you want to repeat the dose or not.
- Average power: in the range 0.5–2 W.
- Power density should be kept low, around 0.1 W/cm².

7.10   Airway

Different respiratory disorders may benefit from LT, as reported in studies on sinusitis, pleurisy, and other conditions. Let's review what's been published, from the upper to the lower airway segments, and the particularities of the treatment techniques.

Rhinitis and sinusitis can benefit both from the anti-inflammatory effect of LT and the response to infections: infectious rhinosinusitis can be helped by decreasing bacterial counts with LT, according to an experimental study in rabbits, in which a 2 log reduction in colony count was achieved.[181] Some time later, a study was conducted by the same researcher in humans, in which LT and topical drugs were used in combination, demonstrating that laser could not only significantly decrease bacterial counts, but also potentially resensitize bacteria to antimicrobials.[257] A pilot clinical study in human patients with chronic rhinitis found significant improvement in patients' ratings of their own symptoms after ten LT sessions, although there was no control/placebo group.[258]

Allergic rhinitis can also be helped with LT according to a mouse model[259] and a pilot study in humans[260] that reported decrease in pro-inflammatory cytokines, lower histological damage to the nasal epithelium, and symptomatic improvement. When treating sinuses, aim the beam from different angles into the sinuses' projection area and nasal cavity and away from the eyes, which should be carefully protected (Figs 7.19 and 7.20). Start with 5 J/cm², and increase to 10 J/cm² if after 2–3 treatments no change is noticed. Keep a power density of about 1 W/cm² and monitor the temperature of the skin, since you will be moving the handpiece over a relatively small area. Ideally, we would treat on a daily basis for 2–3 sessions, but if that is not possible at least three times a week must be the goal. Once a good improvement is achieved, spread visits apart progressively.

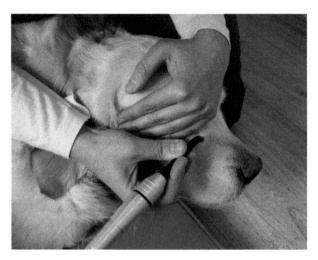

Figure 7.19 Treatment of the nasal sinus with smaller hand-piece while protecting the eye with the hand.

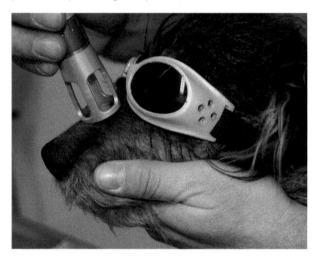

Figure 7.20 Treatment with a longer hand-piece decreases power density.

Another potential application for LT is the postoperative treatment of **brachycephalic** dogs; an analgesic effect after tonsillectomy has been reported in human patients in a placebo-controlled study in which both visual analog scale rating and analgesic consumption decreased in the LT group.[261]

Consider it before they even wake up, so you are able to do a direct open-mouth treatment; treat the palate and pharynx with 1–4 J/cm² using low power density. Treating the larynx from the outside requires you to at least double the dose and power: so use 5–10 J/cm² and 3–4 W. Research in this field is almost nonexistent; however, a study in rats did describe good results in a laryngitis model.[262] Although you don't want to treat directly over the thyroid area for a long time, you will

Table 7.9 Recommended parameters for transthoracic treatments.

	Dose (J/cm²)	Power (W)	Power density (W/cm²)
Cat/small dog	4-10	3-6	1-2
Large dog	6-12	4-10	1-2

occasionally pass over it when treating the larynx, but that will not be a problem.

The list of **intrathoracic** respiratory conditions for which LT could be a helpful adjunctive therapy includes:

- asthma
- pleurisy
- pneumonia
- idiopathic pulmonary fibrosis
- bronchitis
- SIRS syndrome.

Probably the most common respiratory disorders in which LT is used in small animal practice are feline asthma and canine pulmonary fibrosis. Studies in asthma and pleurisy models show regulation of hyper-responsiveness of bronchial and tracheal smooth muscle; decrease in inflammatory cells and mediators, such as circulating histamine, ICAM expression, and Th2-type cytokines; and a reduction in exudate volume. [44, 46, 56, 69]

Although there are no published clinical studies in small animal airway conditions and LT, some have been published on the human side. In pneumonia patients, LT improved peripheral microcirculation, decreased pain and coughing, and helped to resolve clinical parameters and leukocytosis[263, 264]; mean duration of hospital stay was reduced from 19 to 15 days in a study using LT for acute pneumonia,[265] and from 28 to 23 days in another study of elderly patients with pneumonia.[263] This was also described in patients with pleurisy and tuberculosis, who after laser treatment showed a decrease in total amount of exudate and earlier resolution of hyperthermia, in the study by Tiukhin et al.[266]

For transthoracic treatments, use 3–10 W and calculate 4–12 J/cm² to be applied over each hemithorax (intercostal spaces may help you) and also over the thoracic inlet area – include this area in your treatment area calculations! You can start on the lower end of the power and dose ranges: start with 3–4 W and 4–6 J/cm² for a smaller patient, and progressively increase if

needed. Maintain a power density of 1–2 W/cm² (Table 7.9).

With asthma, the clinical goal is to decrease the duration and frequency of episodes; in case of a marked seasonal component, treatments can be spread further apart when the season is over, but others will need high maintenance, such as weekly or biweekly sessions, for a sustained improvement. In the case of pulmonary fibrosis, which is a progressive and fatal disease, our goal with LT is to slow down the progression and improve quality of life by relieving the symptoms. Concomitant pulmonary arterial hypertension (PAH) may develop; make sure this is treated and monitored as needed. Since LT may act on vascular tone (smooth muscle relaxation) via nitric oxide, and the treatment of PAH involves this precise mechanism, with drugs like sildenafil, there could be a potential benefit for this secondary condition, but this has not been investigated. A minimum frequency of three times per week is needed for 2–3 weeks, then twice a week for the same period, followed by treatments once a week and a maintenance regime of at least one treatment every 2–3 weeks. Nevertheless, some patients with asthma or pulmonary fibrosis will require a continued higher frequency of treatment, such as twice a week, in order to maintain the clinical improvement.

Summary from a different perspective

Soft tissue injuries are some of the most popular candidates for laser therapy, mostly because being predominantly superficial, it is relatively easy to deliver a high enough dose to the affected tissue. But as you've read, there are many subdermal issues that can benefit from laser. And for many of these, the other therapeutic options are pharmaceutical and come with highly undesirable (and unfortunately probable) side effects. If you don't suspect cancer, laser.

7.11 Case studies

The following are examples of the clinical use of LT in patients who have been treated by the author (MS). The World Association of Laser Therapy approved a consensus in 2004 about how treatment parameters used in clinical studies should be reported,[267] and although clinical cases are not the same as clinical trials, the guidelines will be followed quite closely. These specify that the following information regarding the description of the intervention should be provided: next to each parameter you can read some notes on how it applies to these cases and also to the ones under the musculoskeletal section.

- **Number of treatment sessions and frequency of sessions per week:** in clinical cases this is not as strict as in a designed trial and may depend on extrinsic factors, such as the agenda or resources of the patient's caretaker. So do not try to compare different cases in this section; one in which full closure of a wound took 20 sessions might not be worse than another that took 10; maybe the patient could be seen less often, or maybe he was removing bandages and licking the wound. "Real-life" cases are different from laboratory studies.
- **Application procedure:** scanning mode vs. stationary or fixed spot; contact mode vs. non-contact mode. All musculoskeletal cases in Chapter 9 were treated in scanning mode, and all wound cases in this section were treated in non-contact mode, unless otherwise specified.
- **Wavelength (nm) or wavelengths:** all cases were treated using a combination of 660 nm, 800 nm, 905 nm, and 970 nm, unless otherwise specified.
- **Average output power of the laser (Pa):** since

cases were treated with a class IV device, watts are used instead of milliwatts.

- **Treatment time (Tx time):** instead of just seconds, minutes (and seconds if needed) will also be used to facilitate understanding of the time (you will probably get a quicker idea of the time if you read 5 min 15 s than if I say 315 s).
- **Energy dose delivered, in J/cm_2:** in a clinical setting, being completely accurate is often not possible, so consider that 4 J/cm^2 could include 3.5 or 5 J/cm^2. Total J per session will be reported.
- **Spot size on the skin in cm_2:** a hand-piece with an adjustable zoom has been used in all cases, which combined with the distance from the patient's surface allows us to modify the spot size and concentrate or disperse the energy over a different area.
- **Power density (W/cm_2):** again, as a class IV laser was used, this will be expressed in W/cm^2 instead of mW/cm^2.
- **Accumulated energy** delivered from all sessions, in joules, can be calculated using the total J per session times the number of sessions (No. Tx).

All treatments included **both CW and pulsed emission**, unless otherwise reported, with about 20% of the energy delivered in CW and the rest within a pulse (mid to very high) frequency range.

The **treatment area** can be calculated using the total energy per session and the J/cm^2; every time a wound is treated, a 2–5 cm margin is included.

Testing of optical output (am I getting the W that the screen says on the surface of my patient?) was performed with the devices used in these cases at several points in time; your manufacturer or distributor will be able to provide you with this service, which is important, as with any clinical device.

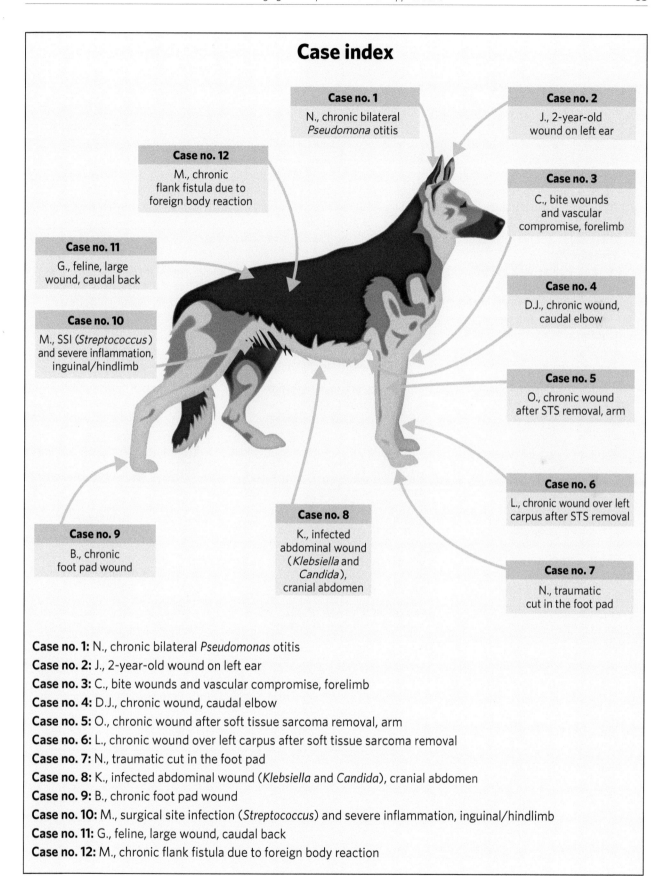

Case index

Case no. 1
N., chronic bilateral *Pseudomona* otitis

Case no. 2
J., 2-year-old wound on left ear

Case no. 12
M., chronic flank fistula due to foreign body reaction

Case no. 3
C., bite wounds and vascular compromise, forelimb

Case no. 11
G., feline, large wound, caudal back

Case no. 4
D.J., chronic wound, caudal elbow

Case no. 10
M., SSI (*Streptococcus*) and severe inflammation, inguinal/hindlimb

Case no. 5
O., chronic wound after STS removal, arm

Case no. 6
L., chronic wound over left carpus after STS removal

Case no. 9
B., chronic foot pad wound

Case no. 8
K., infected abdominal wound (*Klebsiella* and *Candida*), cranial abdomen

Case no. 7
N., traumatic cut in the foot pad

Case no. 1: N., chronic bilateral *Pseudomonas* otitis
Case no. 2: J., 2-year-old wound on left ear
Case no. 3: C., bite wounds and vascular compromise, forelimb
Case no. 4: D.J., chronic wound, caudal elbow
Case no. 5: O., chronic wound after soft tissue sarcoma removal, arm
Case no. 6: L., chronic wound over left carpus after soft tissue sarcoma removal
Case no. 7: N., traumatic cut in the foot pad
Case no. 8: K., infected abdominal wound (*Klebsiella* and *Candida*), cranial abdomen
Case no. 9: B., chronic foot pad wound
Case no. 10: M., surgical site infection (*Streptococcus*) and severe inflammation, inguinal/hindlimb
Case no. 11: G., feline, large wound, caudal back
Case no. 12: M., chronic flank fistula due to foreign body reaction

Case no. 1

N., canine, 6 years old, Maltese, FS, 4 kg

- **Complaint:** chronic bilateral otitis.
- **History:** N. had been adopted 2 years before with a pre-existing otitis and the condition had never resolved. Oral and topical treatments had been used with no result. Last culture was positive for *Pseudomonas*, antibiogram showed sensitivity to marbofloxacin but again there was no response to oral and topical treatment. Both tympanic membranes have been lost and MRI suggested both bullas are affected; owners refused surgical treatment.
- **Physical examination:** severe bilateral otitis, with thick dark secretion, but without significant stenosis of external ear canal.
- **Diagnosis:** chronic bilateral external and middle ear otitis due to *Pseudomonas*.
- **Treatment:**
  - Initial cleaning was performed under sedation due to the severe inflammation and pain (Fig. C1.1).
  - **Laser therapy:** treatment over the pinna covered an area of about 25 cm², while the external ear canal projection area was slightly smaller. But while treating directly over the inflamed epithelium requires a lower dose and power, higher values are used to reach inside the canal from outside.
- **Outcome:** in this case, complete resolution was achieved after 12 treatments (Fig. C1.3); the patient is otitis-free 2 years later. This is not often the result; most patients with chronic otitis need a maintenance regime. The unusual lack of stenosis and other tissue changes in this patient probably contributed to the success.

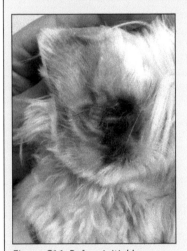

Figure C1.1 Before initial laser treatment.

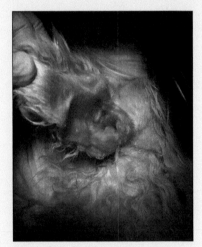

Figure C1.2 Seventh treatment.

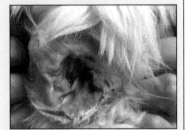
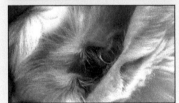

Figure C1.3 (a) Right ear and (b) left ear after 12 treatments.

P$_a$ (W)	Tx time	J/cm²	Total J/Tx	Spot (cm²)	W/cm²	Tx/week	No. Tx
1.5 (pinna), 3 (canal)	66 s (pinna) plus 66 s canal	4 (pinna), 10 (canal)	100 (pinna) plus 200 (canal)	8 (pinna), 5 (canal)	0.25 (pinna), 2 (canal)	3-3-2-2-1-1	12

Case no. 2

J., canine, 15 years old, Belgian Shepherd, FS, 25 kg

- **Complaint:** wound on left ear.
- **History:** chronic wound had appeared for the first time 2 years previously. No conclusive diagnosis could be reached, although vasculitis was suspected. Systemic infections such as leishmaniasis had been ruled out. Several long courses of antibiotics and steroids had been used, with an initial good response, but the wound would reopen as soon as medications were stopped. No response to local treatments. Last dose of triamcinolone had been a week before the case was referred for LT.
- **Physical examination:** 2–3 cm² in size (Fig. C2.1), almost full thickness wound on the distal third of left ear pinna. No granulation present. No exudates.
- **Diagnosis:** chronic non-healing wound due to suspected vasculitis.
- **Treatment:**
  - **Wound management:** lavage with saline if any debris present.
  - **Laser therapy:**
    - The initial treatment used 4–5 J/cm², but after three treatments there was no improvement (Fig. C2.2 and C2.3), so dose was increased to 8 J/cm².
    - After day 10 (6th treatment), the change was very subtle so dose was again increased to 12 J/cm², which seemed to be of significant help; by session 12 the wound was no smaller but the bed was filled with healthy granulation tissue and dose was increased to 16 J/cm².
    - One month after beginning LT, active epithelialization was evident at the edges (Fig. C2.5). Dose was increased to 20 J/cm².
    - On day 40, dose was increased to 25 J/cm². By day 52, only an 8 × 1 mm defect remained.
    - In this case, 2 min of time off were taken between each 4–5 J/cm². So eventually, when 25 J/cm² was being delivered, the session length was around 15 minutes long: around 1 min on, 2 min off.
  - **Others:** no other local nor systemic medications were used during the course of laser treatments.
- **Outcome:** full closure in 2 months (Fig. C2.8) with 22 sessions. This patient would be considered a weak reactor, since it took 2 months to resolve (although the wound was present for 2 years) and needed very high doses of LT. Three more weekly treatments were performed to prevent reopening. The steroid treatment could have contributed to the slow initial response.

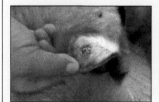

Figure C2.1 Initial wound.

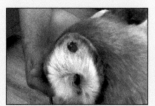

Figure C2.2 Day 1.

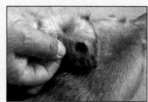

Figure C2.3 Day 4, no improvement.

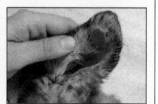

Figure C2.4 Session 12, day 21. Wound bed is granulated.

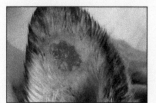

Figure C2.5 Day 29. Margins with good epithelialization.

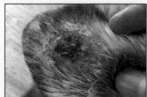

Figure C2.6 Day 40.

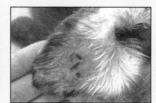

Figure C2.7 Day 52.

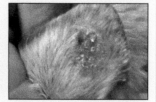

Figure C2.8 Day 60. Full closure.

P$_a$ (W)	Tx time	J/cm²	Total J/Tx	Spot (cm²)	W/cm²	Tx/week	No. Tx
3	66–333 s (5.5 min)	4–20	200–1000	5–6	0.5	3-2-1	25 (22)

Case no. 3

C., canine, 2 years old, mixed breed, MC, 16 kg

- **Complaint:** bite wounds and limb swelling.
- **History:** he had been attacked by other dogs 48 h before. The most severe wound was in the right forelimb and axila. At the emergency clinic they had lavaged the wound, put in several Penrose drains and completely closed with sutures. His regular vet referred him for LT. He was on tramadol, meloxicam, cephalexin, and metronidazole.
- **Physical examination:** C. was brought in unable to stand due to severe pain (9/10). His right forelimb showed severe inflammation, oozing, edema, and progressive tissue necrosis (Fig. C3.1a, b).
- **Diagnosis:** bite wound with severe compromise of venous return of the limb due to primary closure of wounds.
- **Treatment:**
  - **Wound management:**
    - In this case, LT was not the priority. Sutures had to be removed to reopen the wound, release the proximal tension and allow blood to properly flow. Otherwise, tissue necrosis would have compromised the viability of the limb, and potentially the patient's life. Patient was sedated to open the wound and perform a thorough lavage. A hematoma was present over the pectoral area. Analgesic treatment was changed to buprenorphine 0.015 mg/kg q6h during the first 24 h.
    - The procedure was repeated 24 h later, new drains were placed, and LT was started (Fig. C3.2). Alginate dressings were used to evacuate exudates and facilitate debriding and granulation, with changes q48h initially. Patient was comfortable and able to walk from day 2, and drains were removed on day 3. Wounds were kept bandaged at all times.
    - On day 6, only a small portion of moist necrotic tissue remained and the rest of the skin on the limb was visibly viable (Fig. C3.3). The skin around the axila and proximal limb was still detached from underlying tissue.
    - By day 20 (Fig. C3.4) a good granulation tissue was present. The wound was moderately exudative and Manuka honey impregnated polyurethane foam wound dressings were then used. Antibiotics were discontinued.
    - An axial pattern flap from the superficial brachial artery was considered but its integrity was questionable and C. was an extremely active dog for whom bandage protection and rest was very challenging, so it was decided not to graft the defect either and to continue with second intention closure and LT.
  - **Laser therapy:**
    - Initially (Fig. C3.2), a low dose of 2–4 J/cm^2 was used, with power densities around 0.25 W/cm^2, covering all the area from the carpus to the axila and cranial pectoral surface (300 cm^2).
    - As the wound bed became granulated, doses were progressively increased to 15 J/cm^2 and power densities to 0.6 W/cm^2. The treatment area decreased in time, so the treatment time was kept around 4–5 min (dose increased but so did power). For instance, by day 32 (Fig. C3.5) we were using 8 J/cm^2 over 100 cm^2 (total amount of energy 800 J) with an average power of 3 W. With 3 W, it takes 266 seconds (4.4 min) to deliver 800 J.
    - The first week, laser was performed q48h; in the second, third, and fourth week, twice a week. Later on, only once a week.
- **Outcome:** a total of 20 treatments were performed and patient was discharged with a remaining 3 × 10 mm epithelial defect (Fig. C3.6). The new skin was flexible, covered with hair for the most part, and no restrictions in the range of motion were noted.

Case no. 3 (cont.)

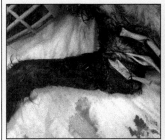
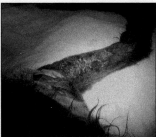
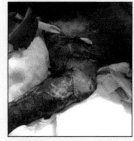
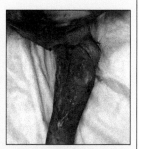

Figure C3.1 (a, b) Initial evaluation. Wound had been sutured 36 h before.

Figure C3.2 Beginning of LT, 24 h after suture removal.

Figure C3.3 Day 6, third treatment.

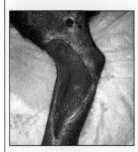
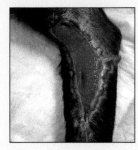
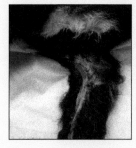

Figure C3.4 Day 20.

Figure C3.5 Day 32, evaluation. Wound had been sutured 36 h before.

Figure C3.6 Day 75, 18 treatments. 24 h after suture removal.

P_a (W)	Tx time	J/cm²	Total J/Tx	Spot (cm²)	W/cm²	Tx/week	No. Tx
2 to 3	240–300 s (4–5 min)	2 to 15	600–1000	8 to 5	0.25 to 0.6	3-2-1	20

Case no. 4

D.J., canine, 1 year old, Briard, MNC, 23 kg

- **Complaint:** wound.
- **History:** he underwent surgery for elbow pseudo bursitis and had dehiscence at surgical incision. After two more attempts to close the wound with tension-relieving suture patterns, it was left to heal by second intention, but was not progressing. Also, D.J. kept licking the elbow area and owner refused to use E-collar. He was referred for LT.
- **Physical examination:** open chronic wound over caudal surface of the right elbow. The skin defect was 20 cm² (Fig. C4.1a), and showed immature granulation, but for at least 2 cm around it the skin was detached from the underlying tissue (Fig. C4.1b). The holes left by the previous sutures were inflamed and had not healed. Small amounts of exudate were present.
- **Diagnosis:** chronic wound.
- **Treatment:**
  - **Wound management:**
    - The day of the first treatment, approximating skin sutures were placed in an attempt to improve the adherence of the skin.
    - Lavage and covering with polyurethane foam as a primary layer.
  - **Laser therapy:**
    - The initial treatment area becomes 150 cm² if we want to include the unhealthy margin plus 2–3 cm of apparently healthy tissue. With an initial dose of 5 J/cm², that becomes 750 J per session. As the skin around the wound healed, the treatment area was decreased but never below 50 cm².
    - Dose was increased to 10 J/cm² in the final stages, so the total amount of energy per session oscillated between 500 and 750 J.
- **Outcome:** wound closure after 18 sessions. A shorter resolution time would probably be expected without the self-trauma component.

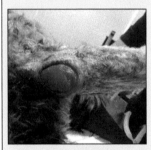 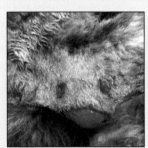 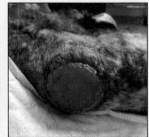 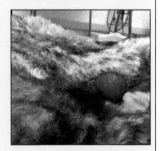

Figure C4.1 Before treatment. (a) Caudal and (b) lateral views.

Figure C4.2 Five days and two treatments later.

Figure C4.3 Day 12.

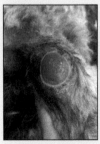 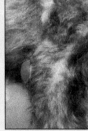 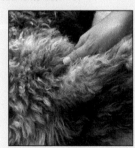

Figure C4.4 Day 25. (a) Caudal and (b) lateral views.

Figure C4.5 Day 40.

P$_a$ (W)	Tx time	J/cm²	Total J/Tx	Spot (cm²)	W/cm²	Tx/week	No. Tx
3	166 s (2.7 min)–250 s (4.2 min)	5–10	500–750	8	0.4	2–3	18

Case no. 5

O., canine, 9 years old, mixed breed, MC, 20 kg

- **Complaint:** wound over left elbow area.
- **History:** Addison's disease, on treatment. Surgery for soft tissue sarcoma with clean margins at the site of the wound 2 months before (Fig. C5.1). Postoperative complications and non-healing wound over the next months.
- **Physical examination:** 6 cm² wound, mildly exudative, over lateral part of cranial right antebrachium. Surrounding skin detached from underlying tissue, no active borders (Fig. C5.2).
- **Diagnosis:** chronic (non-healing) wound.
- **Treatment:**
  - **Wound management:** lavaged with sterile saline and covered with sterile gauze and a non-compressive bandage. No topical treatments were used.
  - **Laser therapy:** treatment area included the open wound and a 2–3 cm margin around it. The initial dose was 5 J/cm² and this was gradually increased to 10 J/cm² during the course of treatment.
- **Outcome:** full closure with a total of 15 sessions spread over 7 weeks. Oral steroids had to be maintained due to Addison's.

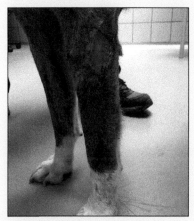

Figure C5.1 Wound after surgery.

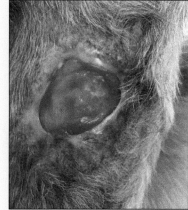

Figure C5.2 Two months after surgery. Beginning of LT.

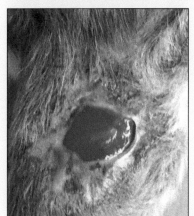

Figure C5.3 Three weeks into LT.

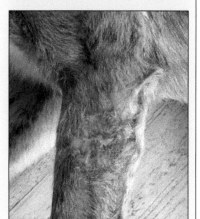

Figure C5.4 15th treatment.

P$_a$ (W)	Tx time	J/cm²	Total J/Tx	Spot (cm²)	W/cm²	Tx/week	No. Tx
3	116–233 s (1.9–3.8 min)	5–10	350–700	6	0.5	3	15

Case no. 6

L., canine, 15 years old, Belgian Shepherd, FS, 23 kg

- **Complaint:** wound over left carpus and lameness from same limb.
- **History:** surgery for soft tissue sarcoma at the referring practice 4 months before. Clean margins according to pathology report. A week after surgery, patient presented with wound dehiscence. The wound size had not changed for the past 11 weeks.
- **Physical examination:** lameness was graded as 2/5 and related to the wound after physical examination ruled out other locations. Despite lack of healing, the wound, which was 35 cm^2 in size, presented a well-vascularized granulation bed with no signs of infection (Fig. C6.1).
- **Diagnosis:** chronic (non-healing) wound.
- **Treatment:**
  - **Wound management:** lavaged with sterile saline and covered with sterile gauze and a non-compressive bandage. No oral or topical treatments were used.
  - **Laser therapy:** on the first day, the patient was treated with 4 J/cm^2; 18 h later, the granulation bed had an exuberant appearance (Fig. C6.2), so a lower dose of 2 J/cm^2 was used that day, using half the previous power and power density. Treatments were then performed q48h, and after the second week, q72–96h.
- **Outcome:** full closure of the wound after 11 sessions in 32 days (Fig. C6.8). Lameness disappeared after the first week.

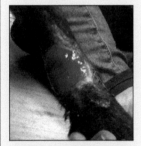

Figure C6.1 Initial aspect.

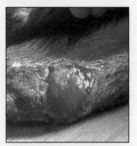

Figure C6.2 18 h after first laser treatment.

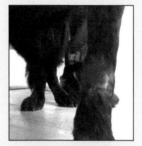

Figure C6.3 Day 7.

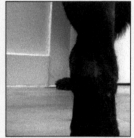

Figure C6.4 Day 10.

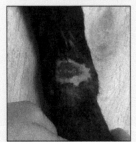

Figure C6.5 Day 17.

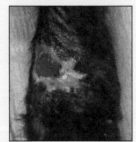

Figure C6.6 Day 21.

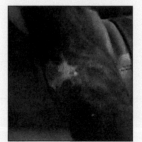

Figure C6.7 Day 28.

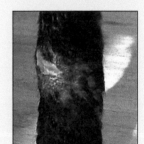

Figure C6.8 Day 32.

P$_a$ (W)	Tx time	J/cm^2	Total J/Tx	Spot (cm^2)	W/cm^2	Tx/week	No. Tx
3	132 s (2.2 min)	4	400	6	0.5	3-2	11

Case no. 7

N., canine, 5 years old, Golden Retriever, FS, 26 kg

- **Complaint:** traumatic cut in the paw.
- **History:** she came home bleeding from the paw 36 h previously. She had probably cut herself on something in the park. Owners had performed initial lavage with copious amounts of water.
- **Physical examination:** cut wound on left forelimb foot pad, raising a flap that ran along the width of the central pad (Fig. C7.1). No signs of infection. No foreign material inside.
- **Diagnosis:** accidental cut wound.
- **Treatment:**
  - **Wound management:** lavaged with 0.05% chlorhexidine and sutured with 3/0 non-absorbable monofilament. Protective bandage.
  - **Laser therapy:** 4 J/cm² over a 100 cm² area, to cover not just the suture line but also the proximal palmar surface and stimulate blood flow to the pad. Wound looked healthy after 48 h (Fig. C7.2) and the scar was barely visible after 1 week (Fig. C7.3).
- **Outcome:** complete healing with good tensile strength and minimal scarring after 2 weeks (Fig. C7.4).

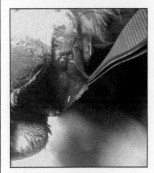 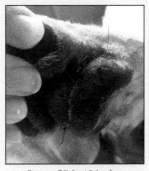 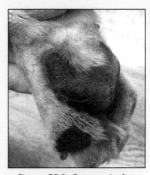 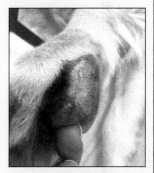

| Figure C7.1 Wound before treatment. | Figure C7.2 48 h after treatment. | Figure C7.3 One week after treatment. | Figure C7.4 Day 14. |

P$_a$ (W)	Tx time	J/cm²	Total J/Tx	Spot (cm²)	W/cm²	Tx/week	No. Tx
3	133 s (2.2 min)	4	400	6	0.5	3	6

Case no. 8

K., canine, 6 years old, mixed breed, FS, 8 kg

- **Complaint:** abdominal wound.
- **History:** surgery for gastric foreign body 3 weeks before. Surgical site infection that required multiple surgical procedures and debriding, performed at referring practice. Wound seemed to penetrate to abdominal cavity last week. Wound was dressed and managed on a daily or twice a day basis. Culture positive for *Klebsiella pneumoniae* and *Candida* spp. Antibiogram shows multiple resistance to all antibiotics tried, including amoxicillin/clavulanic acid, cephalexin, cefovecin, imipenem, enrofloxacin, marbofloxacin, ciprofloxacin, pradofloxacin, gentamicin, doxycycline, sulfadiazine, trimethoprim, and others, except amikacin.
- **Physical examination:** open wound, 6 cm^2, affecting the cranial part of the laparotomy incision plus xiphoid area, sloughing bed, moderately exudative, no active borders (Fig. C8.1).
- **Diagnosis:** chronic infected wound with primary *K. pneumoniae* and secondary *Candida* infections.
- **Treatment:**
  - **Wound management:** lavaged with sterile saline and covered with sterile gauze and a non-compressive bandage, with outer tubular mesh. No topical treatments were used.
  - **Others:** amikacin was administered for the first week by the referring vet.
  - **Laser therapy:** treatment area included the laparotomy incision, the open wound, and a 5 cm margin around them. On the first day, the patient was treated with 4 J/cm^2; 48 h later, the wound bed started to show healthier granulation tissue and less exudate (Fig. C8.2). By day 5 (4th treatment, Fig. C8.3), the wound size was also about 25% smaller. The initial dose was gradually increased to 12–15 J/cm^2 during the course of treatment, with a total of ten sessions.
- **Outcome:** full closure after ten sessions performed over 3 weeks.

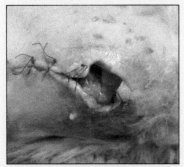

Figure C8.1 Initial wound.

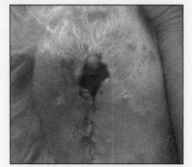

Figure C8.2 Day 2.

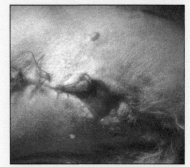

Figure C8.3 Day 5.

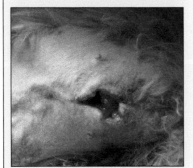

Figure C8.4 Day 9.

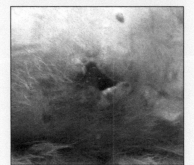

Figure C8.5 Day 14.

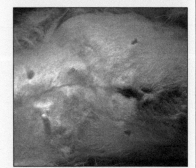

Figure C8.6 Day 18.

P$_a$ (W)	Tx time	J/cm^2	Total J/Tx	Spot (cm^2)	W/cm^2	Tx/week	No. Tx
3	266–500 s (4.4–8.3 min)	4–15	800–1200	6	0.5	3	10

Case no. 9

B., canine, 7 years old, Golden Retriever, MC, 32 kg

- **Complaint:** foot pad wound.
- **History:** B. underwent surgery for fistulous tract 3 months prior. Wound has not changed for 2 months despite different topical treatments.
- **Physical examination:** 9 × 4 mm wound in the right hindlimb pad of the fourth digit (Fig. C9.1).
- **Diagnosis:** chronic non-healing wound.
- **Treatment:**
  - **Wound management:** lavage with 0.05% chlorhexidine. Manuka honey ointment. Protective bandage.
  - **Laser therapy:** 10 J/cm² as a starting dose due to the chronicity and depth of the wound. Although it may seem like a small defect, note the dead tissue around the wound, with excess keratin that is unattached to the underlying tissue. Dose was increased to 15 J/cm² after 1 week (6 × 5 mm). Again, in this case the treatment area included the blood vessels running along the plantar surface of the paw. Before a decrease in wound size was noted, progressive attachment of the keratin layer was observed as well as a more reactive and vascularized wound bed (Figs C9.2 and C9.3).
- **Outcome:** closure after six treatments spread over 1 month (Fig. C9.5).

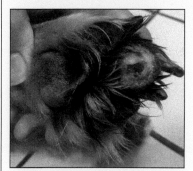

Figure C9.1 Before initial treatment. 9 × 4 mm.

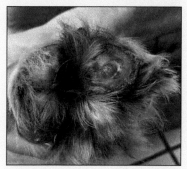

Figure C9.2 After one week. 6 × 5 mm.

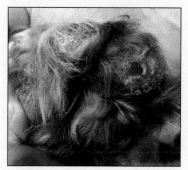

Figure C9.3 Second week. 6 × 5 mm.

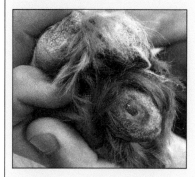

Figure C9.4 Third week. 3 × 1 mm.

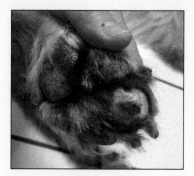

Figure C9.5 Fourth week. Wound closure.

P_a (W)	Tx time	J/cm²	Total J/Tx	Spot (cm²)	W/cm²	Tx/week	No. Tx
3.5	85 s (1.4 min)–128 s (2.1 min)	10–15	300–450	5	0.7	2–1	6

Case no. 10

M., canine, 7 years old, Doberman, FS, 27 kg

- **Complaint:** swollen limb and soft tissue inflammation.
- **History:** 2 years prior, she underwent tibial tuberosity advancement (TTA) for left cranial cruciate ligament rupture. She was also diagnosed with chronic left hip luxation. A year later, she developed surgical site infection (SSI) signs and the plate had to be removed. She had been OK until a week before, when she developed left non-weight-bearing lameness, absolute anorexia, hindlimb edema, tumefaction, and later discharge, starting at the medial stifle. Complete blood count showed leukocytosis with neutrophilia, lymphocytosis, and monocytosis. Her regular vet had her hospitalized for 5 days with intensive medical care, including IV fluids, heparin, meloxicam, furosemide, buprenorphin, marbofloxacin, metronidazole, and cephazolin. Once a slight improvement was noted, she referred her for LT with a differential diagnosis of necrotizing fasciitis/SSI. Once culture of the exudate retrieved *Streptococcus agalactiae*, with some resistances (aminoglycosides and quinolones), cephalexin was continued as antimicrobial therapy.
- **Physical examination:** 3/5 left hindlimb lameness. Soft tissue inflammation and tumefaction over left femoral and lower gluteal (Fig. C10.1a, b), caudal abdominal, and inguinal areas (Fig. C10.1c, d), extending down to the medial stifle, where a 1 × 2 mm open draining tract was present. Limb edema with a diameter of 37 cm at stifle and 24 cm at tarsus. Overall pain score 6/10.
- **Diagnosis:** severe and extensive cellulitis due to chronic *Streptococcus* SSI.
- **Treatment:**
  - **Wound management:** the owner was instructed to keep the skin around the draining tract clean and dry, using 0.05% chlorhexidine and sterile gauzes.
  - **Laser therapy:**
    - An initial low dose over a large area was used: 2–3 J/cm^2 over 600–700 cm^2, with a total of 1800 J. Because the patient was so sensitive at this point, 0.25 W/cm^2 power density was used, which was later increased to 0.5 W/cm^2. After the first session, limb diameters decreased to 32 cm (stifle) and 21 cm (tarsus). Inguinal cellulitis showed a slight improvement but was still very evident (Fig. C10.2).
    - After the second treatment, the soft tissue deformity at the gluteal area had disappeared, and tarsal diameter was 17 cm (Fig. C10.3a). The inguinal inflammation was also decreased (Fig. C10.3b).
    - Treatments were performed on days 0, 1, 3, 5, 7, 10, 14, 18, 23, and 28.
  - **Others:**
    - Oral cephalexin.
    - *Coptis chinensis* powder was applied over the inguinal and medial femoral area; this has anti-inflammatory and antimicrobial properties (berberine alkaloids) and explains the yellow color in the pictures (Fig C10.4 and C10.5).
- **Outcome:**
  - Full resolution of limb edema and soft tissue inflammation, and wound closure (Fig. C10.5).
  - Lameness decreased to 2/5, pain to 2/10 localized at hip joint (chronic luxation). Surgery was considered but postponed due to the risk of infection.
- Necrotizing fasciitis is a very severe and often fatal disease, which in the canine species is usually caused by *Staphylococcus pseudintermedius*, and occasionally from *Streptococcus canis* and *E. coli*. Although initially suspected, necrotizing fasciitis could not be confirmed, since no biopsy was taken, and no necrosis or tissue loss were evident.

Case no. 10 (cont.)

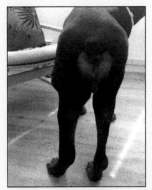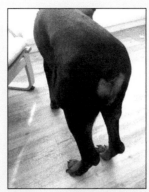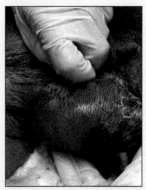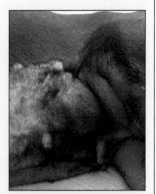

Figure C10.1 (a, b) Initial tumefaction over left femoral area, caudal view. (c) Initial inguinal swelling. (d) Initial swelling in the caudal abdomen, lateral view.

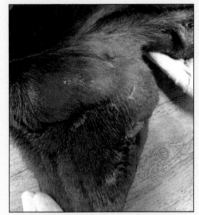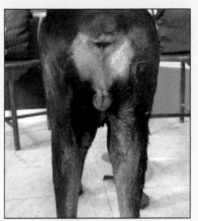

Figure C10.2 After first treatment.

Figure C10.3 Inflammation and edema have decreased after two treatments. (a) Caudal view. (b) Inguinal area.

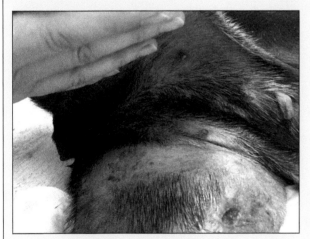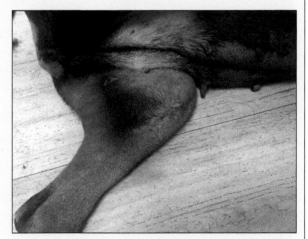

Figure C10.4 Day 5, fourth treatment.

Figure C10.5 After seven treatments.

P_a (W)	Tx time	J/cm²	Total J/Tx	Spot (cm²)	W/cm²	Tx/week	No. Tx
2.5	720 s (12 min)	2–3	1800	10–5	0.25–0.5	4-3-2-1	10

Case no. 11

G., feline, 5 years old, Domestic Shorthair, MC, 5.5 kg

- **Complaint:** wound, skin progressively coming off.
- **History:** G. disappeared for a couple of days and came home with his rear end covered in what seemed to be motor oil. Owners noticed skin in that area started to first harden and then come off.
- **Physical examination:** large burn-type wound over the caudal sacral, proximal coccygeal, right hip, and proximal right hindlimb areas. All the skin in that area was missing or necrotic. All the subcutaneous fat was necrotic (Fig. C11.1). The patient had been started on amoxicillin/clavulanic acid.
- **Diagnosis:** burn wound (suspected).
- **Treatment:**
  - **Wound management:**
    - Initially, surgical debridement was performed in two stages (Figs C11.2 and C11.3) under general anesthesia.
    - A microbial culture was taken, which retrieved *Pseudomonas aeruginosa* resistant to amoxicillin/clavulanic acid but sensitive to marbofloxacin, and therefore the antibiotic treatment was changed accordingly.
    - Alginate dressings (Fig. C11.4) were used as a primary layer in the bandages.
    - As the wound bed and surrounding skin healed, approximating sutures were used at the edges to help wound contraction (Figs C11.3 and C11.5).
  - **Laser therapy:**
    - Initially, 2 J/cm^2 was used (Fig. C11.2), which was then progressively increased to 5 J/cm^2, covering an area of about 250–300 cm^2 initially and 200 cm^2 later on. A low power density was maintained to prevent tissue dehydration.
    - Treatments were performed under sedation, at the same time as wound lavage and dressing changes, three times a week initially, then twice a week.
  - **Others:** marbofloxacin, tramadol, meloxicam.
- **Outcome:** wound progressed to a healthy granulation tissue (Fig. C11.6) and then reconstruction was performed in two steps: an initial advancement flap (Fig. C11.7) from the lumbar skin and then closure of the remaining defect (Figs C11.8 and C11.9).

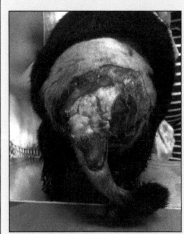

Figure C11.1 Before treatment. Note the extensive fat necrosis.

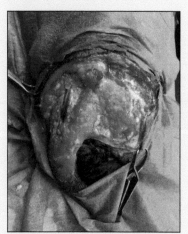

Figure C11.2 Initial debridement and laser treatment.

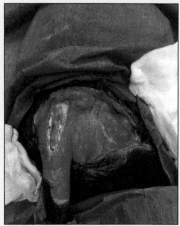

Figure C11.3 Debridement, LT, and suturing.

Case no. 11 (cont.)

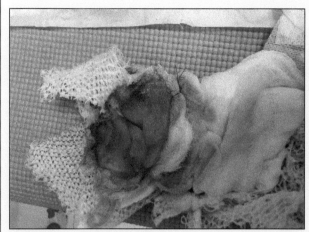

Figure C11.4 Saturated alginate dressing.

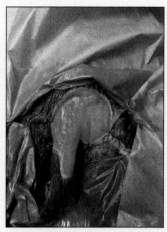

Figure C11.5 Further LT and approximating sutures.

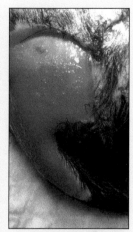

Figure C11.6 Tissue is now ready for reconstruction.

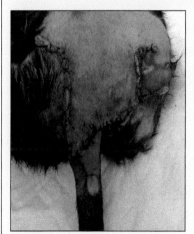

Figure C11.7 Advancement flap.

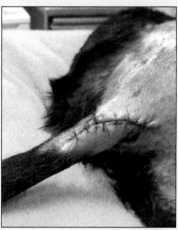

Figure C11.8 Second phase of the flap.

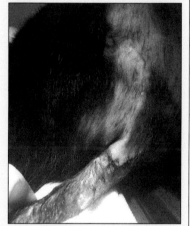

Figure C11.9 Final result.

P_a (W)	Tx time	J/cm²	Total J/Tx	Spot (cm²)	W/cm²	Tx/week	No. Tx
1.5	333 s (5.5 min)–666 s (11 min)	2–5	500–1000	6	0.25	3-2	15

Case no. 12

M., canine, 6 years old, Labrador, FS, 27 kg

- **Complaint:** fistula.
- **History:**
  - M. was referred for surgery for a chronic fistula in her caudal right flank, which had appeared for the first time 2.5 years ago. It had undergone three previous surgeries in other practices. The fistula would improve with steroid treatment, but recur after its withdrawal. Antibiotics did not seem to help. Reopenings of the fistula were sometimes preceded by a clear vaginal discharge.
  - A month ago, she had been treated for proximal ureteral stenosis and mild hydronephrosis, using prazosin and tramadol, with a good response. The initial abdominal ultrasound had evidenced a hyperechoic structure in the proximal ureter, but later on it could not be located and calculi/foreign material had been ruled out.
  - Urinary culture was negative. Blood culture showed leukocytosis with neutrophilia.
- **Physical examination:** open fistula in the caudal right flank, with purulent discharge (Fig. C12.1). Scars from previous draining tracts and surgeries.
- **Complementary tests:** an MRI was performed before surgery, and a connection from the fistula to the caudal area of the right kidney was evident (Fig. C12.2).
- **Surgical procedure:**
  - First, an exploratory laparotomy was performed. Both ovarian and uterine pedicles had braided non-absorbable suture. The fibrosis around the right pedicle had entrapped the proximal ureter. All non-absorbable sutures were removed and the ureter was released (Fig. C12.3).
  - The fistula was opened along the right flank and partially debrided along its main tract. Before closure, two Penrose drains were placed.
  - Culture of the fistula showed no bacterial growth.
- **Diagnosis:** chronic inflammatory fistulous tract due to inadequate use of non-absorbable suture material.
- **Treatment:**
  - **Wound management:** regular cleaning. One of the drains was removed on day 3, the other on day 5.
  - **Laser therapy:**
    - In this case, LT was started 24 h after surgery. Treatment area on the flank was around 300–350 cm^2, and the initial was dose 3 J/cm^2, so a total of 1000 J was used.
    - Treatments were performed on days 1, 3, 5, 7, 10, and 14 (suture removal) after surgery. From day 5 onward, 5 J/cm^2 was used, with a total of 1500 J per treatment. On day 14, contact mode was used, using a 5 cm^2 spot size and therefore a slightly higher power density (0.6 W/cm^2).
  - **Others**: marbofloxacin 2 mg/kg q24h × 3 days (until culture results available), tramadol 3 mg/kg q8h × 3 days, prednisone 1 mg/kg q24h × 5 days, and then progressively weaning off.
- **Outcome:** uneventful healing. Surgery resolved the origin of the problem and LT prevented many of the potential complications of this case, such as seroma, recurrence of the fistula, delayed healing, etc.

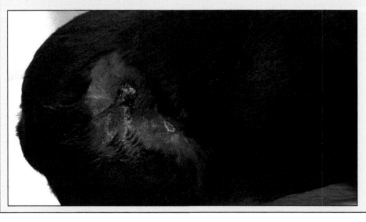

Figure C12.1 Opening of the fistulous tract in the right flank.

Case no. 12 (cont.)

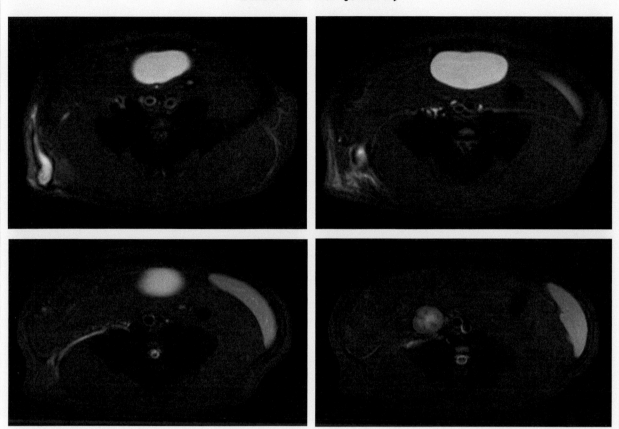

Figure C12.2 (a–d) MRI images showing fistulous tract from the skin and subcutaneous tissue to the caudal pole of the right kidney.

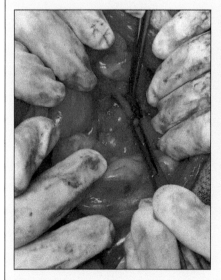

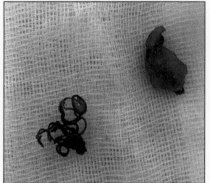

Figure C12.3 (a) Intraoperative image of the suture left in the right ovarian pedicle. Note the fibrosis around the right proximal ureter. (b) Non-absorbable braided suture material extracted from ovarian and uterine pedicles.

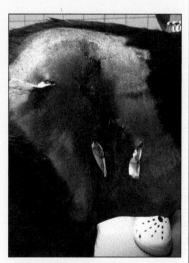

Figure C12.4 Day 1 after surgery.

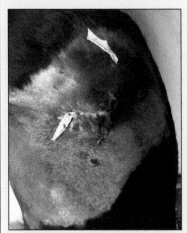

Figure C12.5 Day 3.

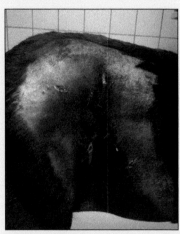

Figure C12.6 Day 7.

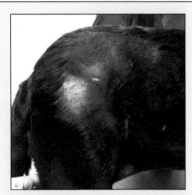

Figure C12.7 Day 14, suture removal and last treatment. Hair is regrowing faster in the treatment area, which is not uncommon.

P_a (W)	Tx time	J/cm²	Total J/Tx	Spot (cm²)	W/cm²	Tx/week	No. Tx
3	333 s (5.5 min)–500 s (8.3 min)	3-5	1000–1500	6	0.5	3	6

CHAPTER 8

Different flavors (frequencies) for different tissues

The real question is not whether machines think but whether men do.

— B.F. Skinner

You are clinicians, so it is overtly intuitive to you that there are some fundamental differences between bone, muscle, connective tissue (tendons/ligaments), dermis, and the other tissue types in the body. It should be equally obvious, then, that you probably need different "flavors" of light to optimally target each of these. Unfortunately, only a minute percentage of the research literature covers these differences. Instead, research is focused on either uncovering new physiological benefits in the laboratory or quantifying known benefits in the clinical setting. For ease of research and to increase sample size, both of these sectors tend to focus their efforts on a single parameter-set, so that they are using the same power, dose, wavelength, frequency, treatment time, etc. Undoubtedly they've referenced some previously successful study to decide which single parameter-set to use. But this leaves the real-world clinician a little wanting ...

8.1 Evidence that tissue type matters

Those that have truly studied laser to the core have noticed a distinct variation in effect as the parameters are modified. First (and most famous) to make this observation was Tiina Karu, who (as you may be able to tell from the numerous references to her work throughout this book) has done the most significant work in this industry (and as a fellow physicist, the "godmother" of laser therapy wins my favor).

At its heart, this is a fairly easy experiment to perform. Narrow down some useful effect whose amplitude can be measured, and then, for a given cell line, "turn one of the knobs at a time" and record the differences. Karu (and others) did this first with the dose "knob," showing lots of peaks and valleys in the response curves from 0.0007 J/cm^2 all the way up to 50 J/cm^2.[203] We talked about this study back in section 6.5 when we discussed the differences between *in vitro* and *in vivo* experiments and how people often mistakenly apply the Ardnt–Schultz law and assume that "too large a dose is harmful."

Her team went one better and repeated this same experiment with a different cell line and saw even more different behavior, uncovering the idea that different cell types react differently to changing parameters.[268] Then she went even further, and started turning different "knobs." This time it was pulse frequency vs. the continuous wave (CW) lasers she had been using.

For a given cell line, they varied the pulse frequency and noted the change in behavior of the measured effect (they used chemiluminescence in one study, cell adhesion in another, and more). And we are not talking about small percentage point differences. They noticed effects that differed by FACTORS OF TWO depending on the pulse frequency of light used. Further down the rabbit hole, they trialed this for several cell lines (mouse, human, etc.) and each time noticed differences in behavior based on pulse frequency used.[269]

This really let the cat out of the bag, from a clinical standpoint. We spent entire chapters in this book showing that dose is ALWAYS going to vary within a given treatment volume depending on the type of anatomy, amount of scatter and absorption, and treatment technique. So the best we can do is make some guesstimates based on the "typical shoulder," for example, to determine an average dose to be delivered to where we expect the pathology to originate.

But when it comes to frequency, depending on how we dial the "knob," we are able to expose the entire treatment volume to a given pulse frequency if we think that frequency might hit a "sweet spot" in the clinical-benefit-effect curve.

IMPORTANT: This book is all about fine-tuning the bits of laser therapy technique you can control. If you take nothing else from this section, it should be that you as the clinician CAN make a difference in the treatment outcomes of your patients, depending on your choice of pulse frequencies that you point at your target tissue.

8.2   Understanding the WHY

Being good scientists (again why I love their work so much), Karu and her team attempted to get down to the why, and from what I've read they have done the best job in simplifying the explanation. And, conveniently for me as I've been writing my sections of this book, the reason boils down to heat, a topic that has come up at least four times so far (I've lost count at this point, so apologies for yet another quick summary here).

Laser absorption results in a very small heat conversion/transfer. The body is quite good at dissipating heat, within certain extremes. And that dissipation takes time, where the amount of time is determined by the amount of heat and the size of the "thing" dissipating it; i.e. whether we are talking about bulk tissue or individual cells. Creating time gaps between when the laser is on (i.e. pulsing) allows time for the cells to dissipate heat. Going back to the macro-example, this is akin to using an ice-pack (or heating pad) for 20 minutes on, then 20 minutes off, then repeat.

While the laser is on, heat is accumulating, and there is some threshold where the body simply saturates. One could make the case that if there is too much accumulation, beyond mere saturation, the body will attempt to take countermeasures to maintain homeostasis, and therefore secrete some enzymes or make its cells' membranes more permeable. Some theories of laser mechanisms of action say this can be exploited as the

stimulus to trigger a chain of chemical signaling reactions or get more nutrients into the cells or simply as a general physical catalyst (as in acupuncture) to initiate a physiological response.

But in either case, whether we are talking saturation or secondary response, there is a period of time after which the local environment changes because of this heat. The way to mitigate this, and potentially get the most out of the therapy, is to allow time in between pulses for the body to dissipate this heat.

This theory is most popular because more of Tiina Karu's work illuminates the mechanism.[268] What was so special about these different pulse frequencies? For a given pulse there are two main components: the pulse width/duration (i.e. how long the beam is on) and the "dark" period in between (i.e. how long between pulses). When her team varied the pulse width from 5 to 1000 ms, they saw a fairly flat behavior, not much difference in the measured effect (cell attachment in this case).

But when they varied the dark period between pulses for this cell line, they saw a significant (almost a FACTOR OF TWO) increase in the effect between its peak and its baseline. Again, we very much care about factors of two. So why the big jump?

The hypothesis, which is substantially more than just a hypothesis by now, was that this particular cell line's thermal dissipation constant was right in line with the peak dark period. In other words, if there was not enough time between pulses for the heat from that pulse to be dissipated, then the physiological effect wasn't as strong as it could be, probably because of this saturation. And if that were the end of the story, there would just be a lower threshold for the dark period such that the effect after that was the same (i.e. as long as you waited longer than that threshold for the next pulse, it didn't matter how much longer you waited).

But that's not what they saw as they dug deeper. It turns out that the curve went back down AFTER the peak. In other words, if there was too much time between pulses, so that the heat was completely gone from the previous pulse, then there was only a more modest increase in effect. Within a "sweet spot" though, a heightened effect (remember, a factor of two increase) was achieved. This means there is some natural thermo-relaxing resonance of cells we can exploit to get the most out of laser therapy ... if we make the right guesses about what we are treating.

8.3   Best guesses

So how can we find the best possible frequency to use for which tissues? After all, that's why you started reading this entire section in the first place.

Disclaimer: here is where a little of the hand-waving starts, simply because, as I mentioned earlier, not a lot of people have put in the time/resources to find the "right" answers. That said, there is some simple, sound science here that should help connect the dots.

The name of the game is allowing time for cells/tissue to dissipate heat between pulses. The most abundant heat conductor in the body is water, which makes up about 80% of the body. But that 80% is a broad average. The number fluctuates more than a little between the different tissue types in the body, with bones having closer to 60% water content and soft tissue having closer to 90% water content.[270] More water (thermal conductor) means more heat transport, which means quicker dissipation.

Theoretically, then, the tissue types that have lower water content (e.g. bone) will need more time between pulses to dissipate heat. More time between pulses means fewer pulses per second, or lower frequencies. Conversely, tissues with higher water content can dissipate heat faster and so can support the use of higher pulse frequencies where there is less time between pulses.

And while tissues such as bone with low water content will, by this logic, not respond well to higher frequencies (not enough time to dissipate heat), lower frequencies (with longer dark periods) can be useful across the board, even in soft tissues. But as the experiment bore out, there seems to be a "sweet spot" where an optimal effect can be achieved, and so to best target soft tissues, higher frequencies could be the "right" choice. Tendons and ligaments, being somewhere between bone and soft tissue in their water content and therefore dissipation times, perhaps respond best to mid-range frequencies.

8.4   Little bit of this ... little bit of that

It's finally time to put your clinician hat back on and realize that, for a given injury, there are probably multiple tissue types affected. An arthritic hip, for example, has the bone (and any calcifications), the connective tissue, and the surrounding soft tissue.

> IMPORTANT: Lasering a given injury will help that injury, regardless of the technique, parameters, treatment frequency, etc. (within a range of extremes, of course). But you are reading this book to find the best way to perform the most efficient treatments that produce the optimum clinical output. So the advice contained here aims to help you make the decisions to achieve just that. The advice is NOT intended to "poo-poo" any ideas or successes you may have previously experienced using parameters/techniques that stray from what you see here. Knowledge is power ... keep that in mind.

So if you have an injury that you know involves multiple tissue types, and if you're convinced that each of these tissues has its own optimal "sweet spot" of pulse frequencies, then wouldn't a blend of frequencies have the best chance of treating that injury most effectively?

I'll leave that question open-ended, even though you know our answer to it. And if you fall in line with that way of thinking, there are several ways to accomplish that. You can use a multi-phase approach where, within a given treatment, you vary the frequencies within the range of "sweet spots" of the target tissues. You can instead do a multi-regimen approach where each treatment in the regimen uses a given frequency throughout the entire treatment, but where the frequency for the following treatment (whether it be the next day or the next week) is one that targets a different tissue. This may be useful in pathologies that require some serious anti-inflammatory response earlier in the regimen before you get to work on the tendons or bones or whatever.

Whapp!!! That was the sound of my co-author cracking my knuckles with her yardstick because I just stepped out of line. She's the clinician. So she's the expert. So she gives the advice on that.

But I will make one more important clarification, which perhaps should have been made earlier. Pathologies do NOT absorb light. Gross anatomies (i.e. a shoulder or a hip) don't even absorb light. Individual cells absorb light. So the flavor of light you point at a pathology within a given anatomy depends on the cellular makeup of that tissue, not the pathology itself.

And groups of cells (up to the macro-level of tissues) are oriented in such a way that they can be affected differently within the timescales of laser pulses. So it is even safe to say you can target individual tissue types.

But if you ever read examples of recommendations in the form of "fractures are best treated with X wavelength of light" or "arthritis responds best to Y frequencies," do me a favor and cringe a little.

You may be able to say that bones, being higher in calcium content and lower in water content, may be targeted with lower frequencies. But you still have to get through dermis and soft tissue to get to that bone, so it is important to keep that in mind.

To talk about arthritis in general terms, though, is entirely too vague. Arthritis is inflammation of the joint, which is composed of bone, cartilage, tendons, ligaments, blood vessels, and even some musculature. Granted, your goal is an anti-inflammatory effect, and to a lay technician you are simply shining light on the stifle and hoping to decrease the size of it, but having read this far into the book, you (we hope) have a better understanding of how the individual tissues respond for the greater good.

Different pathologies can have different therapeutic goals. Tendinitis means a tendon is inflamed, and that it has undergone an acute or heavy force that has led to small tears. So the goal would be to either decrease inflammation and/or make it resolve faster and with a better result. If the body fails to properly resolve this inflammatory state, chronic degenerative changes can happen to the collagen, leading to tendinosis. At this point, rather than treating *inflammation, the goal is to help the tendon generate proper (in terms of amount and type) collagen and blood supply. Although tendon and connective tissue in general would have a higher affinity for medium frequencies due to their water content and structure, with the scientific data available today there is no point in saying 500 Hz will be stimulating collagen synthesis while 2000 Hz will treat inflammation. Or that it won't absorb and make good use of CW. The tendon will absorb the light, improve metabolism, and work in a more physiological way.*

Nevertheless, you may want to keep in mind that an acute tendinitis can be painful and may tolerate lower power density or less pressure/contact during the treatment.

I won't insult your intelligence by offering up a standard lookup table where X pathology gets Y laser parameters. With that said, I can't in good conscience leave this section without giving you at least a ballpark approximation of how best to tailor your treatments to the patient and condition presented.

One last hesitation: literature references for what you are about to see are scarce, again simply because most clinical papers are meant to show THAT a given parameter-set worked, not compare two different parameter-sets. And even then, there are so many more variables to consider than just frequency (dose, wavelength, power density, treatment frequency, etc.) to find the optimum treatment. Please don't email us saying, "but I read a paper that used frequency X on tissue Y and you said that one wouldn't work."

So the final disclaimer is that Table 8.1 shows our opinion – formed from the theory of the fundamental interactions of light with tissue combined with personal experience treating patients with lasers of a wide frequency spectrum (CW and pulsing up to 25,000 Hz) and sprinkled with a little literature review – of the ballpark scale of frequencies suited for the variety of tissue types found in your patients.

Summary from a different perspective

Firstly, a reminder that dose and effect don't have a linear relationship. What's more, different tissue types may respond differently to changes in parameters of dose and frequency of pulsing. The reason why frequency of pulsing and dark phase duration are important seems to be related to the ability of the cells to dissipate the heat, and this is closely related to the amount of water in the tissue. It is therefore hypothesized that tissues with lower water content, such as bone, can benefit more from lower frequency pulses (longer dark phases). But in practice, most injuries/conditions involve different tissue types, so a good strategy seems to combine different pulsing frequencies, either in a single treatment or at least over the course of a series of visits.

Table 8.1 Ballpark values for pulse frequencies to "optimally" stimulate healing in a variety of common tissue types.

Tissue	Relative frequency	Ballpark value	Principal reason
Bone	Low	<500 Hz	Bones are made up of tightly packed, dense cells, with low relative water content, all of which leads to a slower dissipation of heat and therefore a longer time needed between pulses for an optimal response.
Connective tissue (tendons, ligaments)	Medium	500–2000 Hz	The density and spacing of these cells fall somewhere between bone and muscle; they are often surrounded by sheaths that are even more dense.
Muscle	High	2000–10,000 Hz	Muscles are made of more water-rich cells that can dissipate heat faster, and therefore resonate with pulses of shorter down-time, meaning you can use more pulses per second (Hz).
Dermis	Very high	>10,000 Hz	Dermis is very porous and well suited to "ventilating" itself to dissipate heat. Also, conditions of the dermis often involve bacteria, which are smaller and less dense than our cells, thereby dissipating heat even faster. By whichever antimicrobial mechanism, this higher frequency may be the best flavor.

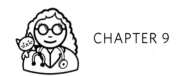

Pointing light at musculoskeletal and neurological conditions: clinical applications

The good physician treats the disease; the great physician treats the patient who has the disease.

— William Osler

Together with wound healing, musculoskeletal pain and inflammation are the most common applications of laser therapy (LT), not only in veterinary practice, but also in human physiotherapy and sports medicine. The reasons can be summarized as follows.

- **Enhanced healing of the affected tissues:** LT can stimulate osteoblasts, fibroblasts, and muscle cells to replicate more and be more metabolically active. These cells will not do something they are not supposed to do; they will just work more efficiently.
- **Modulation of the inflammatory response** in all tissues involved: even in fractures, arthritis, or tendinitis there are usually several types of tissue involved, whether this is due to nearby trauma, overloading, or other causes. For instance, osteoarthritis affects the bone/cartilage articular surfaces, the synovial membrane, surrounding ligaments, etc.
- **Pain reduction:** although LT can also reduce soft-tissue and skin pain, its analgesic properties have been studied more in the field of musculoskeletal pain; the World Health Organization included LT among the recognized therapies with proven efficacy for the relief of non-specific low back pain and osteoarthritic pain.[271, 272]
- **Improvement of functionality:** this is a direct consequence of the above effects, with a great impact on quality of life and sports performance.

And all these benefits come with no side effects or positive results in doping tests. Next, we will review the parameters and particular considerations for treating musculoskeletal conditions, the actions of LT in these tissues, and their most common ailments, followed by sections on outcome improvement and assessment and clinical tips for treating different areas of the body.

But first, the following are examples of the wide range of LT applications in musculoskeletal problems:

- muscle tears
- myositis
- ligament rupture
- tendinitis
- postoperative treatment of fractures and orthopedic procedures such as tibial tuberosity advancement (TTA) and tibial plateau leveling osteotomy (TPLO)
- partial fractures
- delayed healing fractures
- osteoarthritis
- general pain management
- trigger point treatment.

9.1 General treatment considerations

A major practical difference when treating wounds or skin vs. musculoskeletal conditions is that in the first case we avoid contacting the surface of the patient, while **treating in contact** is usually preferred in musculoskeletal problems. Actually, not just in contact but with a variable degree of pressure. There are several reasons for this.

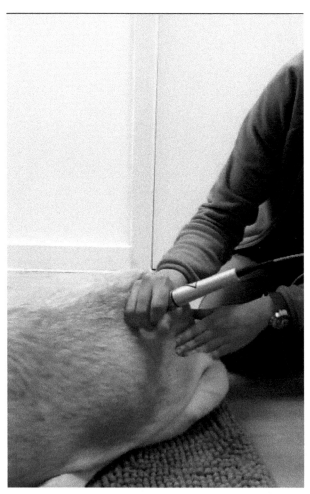

Figure 9.1 Treating in contact and with a degree of pressure that is comfortable to the patient improves penetration of light. Remember to keep the hand-piece perpendicular to the surface.

- While applying pressure we decrease the distance from the probe to the depth of tissue.
- By mobilizing the vascular bed we push away blood, therefore it will absorb less energy and allow more photons to travel deeper, so we improve penetration.
- If the tip of the probe is being held and surrounded by your hand (Fig. 9.1), contact also lets you know if there are tender, fibrotic, or other abnormal areas, and gives real-time feedback about the surface temperature.

The non-dominant hand can help separate the coat, which will also improve penetration, although not as much as the alternative of shaving/clipping the area. In practice, clipping is possible if only one or two areas are affected; but if the patient needs to have the spine,

hips, and stifles treated, clipping is not likely to be an option, and although preferable, is not indispensable in most cases.

The exceptions to treating in contact would be recent fractures or conditions with concurrent skin damage. If the animal is in pain when touched, contact can be avoided during the first sessions at least; to avoid losing power density (which can be significant for pain management and crucial to achieve significant penetration) you will need a hand-piece with an adjustable spot size, or an extra hand-piece with a smaller tip, able to concentrate the beam from a distance.

9.1.1 Dose (J/cm²)

The range of appropriate doses or energy densities for most cases will be from 4 to 15 J/cm² (Table 9.1), and as in the soft-tissue applications described in Chapter 7, this will vary according to the following factors.

- **The depth of the condition:** a calcaneus tendon is quite a superficial target, especially if we compare it with an iliopsoas or the caudal cervical muscles. Remember that most of the dose will be absorbed in the more superficial tissues, but a higher starting dose still means more energy will be left at a certain depth.
- **The chronicity of the process:** chronic conditions need about a 30–50% higher starting dose. So after an acute trauma to the hip area, the initial dose will be about 5–6 J/cm², but a chronic osteoarthritis will require around 8–10 J/cm² to begin with.
- **The amount of inflammation present:** managing inflammation may need a lower dose than treating pain. What is more important is that whatever dose you choose should not be delivered with a high power density.[37]

It makes sense to treat an area that is proximal to the injury, not just for the blood flow – although this will be improved if there is a lack of it – but for the segmental analgesia. In painful conditions, especially in chronic ones, the nerve roots supplying that area may be sensitized. Consider the associated spinal segments as extra treatment areas if necessary, especially in chronic and refractory pain. For instance, consider treating the lumbar area together with the knee area if a case with chronic osteoarthritis of the stifle is not improving. These extra treatment areas need to have

Table 9.1 Recommended parameters for musculoskeletal conditions.

	Example	Dose (J/cm²)	Power (W)	Power density (W/cm²)
Acute superficial	Tendinitis	2–5	3–5	0.2–1
Acute deep	Closed fracture	4–8	4–8	0.5–1.5
Chronic superficial	Chronic tendinitis	4–15	4–6	0.5–1
Chronic deep	Spondylosis, hip dysplasia	8–20	6–15	1.5–3

their own treatment energy calculated, i.e. if you were going to deliver 800 J to the stifle, do that and then calculate what amount you would need for the spinal area.

9.1.2   Power (W)

The power used usually ranges from 3 to 15 W, and as we explained in Chapter 7, it will influence the following.

- **How long it takes to treat an area:** as for wounds, decide in the first place the area you want to include

and the dose you want to apply. The AVERAGE power, not the peak power, will tell you how long the treatment will take.

- **What density of photons penetrates the surface:** this becomes even more important if our target tissues are not on the surface. When working with musculoskeletal pain, though, we target not just deep articular surfaces of synovial membranes, but also more superficial nociceptors. This is good news, since photon density will always be higher close to the surface, and pain management usually requires this higher dose, while tissue healing and inflammation will likely use less.

Calculating your treatment in four steps

1. Decide the dose (J/cm²) you will deliver, based on reference values and clinical progression of that particular case.
2. Estimate or measure the treatment area (cm²).
3. Multiply those two values to calculate how many J you want to deliver in that session, in that area (J/cm² × cm² = J).
4. The average power you work with (W) will determine how long it takes to deliver those J (time in s = J/W).

Example

1. You have decided to deliver a dose of 10 J/cm² over the thoracic and lumbar area of a dog.
2. The treatment area covers 40 cm from cranial to caudal, and 10 cm from side to side, so it has an area of 400 cm².
3. Therefore, you want to deliver a total amount of energy of about 4000 J in that session.
4. If we work with an average power of 1 W, it will take 4000 J/1 W = 4000 s (almost 67 min). Those same 4000 J using 12 W of average power will take 4000 J/12 W = 333 s or less than 6 min, and working with 10 W will take slightly longer: 4000 J/10 W = 400 s (6.6 min).

If your device does not state the joules used, multiply the average power by the treatment time. By dividing those final joules by the treatment area, you can then calculate the dose that is being delivered (J/cm²). For instance, your device tells you it is going to treat the hip for 3 min (180 s). You know the average power it is using is 1 W. Then you can calculate that the amount of energy delivered is J = 1 W × 180 s, so it will deliver 180 J. In this example, if you are treating a hip area of 180 cm² with that program, you would only be applying 1 J/cm², which is very insufficient.

This is one of the reasons why if you plan to treat musculoskeletal conditions or large surface areas, and you want to scan them uniformly, a well-powered class IV laser is preferred over a lower power (or class of) device – and why a 12 W device is more suitable than a 2 W one.

- **How warm the surface gets:** since we will be using more power and power density than in skin problems, this is something you need to keep in mind.

Remember, it is not just power that influences how warm the surface gets, but also the wavelength used, the color of the patient, how fast you move the hand-piece, and power density, meaning how that power is concentrated (W/cm^2). Usually musculoskeletal conditions are treated with higher power than wounds, and also in contact with the patient, to improve penetration. So keep that in mind: do not exceed 2–3 W/cm^2 unless you are moving the hand-piece relatively fast. If your hand-piece has an adjustable spot size, use the maximum available size if you are working in contact mode.

Power density is quite similar to the strength of a massage: a higher power density feels like a stronger manipulation. When you have a sore muscle or back, sometimes you may need a stronger massage to alleviate it. But if the main problem of a tissue or area is acute inflammation, you definitely don't want any strong manipulation there. In the same way, some painful conditions need a more intense approach to reduce pain, but usually your patient with severe acute inflammation will prefer a more subtle approach.

Continuous wave (CW) is always the fastest way to deliver the calculated energy, but is also more warming (there are no dark periods between pulses to allow for thermal dissipation in the tissue), and when working with higher power densities, as happens with musculoskeletal conditions, warming can become significant, especially for darker coats. If there is significant erythema in the treatment area, try not to use a lot of CW, since it has a stronger vasodilating effect than pulsed radiation. Pulsing the light will allow you to do the following.

- **Use a higher power.** Average power (Pa) will be the result of peak power (Pp) times the duty cycle (DC), which represents the percentage of each second that the light is "on." DC can be calculated by multiplying the frequency of the pulsing (Hz) times the duration of those pulses (ton). The range of effective pulses described for pain is very broad, though, from 2 to 8000 Hz.[48, 201]

$$P_a = P_p \times DC$$
$$DC = Hz \times \text{pulse duration } (t_{on})$$

"Can I burn my patient? Can I burn them without even knowing it?" These are questions many practitioners have in mind when they start using LT. The answer is of course a bit more complex than yes or no. Let me start with the second question.

- "Can I burn my patient without even knowing I am doing so?" NO, unless the patient or the area you are treating is anesthetized or has no pain perception. If the patient is awake and the area has pain perception, there is no way you could be burning him and not realizing. The feeling for the patient would first be discomfort, and if you persisted, the patient would feel pain and try to run away/bite/scratch you. There is no way you would not notice.
- "Can I burn my patient?" If you try really hard, maybe. Burning comes from an accumulation of energy, or heat, in a tissue that goes beyond its capacity to disperse that energy or cool off. The way to "try hard" to burn your patient is by using too high a power density, especially

if you do not move the hand-piece and treat in contact. That would mean treating with a high power, using a small hand-piece or concentrated spot size, while not moving.
- "What if I make a mistake?" A Class IV laser can produce heat on the surface of the patient, especially those with dark and/or thick fur. It is unlikely and easy to avoid if you are treating properly, but if on some of the larger-body-part protocols (which call for higher power) you stay in one spot for too long, heat can accumulate, even to the point of singeing the hair. This will cause an unpleasant smell and will probably scare your staff (and the pet owner), but the good thing is that it likely won't hurt the patient. To prove this to yourself, take some hair clippings from a dark dog, put them on your palm, and start to treat that hair until it singes. You'll notice that your palm didn't burn. Another exercise may be to take those clippings and start treating them, but move the hand-piece around as you do so. You'll notice that you won't singe the hair, because you are spreading the power around.

Here are some examples of these calculations.

- If your peak power is 18 W and your average power is 12 W, that means you are working with a 66.67% DC.
- If you know you are operating with a DC of 50% and the screen tells you the peak power is 6 W, you know your average power is 3 W.
- If you want to know how long your pulses are, and you are working at 100 Hz with a duty cycle of 30%: 0.3 = 100 Hz × pulse duration, so pulses are 0.003 s or 3 ms. With that same DC, if you were pulsing at 2 Hz, those pulses would last 150 ms or 0.15 s.
- **Target different cell lines.** Osteoblasts seem to respond better to lower frequencies, for instance.

Therefore, a good strategy seems to combine both CW and different pulsing frequencies (as we talked about at length in Chapter 8), which will also avoid a potential saturation of the biological response.

9.1.4   How often?

As in wound management, **acute** conditions need lower doses but more often initially: daily for 2–3 days, then q48h for two to three more treatments, and then twice a week if needed until resolution. And chronic conditions need higher starting doses but they can be treated less often, although initially at least three treatments a week are recommended.

When dealing with a wound, a full resolution is the clinical expectation, but in many **chronic** musculoskeletal problems the goal is to achieve a significant improvement, then decrease the frequency of visits, and find a maintenance regime that will ideally prevent relapses and improve the quality of life of the patient, but will not cure or reverse the basic underlying process. These phases are often named induction (we achieve the clinical effect with more frequent treatments), transition (we maintain that but decrease the frequency), and maintenance. So after treating three times a week (or q48h), usually for 1–2 weeks, and once an improvement is noted (not before!), LT can be delivered twice a week (usually for 2–3 weeks), then once a week for 2–3 weeks. The maintenance regime after that will vary with the patient. For instance, an old Labrador with degenerative joint disease (DJD) of the hip may need to come again more often in the next cold/humid season, when his hips hurt more, but may

do well without treatment for a couple of months in the warmer season. Others will do best when treated every 3–6 weeks for maintenance.

Most musculoskeletal conditions will need longer sessions or appointments than wounds, since very often there is more than one body area affected or sore because of overload. Good orthopedic, neurological, and biomechanical exams are essential to plan how many areas, how often, and how long will it take to apply the desired doses over the planned areas. This will influence the appointment length, and probably the fee that is charged.

9.2   Laser therapy for fractures and osteotomies

Animal models have demonstrated that LT can increase bone mineralization. It stimulates osteoblastic activity by modulating bone morphogenic factors. The tissue will have a higher number of active osteoblasts and they will be secreting more collagen matrix, so LT can help fractures and osteotomies heal faster and produce a better organized and less exuberant callus.[160, 273–276] This will lead to stronger bone formation; animals treated with LT show higher maximum loads at failure in bone bending tests.[276, 277] When we use LT in fractures, the aim is to enhance biological processes that contribute to bone healing; we can influence growth factor release, vascularization, osteogenic activity, and inflammation. Research and experience have proven how important preserving the soft tissue and blood supply is to fracture biology, and LT contributes to this.

If bone grafting is to be used in the fracture repair procedure, LT can improve bone graft survival. Animal models show that LT improves incorporation at the graft–host interface, filling of osteocyte lacunae, and collagen deposition, while it decreases the inflammatory infiltrate in the early postoperative period.[275, 278, 279]

These, together with the anti-inflammatory and analgesic effects, are the reasons LT can improve fracture repair and patient's quality of life. Clinical studies (again, very few have been published) in humans show that patients achieve better analgesia and functional recovery in closed fractures of the wrist and hand.[280] Also, LT helps bone formation and healing after mid-palatal suture expansion in children[281] and in dogs,[161] and may decrease orthodontic correction time.[282]

Nevertheless, the body's resources, even with the help of LT, can be overwhelmed by other factors, some of which we should at least mention.

- **Nonviable bone at the fracture area:** in this situation the edges have become atrophic, necrotic (sequestrum), or have lost vascularization, and need to be removed.
- **Excessive gaps:** how much of a gap is considered too much? This is still under study, but it has been suggested to avoid approaching the diameter of the bone.[283] When a gap persists, it gets filled with fibrotic tissue and/or muscle, which then has to be surgically removed.
- **Deficient realignment or fixation:** LT will enhance neovascularization, but if the fixation is insufficient, excess motion will perpetuate damage to capillaries and poor blood supply, plus the excessive strain will promote fibrous tissue rather than new bone formation. Strain increases fibrous tissue formation and some compression stimulates bone formation; that is one reason why we use dynamic compression plates in orthopedic surgery.
- **Osteomyelitis:** LT may help in osteomyelitis due to the effect on blood supply and metabolism; ischemia is both a predisposing factor and a consequence of osteomyelitis. In an experimental osteomyelitis model in rats by Kaya et al., LT reduced bacterial counts.[188] Of course, in osteomyelitis you should include other therapeutic interventions.

It is mandatory to address these mechanical and biological factors ASAP. LT cannot fix them by itself, and if these problems are present, we still need to use bone grafts, make sure there is adequate fixation, debride, provide 6–8 weeks of proper antibiotic therapy, and perform any other necessary actions. Control radiographs should be taken every 3–4 weeks.

Osteotomies may also benefit from LT. A blinded, randomized, and controlled clinical study on TPLO and LT preconditioning, in which patients received a single treatment before the procedure,[284] showed a difference in the peak vertical force 8 weeks after surgery (measured with a force plate) between the laser and control groups. Vertical impulse was unchanged. Eight weeks after the surgery, 62.5% of animals in the LT group showed radiographic signs of osteotomy healing, compared to 25% in the control group, although this difference was not statistically significant and eventually all

osteotomies healed well. But think – that was just ONE treatment, whereas in clinical practice at least half a dozen would have been prescribed. The first treatment should ideally take place in the operating room. The usual treatment regime would include 2–3 treatments a week for 2–3 weeks, and a control radiograph every 3–4 weeks.

A more recent study again showed a potential benefit of LT for canine TPLO patients. This randomized, placebo-controlled trial included 95 dogs, receiving three treatments (or placebo ones) during consecutive days in the perioperative period. When rechecked 8 weeks after the surgery, those treated with LT had an improved gait.[285] In these dogs, not only the area of the osteotomy was treated, but also the ipsilateral lumbosacral area.

Both fractures and osteotomies will have a concurrent skin wound over them (well, open fractures have more than that). That part should be initially treated as a wound, i.e. with lower power, dose, and power density than the rest of the perimeter of the limb. For the wound area, a dose of about 4 J/cm^2 or less is used, while the rest of the treatment area will require 6–10 J/cm^2 that can be applied with more power. Lower dosages have been used for more superficial targets – a cat mandible can be treated with 4 J/cm^2, but most cases will require more – unusually, even 20–30 J/cm^2 has been reported in a rat model.[164]

Opaque bandages, such as Robert Jones or its modifications, do not allow red or infrared light to penetrate, so they have to be removed for the session – if that is the case, schedule both events for the same day. If a fiberglass cast is used, a window can be created to allow laser treatments without a full bandage change, although this option limits the area that can be treated to a small portion.

9.2.1 Laser therapy in growing animals

There is some legitimate debate on laser use in growing animals. The main concern is that if LT stimulates new bone formation and increases the overall metabolic activity of the tissues, could it induce a premature closure of growth plates? It is indeed a good question. But let's review if it is based on any data or if there have been any clinical reports about it.

An experimental model showed premature calcification and shortened bone growth,[286] but it is worth mentioning that the dose used was 10 J/cm^2 in a RAT on a DAILY basis for 21 DAYS, which is very far from what we would do with a real patient. Cressoni et al. described changes in epiphyses and increased numbers of chondrocytes but the same final bone length using 830 nm, with 5 and 15 J/cm^2 applied ten times every other day.[287]

Others have not found these risks. For instance, Cheetham et al. used 820 nm, 5 J/cm^2 three times per week in rats, and histological examination at the 6th and 12th treatments did not show any changes in growth plates.[288] Another research group found no differences on X-ray or cartilage pathology 14 weeks after using 670 nm, at 4, 8, and 16 J/cm^2 at one point over the medial epiphysis, daily for ten days. However, the wavelength used and the fact they irradiated only one point could have meant there was limited penetration and effect.[289]

There is a case report that documents premature closure of a physeal growth plate in a child, with subsequent bone deformity, after using what they call "laser therapy." But in the full text of the report, what they actually talk about is a third-degree burn with a surgical CO$_2$ laser,[290] which works at much higher power densities, with the primary photo-thermal aim of ablating/coagulating/vaporizing tissue, not stimulating its metabolism via photochemical reactions.

So what I do in practice is to encourage LT use, while keeping in mind that younger animals respond faster. If your aim is to help with superficial wounds, the power and dose you will be using are probably not a concern to the deeper bone. If you are dealing with a Salter–Harris fracture, the problem for the growth plate is the fracture, not your laser (Fig. 9.2). Just don't use too much power over an open growth plate. Young animals already have a higher metabolic rate, so try to keep doses and frequency of sessions on the conservative side. Nevertheless, you know that shortening the post-operative recovery period in a growing animal can be extremely valuable, to decrease the risk of pathological fibrosis, atrophy, compensating injuries, and the long-term consequences these may carry. And despite the extensive use of this modality, not a single case (to our knowledge) of angular deformities after laser therapy has been reported in human or veterinary practice.

9.2.2   Laser therapy and metallic implants

Internal metallic implants do not act like a hot iron on the bone. Unlike ultrasound, animals with such osteo-synthesis devices can be treated with LT (Fig. 9.3). And unlike ultrasound, which stimulates osteoclastic activity, laser stimulates new bone formation. When human osteoblast-like cells derived from human mandibular bone are irradiated *in vitro* with LT, they tend to

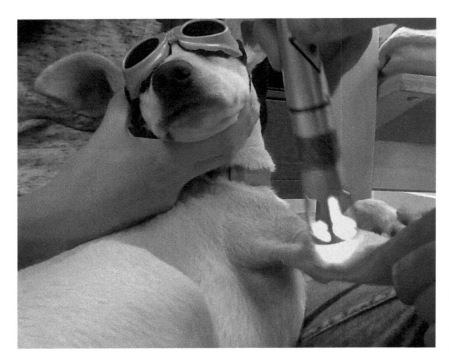

Figure 9.2 Treatment of a puppy in the postoperative rehabilitation of a distal humeral fracture (see Case no.13 in this chapter).

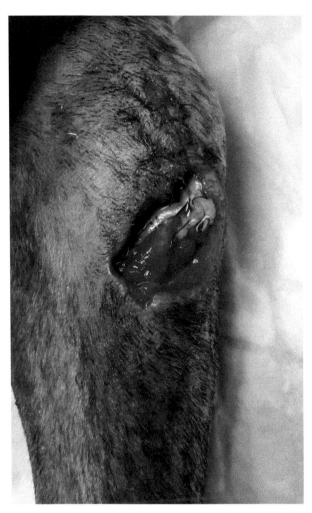

Figure 9.3 Surgical site infection and wound dehiscence over a metallic implant. Laser is indicated (see Case nos. 20–22 in this chapter).

proliferate, differentiate, get more attached to the titanium implant, and produce more TGF-β.[235] In animal models of normal and osteopenic bone, LT can accelerate implant integration and new bone formation.[163] It enhances osteogenic mediators such as bone morphogenic protein, and even one session has been proven to increase the bone–implant interface strength.[291] The sooner an implant is integrated and vascularized, the less likely it is to be colonized by bacteria. So using LT to treat patients with osteosynthesis implants is not just possible, it is advisable, and could help prevent osteomyelitis (you can read more about LT in infected tissue in section 5.6).

If there is a metallic plate placed on the bone, laser will not penetrate the plate to reach the bone, which has two immediate implications.

- If you want to stimulate healing of a fracture or an osteotomy, treat that area as just the wound that lies over it and focus most of the energy around it. For instance, if a TTA plate has been placed on the medial surface of the proximal tibia, treat the surgical wound over it as a regular acute wound and treat more intensely proximal and distal to it, as well as on the cranial, lateral, and caudal side of the tibia. Once the wound has healed you may treat the whole area with similar higher parameters, but not focusing over the implant, rather around it for a better penetration into the fracture/osteotomy line.
- If and when osteomyelitis develops, LT may help decrease bacterial counts as described in an experimental model.[188] You will improve the metabolism of the area, and almost certainly see an improvement, but if you are dealing with osteomyelitis between the bone and the plate, your chances of success are limited and a full resolution is unlikely unless other therapies are combined with LT.

9.3 Tendon and ligament injuries

Fibroblast replication and collagen production provide the base for tendon and ligament repair. LT helps to produce proportionally more type I collagen, which has a better spatial arrangement, and leads to greater final tensile strength of tendons and ligaments, as has been consistently demonstrated in several experimental models.[138, 140, 143, 292, 293] And blood flow, one of the major benefits of LT, is also a critical factor in the repair of these already poorly vascularized structures – if you are an orthopedic surgeon, this is one of your usual concerns.

There have been some animal models studying LT in inflammation after tendon and ligament injuries. The mechanism is similar to other tissues: there is a reduction in the expression of pro-inflammatory mediators, such as COX-2, in both acute and chronic inflammatory phases.[294] Models also show the effect of LT in the surrounding tissues: in rats, 15 sessions of laser therapy at 10 J/cm^2 were able to prevent some of the morphological degenerative changes and proteoglycan loss that occurred after cruciate ligament transection, although in this particular model IL-1 did not decrease.[295] Another placebo-controlled experimental study, using a model in rabbits that developed progressive osteoarthritis (OA) after cranial cruciate ligament transection, described how LT could decrease knee pain, synovial inflammation, and inflammatory mediators related to the inflammatory and catabolic process of OA, such as IL-1 and metalloproteinases.[296] The treated group received a low dose (1.5 J/cm^2 of 830 nm light) three times a week; effects were seen after 6 weeks of therapy.

The pain associated with ligament and tendon injuries can also be alleviated with LT. A placebo-controlled, double-blinded clinical study in human patients with lateral epicondylitis reported significant improvement in pain and functionality scores. They used 6–7 J/cm^2, treating at 10 W and with around 0.5–1 W/cm^2 of power density.[111] Using lower doses and power, another randomized, placebo-controlled clinical trial found an analgesic and anti-inflammatory effect of LT in Achilles tendinitis, also describing a fast decrease in peritendinous prostaglandin E_2 (PGE_2) concentrations. [297]

The above are just examples of experimental and clinical studies about the benefits of LT in tendon and ligament injuries. One of the reasons these transection models cannot be directly extrapolated to the dog is that in our canine patients, although sudden and complete cranial cruciate ligament rupture (CCLR) can occur, it is usually a chronic condition that starts with a partial tear that progresses after an initial period of apparent stabilization and improvement. Breed conformation is also involved.

Another clinical study is relevant here: although it did not have the aim of investigating the effect of LT, the study described excellent results in dogs with partial CCLR using bone marrow aspirate concentrate or adipose-derived progenitor cells in combination with platelet-rich plasma therapy. These patients had at least 50% of the craniomedial band of the ligament intact, as diagnosed by arthroscopy, and together with the stem cell treatment, they underwent a rehabilitation program in which LT was included, and wore a customized stifle orthotic. Not only did pain ratings improve, but in more than half of the cases that were re-examined arthroscopically, the cranial cruciate ligament had fully regenerated.[298]

To treat tendon and ligament injuries, 4–10 J/cm^2 are used, staying at the lower end of the range for relatively superficial structures such as the calcaneal tendon; 3–10 W can be used, but for superficial and/or very inflamed and tender areas keep the power density within 0.5–1 W/cm^2. Initially, treatment should be performed at least three times a week (see section 9.1, "General treatment considerations"). It is recommended to also treat other structures that might be secondarily affected, such as contracted muscles or stiff joints. Rest and proper immobilization or support remain important measures for tendon and ligament injuries; don't let the patient put too much strain or tension on the tendon/ligament despite the initial clinical improvement it may show in terms of pain.

9.4 Muscle and laser therapy

Muscular conditions and injuries can also be treated with LT. The proangiogenic effect of LT enhances muscle repair; the biochemical activity of muscle cells increases and more myofibers differentiate. As in other tissues, inflammation and regeneration/proliferation are related in muscle repair: prolonged inflammation interferes with healing and recovery, and can lead to muscle fibrosis. Functional muscle contractures are also rewarding to treat, since the patient tends to experience a relatively fast relief (Fig. 9.4).

Animal models show LT can help prevent muscle fibrosis and atrophy and suggest its use should be investigated in patients with disuse atrophy, atrophy due to peripheral nerve injury, and even as part of the treatment of Duchenne dystrophy.[148, 149, 299] Genetically manipulated mice that undergo a similar process of muscular dystrophy show less muscle damage and less muscle inflammation when treated with LT.[299] An experimental model of induced myositis showed LT (3 J/cm^2) reduced the number of inflammatory cells and amount of edema[300]; a similar dose was used to prove increased regeneration and decreased inflammation after muscle contusion in rats.[301]

Alves et al. concluded in 2014 after a systematic review of the literature that LT should be considered "an excellent therapeutic resource for the treatment of skeletal muscle injuries in the short term"[8]; but more clinical studies on LT and muscular conditions should be performed, ideally comparing different treatment protocols. There are, however, some trials in sports medicine reporting that LT inhibits the post-exercise increase in creatinine kinase levels and accelerates post-exercise lactate removal,[302] which would mean a faster post-exercise recovery. On the other hand, others found no effect on the recovery of strength performance despite the attenuation in creatinine kinase activity.[303]

Treating large muscle groups can take some time, and should be well planned to include all the area of

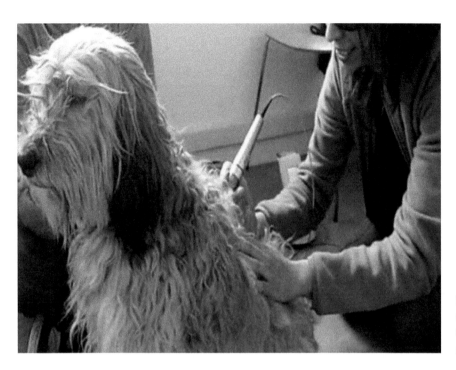

Figure 9.4 Paraspinal muscle contracture treatment in a patient with chronic intervertebral disk disease (IVDD) and spondylosis.

the muscle from different angles, as well as its tendons. For instance, if you are treating the gracilis muscle for contracture, you have to include the area from its origin in the pubic symphysis to the insertion in the cranial border of the tibia. And for this particular treatment, you probably also want to include the semitendinosus muscle, from the tuber ischiadicum to the medial surface of the tibia. You may even want to treat both hindlimbs. Measuring the area – or making a good estimate of it – will give you an accurate idea of how much energy you need if you want to stay within a certain dose range. In this example, if the area is 600 cm^2 and you want to use a dose of 8 J/cm^2, you should probably create or customize a program that will eventually deliver around 4800 J – the preset programs for the knee or the hip usually deliver only around 700–2500 J since they are designed for smaller areas.

9.4.1 Trigger points

During soft-tissue palpation, you may find trigger points (TPs), which are considered a form of myofascial pain. A TP is felt as a taut tender band or nodule, which elicits a local twitch on palpation and a pain response (called the "jump sign" in humans) either in that spot or in a referred area. TPs and their corresponding areas of referred pain have been mapped in humans, but this inter-area link is not usually described in veterinary

medicine – an exception would be traditional Chinese veterinary medicine, especially for equine patients.

Myofascial pain is often underestimated and undiagnosed, and has implications in patient biomechanics and quality of life. These "contraction knots" may cause lameness, restriction of range of movement, and autonomic signs. So although treating the TPs may not be enough for the patient, it is necessary to treat them if we want to provide the best analgesia. Laser therapy is one of the therapeutic modalities that can help alleviate this pain. Let's have a quick review of how TPs are formed to understand why.

Local factors, as well as central and biomechanical factors, are considered in the etiopathogenesis of TPs. Locally, they are the result of abnormal depolarization of motor end plates. Just to refresh a little bit, in the motor end plate we have a presynaptic neuron, a synaptic space, and a postsynaptic muscle fiber. The neurotransmitter of this connection is acetylcholine, or Ach. So increased contraction may be due to increased liberation of Ach in the presynaptic neuron, or to excess activity or number of postsynaptic Ach receptors. Any of these will lead to spontaneous electrical activity, which is actually measurable.[304]

Sustained contraction leads to compression of local sensory nerves and vessels, with subsequent hypoxia. This, together with the increased adenosine triphosphate (ATP) demand (because the muscle is contracted) leads to a local ATP deficit, and this little crisis leads to the release of inflammatory mediators. The persistence of nociceptive stimuli or such mediators can result in central nervous system (CNS) sensitization and hyper-algesia. From a biomechanical point of view, TPs can be the result of or can be perpetuated by trauma, whether this is acute or a series of repetitive microtraumas due to nearby articular dysfunction and postural disorders. All of these will generate more muscle stress. Other factors have been proposed, such as psychological stress, poor diet, visceral pain, and coldness.[305] So, together with its effect on inflammatory mediators and pain modula-tion, the efficacy of LT in treating TPs could be related to its effect on blood flow, oxygenation, and ATP pro-duction, which lie at the core of TP pathogenesis.

Palpation is the most common tool for assessing TPs and it's not a bad one: 73% of clinicians were in agree-ment according to an inter-rater reliability study carried out in humans.[306] Other methods have been described, such as measuring spontaneous electrical activity, or mechanical pressure thresholds, but let's focus on the tools you have closer to hand in your practice.

TPs are most commonly found in stable anatomic locations, most of them in well-known acupoints. Several TPs have been described in the dog, excluding paravertebral TPs. The diameter can range from a few millimeters to several centimeters (Fig. 9.5).[307]

Different treatment modalities can be used for TPs, including LT, needling, and massage with essential oils such as valerian, kava kava, and lemon balm. There are several clinical studies with LT and myofascial pain in humans and some experimental models. One of them found higher doses (27 J/cm² vs. 4.5 J/cm²) applied over the biceps femoris of rabbits were more effective in elevating β-endorphins, while lower doses were more effective in decreasing COX-2 and tumor necrosis factor (TNF).[86] On the other hand, a clini-cal study in humans reported LT with 795 nm using 4 J/cm² improved pressure algometry in the masseter trigger point, while 8 J/cm² over the contralateral point did not.[309] A double-blind and randomized-controlled clinical trial performed in people with chronic myo-fascial pain in the neck showed that LT of TPs could significantly alleviate pain and improve quality of life. They described a dose range of 2–20 J/cm².[310] These data are dose examples, but not necessarily transpos-able to our patients; remember both rats and humans usually have less hair and melanin than cats and dogs, so penetration can be very different.

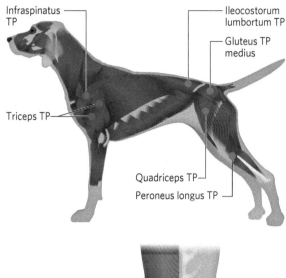
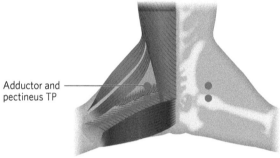

Figure 9.5 Common trigger points in the dog.
Illustrator: Elaine Leggett; adapted from Janssens.[308]

When treating TPs, there are two important things to remember: first, you will be treating in contact; second, you will not be moving the hand-piece, or at least not nearly as much. This means you have to be aware of power density, treatment time, and tissue heating. If you are not sure how your program for treating TPs feels to the patient, try it on yourself first to get an idea.

Rather than just using a fixed-spot technique (or after doing that), follow the muscle band where the TP is felt in a longitudinal direction, and combine LT with stretching techniques. For a fixed-spot technique (a few seconds), consider avoiding CW, since it will have a stronger heating effect. Moving the hand-piece will also allow some tissue cooling and you will be able to use more power density to improve penetration.

9.5 Arthritis

The most common presentation of arthritis in small animal practice is osteoarthritis (OA), also known as degenerative joint disease (DJD). Rather than just degeneration, osteoarthritis is a progressive inflammatory and degenerative disease that involves several structures and tissues. The articular cartilage degenerates and is progressively lost, the bones undergo hypertrophic changes, there is inflammation and fibrosis of the synovial membrane and periarticular structures, as well as qualitative and quantitative changes in synovial fluid. Nearby ligament attachments are eventually affected too, and the patient suffers pain and loss of functionality. About 20% of dogs that are older than 1 year suffer from OA and this percentage increases to 80% if we consider dogs over 8 years.[311, 312] It is the most common source of pain and loss of mobility in older dogs. The impact on our feline patients is often underestimated; although there is no direct correlation between radiographic signs and pain, a study in 100 client-owned cats over 6 years of age found radiographic evidence of appendicular OA in more than 60% of them.[313] Another report increased this number to over 90%,[314] with an increase of 13.6% in expected total DJD score for each 1-year increase in the age of the cat. OA also has a huge financial impact; it is the most common reason to prescribe non-steroidal anti-inflammatory drugs (NSAIDs), which represents a market of over 400 million USD per year,[315, 316] with millions of pets being treated every year.[317]

A lot has been written about OA treatment, and it is very clear that its management has to be multimodal. There is no such thing as a cure: the focus is on controlling the painful and limiting consequences and trying to slow down cartilage degradation, using pharmacological analgesia, physical modalities, and nutraceuticals. And we can't forget weight control, a MUST with or without laser: diet restriction clearly delays the onset and decreases the severity of OA.[318] Weight reduction by itself can reduce clinical signs of lameness in dogs with osteoarthritis.[319]

Other forms of arthritis we may find in small animal practice include septic and traumatic etiologies, rheumatoid arthritis, or those related to systemic infections that lead to arthritic pain, including *Leishmania* and *Rickettsia*, among others. But all forms of arthritis share the fact that the levels of pro-inflammatory mediators are increased and this changes the metabolism of chondrocytes and other cells.

Three groups of canine synovial fluid biomarkers have been investigated: pro-inflammatory mediators, enzymes and their inhibitors, and extracellular cartilage degeneration products. We have previously discussed how LT can decrease the expression of certain mediators, such as IL-1 and TNF. Among the enzymes, the most important are matrix metalloproteinases (MMPs), which are released by chondrocytes, synoviocytes, and inflammatory cells, contributing to cartilage degradation. Although some MMPs have physiological functions, others increase during inflammation (and cancer), serve as biomarkers, and are related to the severity of cartilage damage.

Different etiologies may present different profiles of mediators – they all have inflammatory soups but the amounts of the ingredients may vary. For instance, MMP-1, MMP-2, and MMP-9 are clearly increased in dogs with OA,[320–322] although some MMP-2 activity can be detected at lower levels in healthy joints.[323] Canine immune-mediated arthritis displays an even higher increase in IL-1 and TNF than OA,[324] which correlates with the amount of MMP-3, also elevated in the synovial fluid of dogs with rheumatoid arthritis when compared to OA patients.[325] Unfortunately, these biomarkers are not yet used in practice due to the lack of molecular diagnostic tests. Hopefully in the future these will be available to improve diagnosis and monitoring of the disease.[326]

The reason I'm kind of torturing you with the molecular basis of articular inflammation is because LT has consistently been reported to act at this level. Acute joint **inflammation** decreases with LT due to the reduction in the pro-inflammatory mediators IL-1, COX-2, TNF, and IL-6.[37, 41, 78, 296, 327–329] LT can also reduce the inflammatory infiltrate; in osteoarthritis models, for instance, it decreases polymorphonuclear cells in the synovial fluid and capsule.[41, 73] The resolution of the inflammation is further enhanced with the production of substances such as TGF-β, both in healthy and experimentally-induced diabetic models.[330] Besides, LT can decrease the above-mentioned MMP levels to inhibit cartilage degradation – specifically MMP-2, MMP-3, MMP-9, and MMP-13.[8, 78, 295, 296, 331, 332]

More recently, the role of nerve growth factor (NGF) in joint inflammation and cartilage degradation and its use as a therapeutic target has been described with very promising results.[333, 334] The effect of LT on this particular mechanism should be investigated, since some studies suggest LT could promote NGF release,[89] which would theoretically enhance inflammation. But after reading Chapter 3, you know that the course of inflammation definitely does not depend on just one ingredient.

Table 9.2 Examples of recommended parameters for chronic joint disorders.

Area	Patient	Dose (J/cm²)	Power (W)	Power density (W/cm²)
Carpus, tarsus	Cat, small dog	4–8	3–4	0.5–1
Elbow, stifle	Mid-sized dog	6–12	5–8	1–2
Spine, hip	Large dog	8–20	8–15	1.5–3

So there are well-established grounds for the use of LT in different forms of arthritis. But the question once again is, can these results somehow be transposed to clinical cases? A large and growing number of clinical trials in humans seem to answer "yes" to that question.

- In women with OA of the hand, LT was able to decrease pain and interphalangeal joint perimeter after five and seven twice weekly treatments, respectively. In this study, adding three more treatments did not bring a significant benefit, and the improvement achieved was maintained for 8 weeks.[335]
- In other clinical trials, LT was able to decrease synovial thickness of the knee (as measured by ultrasound) in male patients with OA,[336] as well as pain and MMPs levels.[337] Actually most trials concerning LT and OA refer to knee OA, and it has been proposed that LT should be included in standard conservative care, since the clinical improvement can delay the need for surgical intervention.[338]
- Adding LT to stretching exercises for people with ankylosing spondylitis can improve pain and function scores.[339]
- In temporomandibular OA and pain, LT improves pain and function – even more than ibuprofen according to one study.[340]
- A review of the use of LT to treat rheumatoid arthritis concluded that treated patients experience reduced pain and stiffness and improved joint flexibility.[341]

To the authors' knowledge, there are still no published clinical trials on the use of LT to treat arthritis in dogs or cats, but without a doubt this is among the top five uses of the therapy in small animal practice, so hopefully some will come to light sooner rather than later.

While acute arthritis may respond to lower power and doses, chronic forms often need 10–15 J/cm², 10–15 W, and 2–3 W/cm², especially to treat deeper tissues, for example in spondylosis or the hips in large

dogs. Start treating hips with 8–10 J/cm², but if after a couple of sessions there is no noticeable improvement, increase the dose – up to 18–20 J/cm². Table 9.2 is just a starting point for you to work with. In a cat or a smaller dog, for instance, the initial dose for a carpus would be 4–6 J/cm², and only 3–4 W would be used.

Consider increasing power, especially for obese or large patients. Since you will be working with higher settings and in contact, proper hand speed has to be maintained to avoid thermal saturation (see section 9.1 "General treatment considerations").

Patients with multiple affected joints are going to need longer appointments; plan the time and place to perform it in a proper and comfortable way for everyone (Fig. 9.6). Whenever possible, treat every 48 h or three times a week until you see a clinical response, and do not decrease the frequency of sessions until then. Explain to owners that they may have to come quite often for the first 2–3 weeks, but if after 2 weeks of intensive treatment you see no improvement, reconsider your diagnosis and treatment (see section 9.7, "How to improve results").

9.6   How to assess clinical progression

Part of improving results is assessing your patients and keeping good track of clinical changes and treatment

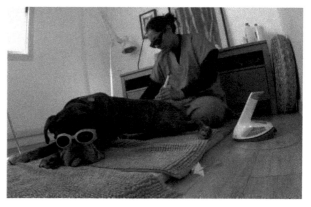

Figure 9.6 Multiple joint treatment in an elderly patient.

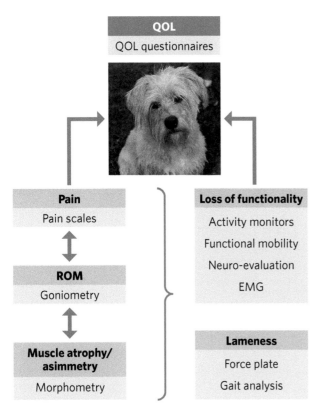

| QOL |
| QOL questionnaires |

Pain	**Loss of functionality**
Pain scales	Activity monitors
	Functional mobility
ROM	Neuro-evaluation
Goniometry	EMG

| **Lameness** |
Muscle atrophy/	Force plate
asimmetry	
Morphometry	Gait analysis

Figure 9.7 Representation of clinical changes and their assessment. *Illustrator: Elaine Leggett; photo: Marc Gelbke*

parameters. Together with imaging changes, such as radiographic progression of fractures and osteotomies, we should be able to answer three main questions about our patients and have a system to quantify and record these answers (and not just when it comes to laser therapy).

- Is my patient more comfortable, with less pain?
- Is she able to move more and be more functional and independent?
- Has her quality of life improved?

These questions can be answered based on scientifically validated scoring and assessment systems, and relate to physical and functional changes that can also be measured (Fig. 9.7). Some of the following tools are available for every clinician:

- **Pain scales**: once you start working with them, you become quite fast at scoring pain, provided you are consistent in your methods. Section 9.6.1 is dedicated to musculoskeletal and chronic pain scoring.

Check Table 4.2 for an overview of these pain scales, some of which are included in Appendix A.

- Of course, **force plate stance and gait analysis** is the gold standard for evaluating lameness, due to its accuracy and objectivity. The two most common variables analyzed are vertical impulse and peak force, which is the maximal force applied in stance. Nevertheless, it is not available for every practice, and interestingly, does not always correlate with functional mobility and with how much the pain interferes with the patient's willingness to exercise and move.[342]

- **Assessment of functional mobility**: this includes the usual movements and postures and the transitions between them, balance and propioception, as well as daily activities such as eating, drinking, or eliminating. Sometimes the first noticeable sign of pain is a reduction in grooming, a change in the eliminating posture, etc., and regaining such activities or normalizing the posture is part of the patient's improvement. We can make up our own questionnaire for this, or even better, use one of the scales that includes questions about daily activities, like the Canine Brief Pain Inventory (CBPI) or the Hudson Visual Analogue Scale (VAS),[343] or add a functional score such as Canine Functional Independence Measure.[344]

- **Goniometry** of the range of motion (ROM) of joints, which can be a source and/or a consequence of pain (see section 9.6.2 for more on goniometry).

- Check for **morphological change**s in muscles or muscle groups. Morphometric or circumferential measuring of different muscle groups gives us an idea of the muscle mass. It is most commonly performed at the femur, but can also be applied to tibial muscles and the forelimb. Measures should always be taken in the same position and at the same point: for instance, at 70% of the length of the femur, in lateral recumbency, and with the coxofemoral joint in a neutral position. Don't forget to measure bilaterally. We frequently find atrophy with compensating contralateral hypertrophy, and the % difference should decrease as the condition improves, the animal is more comfortable, and regains weight-bearing and motion.

- Recently, a new instrument to **stage and monitor osteoarthritis** was developed, the Canine OsteoArthritis Staging Tool (COAST).[345] This system takes into account dog comfort, motion and posture, clinical findings in the orthopedic exam, and radiographic changes, among others, to stage the disease and make therapeutic decisions.

• Another tool to assess the outcome of therapeutic measures in clinical trials in orthopedic patients is the **Canine Orthopedic Index (COI)**. It is designed to be used by owners, evaluating stiffness, gait, function, and quality of life.[346–348]

• **Electromyography**: this is not as readily available to all clinicians, though.

• Assessment of **quality of life** is probably the most comprehensive way to evaluate clinical progression. Having a scientifically validated way to measure this is an extremely valuable tool for practitioners. There are several disease-specific tools, but only one validated generic scale that measures the impact of chronic pain on quality of life, which was published in 2013 by Reid et al.[349] It includes scores in four domains: vitality, pain, distress, and anxiety. The original scale had 46 items, but recently a shorter form, comprising 22 items, was validated and published[350] and is now available for use by practitioners and owners online (www. newmetrica.com). There is also a 20-item questionnaire for cats.

• To keep track of how much an animal is moving, body-mounted, accelerometer-based **activity monitors** are gaining popularity, easily available in practice, and the results can also be monitored by the owner. They are currently being included in clinical trials, and represent a valuable tool to objectively monitor feline activity changes associated with pain and its relief.[334, 351]

9.6.1 Musculoskeletal pain assessment

Several scales have been developed for chronic and **musculoskeletal pain assessment.**

• **Canine Brief Pain Inventory (CBPI)** (available at https://www.vet.upenn.edu/research/vcic-clinical-trials/our-services/pennchart): uses a numerical rating scale in an 11-item questionnaire to describe the pain over the last few days, and how much that pain affects the ability to perform different activities[352, 353] (see Appendix A3). A clinical study compared the owner's assessment using the CBPI and changes in force plate kinetics in dogs treated with

carprofen; although there was improvement noted using the two assessment methods, there was no direct correlation between them,[342] and the reason according to the authors could be that as an owner, the most valued progression is the ability to move and walk, rather than single limb use. However, another study found a correlation between LOAD and CBPI scores and also between these scores and force plate kinetics.[354]

• **Hudson Visual Analogue Scale (VAS)**: developed at Texas A&M University and used to assess mild-to-moderate lameness in dogs; includes questions about behavior and mobility, and the owner's assessment. The answer to each is marked on a 10 cm line. Results of this scale correlate with force plate kinetics.[343] Check it out in Appendix A4.

• **Helsinki Chronic Pain Index (HCPI)**: uses an 11-item questionnaire, originally in Finnish, including ratings about general mood, willingness to play and exercise at different paces, complaining vocalizations, ease of lying down/rising up and ability to perform daily movements.[355, 356]

• **Liverpool Osteoarthritis in Dogs (LOAD)**[354]: includes questions about the patient's background, lifestyle, and mobility.

• **Feline Musculoskeletal Pain Index (FMPI)**: developed by Benito et al. in 2013 at the Comparative Pain Research Laboratory of the North Carolina State University,[357, 358] uses a 17-item questionnaire (was initially 21), and rates each item from 0 (impossible to perform) to 4 (normal). Questions are about mobility, daily activities, and willingness to play and interact. So total scores can range from 0 (impossible to perform any of the activities) to 68 (all normal). A change of about 10% has been proposed as the relevant threshold. This scale has been further validated in several studies and is easy to perform.[334, 359, 360] You have the full questionnaire in Appendix A5 and you can also download it from https://cvm.ncsu.edu/research/labs/clinical-sciences/comparative-pain-research/labs-comparative-pain-research-clinical-metrology-instruments-feline-musculoskeletal-pain-index/.

The placebo effect has to be considered for any pain treatment. It can actually be present to some extent when you interview the owner about the animal's progression. This has been noted in clinical trials evaluating the efficacy of different drugs, supplements, and diets. The phenomenon is more frequent among cat owners than dog owners. And unfortunately, when somebody experiences the placebo effect in his own body, he is really feeling less pain, but when he experiences a placebo relating to the pet's condition, the animal is not getting any relief. So keep examining the patient, do not just rely on the owner's assessment – although you could be experiencing the same effect, beware of your own potential placebo! A worsening of the condition after treatment withdrawal (or when laser sessions are spaced further apart too soon) is also a good indicator of its effects.

9.6.2   Goniometry

Range of motion (ROM) is the entire physiological range through which a joint can move, measured from a neutral or zero position. A decrease in ROM can be due to multiple factors, including pain, joint capsule and muscle fibrosis, tendon shortening, neurological disorders, trigger points, and osteophytes. While LT is not going to make osteophytes disappear, other factors can improve partially or totally with LT, alone or in combination with other therapies, depending on the case.

Goniometry measures change in the passive ROM of limb joints. It is one way of objectifying the evolution of these patients; it is non-invasive and available for everyone with a simple goniometer, and useful both when different clinicians follow the case or when we check the patient over time ourselves. We can monitor the angle the joint achieves and the angle at which pain or discomfort appears. Such angles, depending on the joint and its physiological movements, can refer to flexion/extension, abduction/adduction, or internal/external rotation, and comprise both the neutral and the elastic zones, since both are within physiological limits. It is necessary to have standardized bony landmarks with which to align the arms of the goniometer, then once your arms (fixed and mobile) are aligned, the fulcrum of the device is placed (Fig. 9.8).

Of course, in veterinary medicine we have to consider

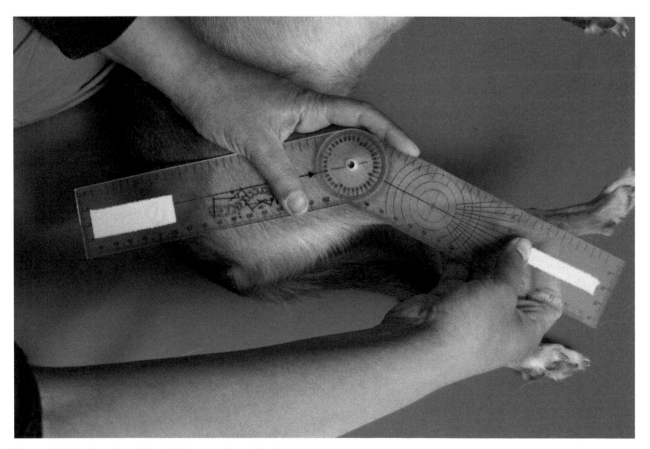

Figure 9.8 Goniometry of the stifle in a canine patient.

the differences between species and breeds. Goniometry has been validated in Labrador Retrievers[361] and cats,[362] but significant differences between breeds have been reported,[363, 364] and there is no universal table of normal ROM measurements; what is normal for one breed may be joint instability for another. That is why it is crucial to do bilateral measurements, so we can compare the pathological limb with the contralateral one.

Table 9.3 is for reference. It is based on data published by Millis and Levine,[365] Cook et al.,[366] Mann et al.[363] (dogs under anesthesia), Jaegger et al.[361] (Labradors), Thomovsky et al.[364] (Dachshunds), and Jaeger et al.[362] (cats). You can check Appendix B for a more visual and graphic reminder of ROMs.

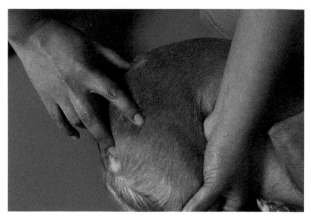

Figure 9.9 Anatomical references of the hip area: tuber ischiadicum, tuber sacrale, and greater trochanter.

9.7 How to improve results

9.7.1 Asking the right questions

Generally speaking, your chances of getting the clinical improvement you expect depend on the initial situation, the type of patient, and the therapeutic approach. Although the following points should be considered from the beginning, they should be reassessed if the progression is not as good as expected.

- **Is the diagnosis correct**? This also includes:
  - What is the diagnosis based on? Have X-rays/magnetic resonance imaging (MRI)/other tests been performed if necessary?
  - Have malignancies been ruled out?
- **Is the diagnosis complete?** Make sure you perform a good general, neurological, and orthopedic exam. Assess compensation and overload areas. A biomechanical change in the body affects other areas, as in a chain reaction. Many patients with hip problems will have soreness in their backs, or the neck and shoulders may be overloaded if the animal is putting less weight on the caudal extremities. If a cruciate ligament is damaged, the contralateral one will be under more strain. All of these situations or extra sore areas need to be addressed in the treatment plan for your patient.
- **Is the right area being treated?** A perfect diagnosis on the report does not mean the person who is delivering the therapy has a good knowledge of the anatomy. For instance, if you are trusting the treatment of a patellar ligament to your new technician,

make sure he/she knows how to find it, and the area around it you want to be treated.

- **Is the size of the treatment area consistent?** If the hip is going to be treated, focusing a particular number of joules over the greater trochanter is very different from spreading that same amount of energy from the sacroiliac joint to the proximal third of the femur; in the second case, your J/cm^2 will decrease. Having clear anatomical references is important (Fig. 9.9). Also, covering the entire area you want to treat will give you better results than just treating some points within it.
- **Are dose and power enough?** Some refractory painful conditions need an increase in both of these parameters. Treat chronic conditions with higher doses: for a hip, 8–10 J/cm^2 is a good starting dose, but increase it by 20–30% in following treatments if there is no improvement after 2–3 sessions. Increase power density in obese animals, to compensate for the subcutaneous fat. As usual, be aware of the power density (W/cm^2) being used and how it increases local temperature; you may need to use a higher hand speed. This is especially true for darker coats. If the coat is also long and frizzy, as in some Belgian sheepdogs (Groenendael), for instance, it may be advisable to stop the treatment every once in a while to remove the hair that may have got stuck in the hand-piece.
- Again, **are you sure of the dose you are applying?** Depending on the patient, you may decide to include a larger or smaller area for each joint. For instance, to treat an elbow, some will include all the area from the distal third of the humerus to the proximal third

Table 9.3 Range of motion (ROM).

Joint	Osteokinematic motion	Range of motion (degrees)					
		Millis and Levine[365]	Cook et al.[366]	Mann et al. (under general anesthesia)[363]	Jaegger et al. (Labradors) [361]	Thomovsky et al. (Dachshunds)[364]	Jaeger et al. (cats)[362]
Shoulder	Flexion	30–60			57		32
	Extension	160–170			165		163
	External rotation	40–50					
	Internal rotation	40–50					
	Abduction	40–50	32				
	Adduction	40–50					
Elbow	Flexion	20–40			36		22
	Extension	160–170			165		163
Radioulnar	Pronation	40–50					
	Supination	80–90					
Carpus	Flexion	20–35			32		22
	Extension	190–200			196		198
	Lateral (ulnar) deviation	10–20			12		10
	Medial (radial) deviation	5–15			7		7
Hip	Flexion	55		46	50	50	33
	Extension	160–165		164	162	155	164
	External rotation	50		50			
	Internal rotation	55		55			
	Abduction (flexed hip and 90° stifle)	120		118			
	Adduction (flexed hip and stifle at 90°)	63		64			
Stifle	Flexion	45		28	42	50	24
	Extension	160–170		172	162	160	164
Tarsus	Flexion	40		40	39	40	21
	Extension	170		175	164	167	167

of the antebrachium, and others will stay closer to the elbow joint. Whatever area you decide to work on at the beginning of a session, stick to it. Treating other areas within the same program will disperse your total energy, decreasing the J/cm². If you want to include other areas, treat them separately and with their own dose.

- **How effectively are you delivering the energy?**

Consider shaving the area to improve penetration, especially for breeds or areas with thicker hair coats. It might not be possible to shave six body areas, but do shave or at least trim the hair if you want to focus on the elbow of a Chow Chow, the hip of a German Shepherd, or the sacrum of a Husky. The owner may be a bit reluctant, but it does make a big difference in terms of light penetration.

- To avoid increasing temperature at the surface, **use pulsed light,** at least in part of the treatment (see box on the right); the dark phases between pulses allow tissue cooling. Remember, though, that sufficient average power has to be maintained.

- **Is the frequency of treatment enough**? Some chronic problems may respond well to a 3–2–1 regime, but others need to be treated every 48 h, or three times a week, until a change is observed. If after 8–10 treatments there is no significant improvement, other factors should be considered, or other therapeutic modalities chosen or combined with LT. Do not suddenly space treatments out too much, as the cumulative effect of the induction phase may be lost.

- Has the patient **changed its physical activity**? Exercise should be controlled as prescribed; some animals may feel better and over-exercise. Discuss this with the owner.

- Has there been any **change in medication** (if there is any)? Unless there is a clinical contraindication, medication should be continued until an improvement is noted. Chronic cases may take longer to respond, and a sudden pharmacological withdrawal before LT has had an effect may give rise to a pain crisis.

- When dealing with very old or debilitated patients that need to have many large areas treated (such as all the back, hips, shoulders, etc.), try not to treat all of them the first day or at least moderate the dose; the vasodilation, endorphins, and other effects might be a bit too much and the patient may feel weak for a couple of days. Increase your local and total dose progressively, according to the patient's response and tolerance. I usually treat no more than 4–5 areas the first day: for example, the thoracolumbar spine, lumbosacral spine, both hips, and a hock.

9.7.2 Some anatomical considerations: tips for different areas

The following descriptions of how to treat joints include the tissues conforming and surrounding them, since painful/inflammatory conditions do not affect just the articular surfaces and bones. The whole circumference of the appendicular joints should be treated, although this is more difficult and not always performed in the shoulder and hip. In the metacarpal/metatarsal areas and digits, the dorsal and palmar/plantar surfaces should be treated.

When treating the patient in recumbency, it is often convenient to treat one side of a joint in lateral recumbency and then let the patient roll onto the other side to treat the medial aspect; this way we can avoid treating with the beam toward us. So if you are going to treat both elbows, for instance, treat the lateral half of one and the medial side of the other, then roll the patient over to its other side and treat the other two halves. Your total energy calculations for each of the articular halves will be easier, based on just two dimensions. Otherwise, calculating the treatment area for the limbs, when treated circumferentially, can be a bit more challenging at the beginning. Having a measuring tape in your "laser kit" is really helpful.

 If your laser employs multi-phase treatments, be sure not to divide the treatment into two halves in such a way that you have different parameters (usually frequencies) in each half. Instead, divide the total treatment time per protocol in half, then repeat the entire (shortened) protocol on each half of your anatomy. This way you get the benefits of all the frequencies on the entire anatomy.

If the patient tolerates it, move the joint you are treating through its passive ROM while you treat, at least during the second part of the treatment – they will relax and accept it more easily than at the very beginning. This will expose a bit more of the articular surfaces you want to include.

Temporomandibular joint

Treat this from different directions, but always aiming the beam away from the ocular globe when working from cranial to caudal. You may need to remove doggles

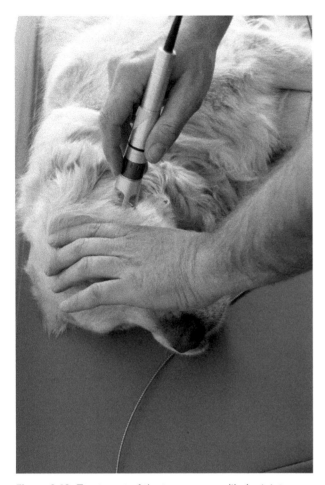

Figure 9.10 Treatment of the temporomandibular joint.

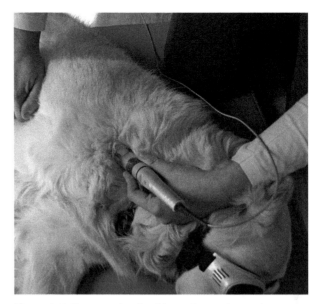

Figure 9.11 Treating the shoulder and cranial scapula.

to properly treat, since they will be in your way; protect the eyes with your other hand (Fig. 9.10). Consider including the masseter, temporal, and zygomatic muscles; you can follow the direction of the fibers: craniocaudal, dorsoventral, and oblique, respectively.

Shoulder

Include a margin around the greater tubercle of the humerus, and consider including the whole scapula in your treatment area if there is tension or tenderness around it. Follow the inter-tubercular groove up to the cranial border of the scapula (Fig. 9.11). It is often beneficial to include the deltoid muscle (both scapular and acromial parts, as well as the supraspinatus). Check for trigger points in the infraspinatus and triceps muscle, caudal and distal to the deltoid. Palpate their tendons for any abnormalities and, if present, treat the whole length of the tendon carefully.

Elbow

Include the distal humerus and proximal antebrachium if necessary (Fig. 9.12). Check for trigger points in the extensor carpi radialis and the common digital extensor muscles. Make sure you treat the medial side properly; many conditions affect the medial compartment to a greater extent.

Carpus

Treat from the styloid process dorsally to the accessory carpal pad ventrally. A flexion–extension motion can be applied, exposing a bit more the interosseous spaces.

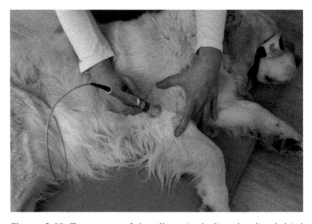

Figure 9.12 Treatment of the elbow, including the distal third of the humerus and proximal antebrachium.

Spine

To help you know what vertebral space you are working over, remember that with the dog standing up, if the last rib is followed dorsally, perpendicular to the spine, you will locate L2–L3. And a change in the direction of the spinous processes can be easily felt at T10/T11. You can also locate the lumbosacral junction and count cranially.

Check for tenderness just cranial to the wing of the ilium; the iliocostalis lumborum may contain a trigger point here. Include the epaxial muscles on both sides. It will be more comfortable for the patient to follow the muscles longitudinally, especially if there is any contracture. Angle the hand-piece to get the beam perpendicular and pointing lateromedially. To try to align the beam with the articular facets, angle it perpendicular in the caudal thoracic spine (from T10/T11) and lumbar spine. Cranial to T10, the angle is 45° (Fig 9.13).

In the caudal cervical spine, pulling the shoulder caudally (Fig. 9.14) will help you access caudal cervical vertebrae better. Consider that treating deep tissue conditions in the cervical area often requires a relatively high dose and power (because of the thick muscle layers), and the treatment may affect blood flow to the head, especially over the carotid area. This is especially

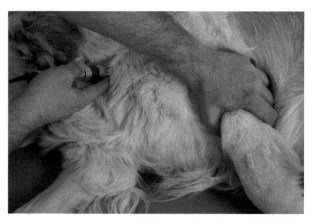

Figure 9.14 Treatment of the caudal cervical spine.

important in patients with epilepsy and other CNS diseases, in which LT is contraindicated (although increasing blood flow to the brain can be indicated in other CNS conditions).

When dealing with appendicular joint disorders, treating the associated spinal roots can be a good strategy, especially in chronic painful conditions, since they will develop a certain neuropathic pain component. So most chronic hips and stifles, for instance, will benefit from treating the lumbar area.

Hip joint

To work from the lateral aspect of this area we locate three anatomical landmarks: the crest of the ilium, the greater trochanter of the femur, and the tuber ischiadicum (see Fig. 9.9). A screening of the area delimited from the upper third of the femur dorsally to the ilium and caudally to the tuber ischiadicum can be the first approach. Then, more emphasis can be given to the greater trochanter area and along the path of the sciatic nerve, following the caudal aspect of the greater trochanter and down between the biceps femoris and semitendinosus muscles. Palpate the quadriceps muscle to check for a trigger point.

When working over the lateral aspect of wing of the ilium, we are directly over the gluteal muscles. In acute conditions, they will likely be reactive and tender (the gluteus medius is another frequent place for a trigger point). In chronic pain, they will likely feel depressed, atrophic, and the reactivity, although it may be present, will be less. It is actually easier to deal with a contracted muscle than with an atrophic one, but in the first case the pressure tolerated will be less.

Also consider treating from the medial side (Fig.

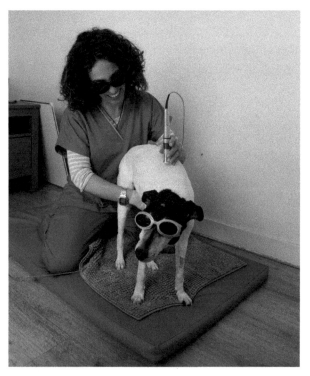

Figure 9.13 Treating T3–L3 segment.

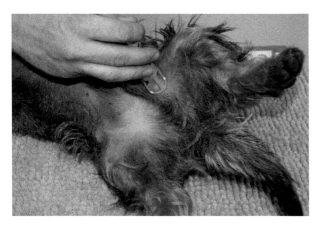

Figure 9.15 Treatment of the medial side of the hip area.

9.15). A good way is to follow the pectineus muscle; start with gentle pressure as this muscle may hold a trigger point. If there is a contracture of the iliopsoas muscle or other hip flexors, the patient will experience discomfort with hip extension, and you should address this. The iliopsoas contracture is a common problem both in sports dogs and in older patients with limb weakness who fall on slippery floors. The whole lumbar area up to the last rib should be treated, calculating a dose of about 8–10 J/cm².

Stifle

When calculating your area of treatment, include at least up to the femoral condyles and down to the head of the fibula. In cases of CCLR it is likely that the medial side (Fig. 9.16) will be more sensitive, especially if there is any damage to the meniscus. Check for trigger points cranial and distal to the head of the fibula (peroneus longus TP).

Tarsus (hock)

Include the distal tibia from the level of the calcaneus to the proximal part of the metatarsal bones. Palpate the calcaneus tendon for any fibrosis and, if present, treat it as well.

9.8 Laser therapy in neurological patients

Small animals can present with conditions affecting both the CNS and peripheral nerves that may be helped with LT. Probably the most common examples are intervertebral disk disease (IVDD) and neurapraxias.

9.8.1 Intervertebral disk disease

A definitive diagnosis of IVDD requires diagnostic imaging; nowadays computed tomography (CT) and magnetic resonance imaging (MRI) provide the best and most accurate information. But even before these are performed, location of the lesion must be clinically determined, in terms of spinal segment, since clinical signs are different. So even if MRI is not a possibility for that patient, we know if we should focus over T3–L3 or caudal to it, for instance. Scoring the severity is necessary both at initial evaluation and during treatment course, to assess results objectively.

The Modified Frankel Score (MFS) is often used to categorize the severity of neurological deficits (Table 9.4). An alternative scoring system was published by Texas A&M University, named the Texas Spinal Cord Injury Score (TSCIS) for dogs (Table 9.5). Both systems correlate with each other and with MRI findings, have a high degree of inter-rater agreement, and show a predictive value in canine patients with thoracolumbar IVDD.[367]

Patients with acute signs who are non-ambulatory but retain pain perception are often surgical candidates, and loss of pain perception makes this a surgical emergency. This does not change even if we can use LT; however, keep the following in mind.

- LT can help in postoperative recovery: animal models show LT can help in acute damage to the spinal cord by modulating the immune response and improving axonal and functional recovery.[171] A clinical study with dogs suffering from thoracolumbar IVDD with acute signs and neurological deficit graded 0 to 3 revealed a significant (four

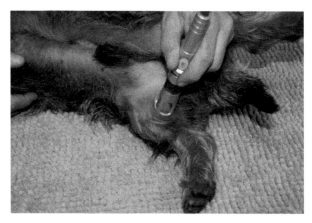

Figure 9.16 Treatment of the medial aspect of the stifle.

Table 9.4 Modified Frankel Score (MFS).

Grade	Neurological deficit
0	Tetra/paraplegia with no deep nociception
1	Tetra/paraplegia with deep nociception but no superficial nociception
2	Tetra/paraplegia with entire nociception
3	Non-ambulatory tetra/paraparesis
4	Ambulatory tetra/paraparesis and/or ataxia
5	Spinal hyperesthesia only (no dysfunction)

times faster!) shortening of the recovery time after hemilaminectomy in dogs who received LT after the surgical procedure[368]: 3.5 vs. 14 days until return to ambulation, in dogs with a similar baseline assessment, and independently of age, weight, and duration of clinical signs at presentation.

- When surgery is not the best option, as in many mild chronic IVDD cases, or is not even an option for some reason, LT can be a great tool to add to the multimodal conservative management. And maybe not just because of the anti-inflammatory and analgesic effects; in a retrospective double-blind clinical study in people who underwent diskectomy, those patients who received LT in the weeks before the procedure had more mucopolysaccharides and newly formed elastic fibers in their intervertebral disks.[369] A clinical trial in people with chronic lower back pain found LT to be more effective as an analgesic treatment than magnetic field therapy.[370] In practice, this combination of LT and magnetic field therapy is quite common and seems to have an additive effect.

Consider shaving or trimming the hair to improve penetration, especially with very thick dark coats. At least 2–3 vertebral spaces should be treated both cranial and caudal to the affected one. Very often, larger areas of the back will benefit from being included in the treatment area, since it is not uncommon to find other reactive or tender segments. Treating the paravertebral muscles in a longitudinal direction feels more comfortable to the patient, but you can also spend an extra 1–2 seconds in the intervertebral spaces (unless you feel the fur/skin gets a bit too warm), aiming the beam perpendicularly to the muscle or in a slightly lateral-to-medial direction.

Use 5–20 J/cm². The values that reach the spinal cord and roots will be much lower, and will more likely have an anti-inflammatory and stimulating effect. In a study with 200–300 g rats, only 6% of 810 nm light reached the spinal cord, located at 10 mm depth, using 0.53 W/cm².[171] Again an important factor here is how fast we

Table 9.5 Texas Spinal Cord Injury Score (TSCIS) for dogs.

	Gait
0	No voluntary movement seen when supported
1	Intact limb protraction with no ground clearance
2	Intact limb protraction with inconsistent ground clearance
3	Intact limb protraction with consistent ground clearance (>75%)
4	Ambulatory, consistent ground clearance with moderate paresis–ataxia (will fall occasionally)
5	Ambulatory, consistent ground clearance with mild paresis–ataxia (does not fall, even on slick surfaces)
6	Normal gait
	Propioceptive positioning
0	Absent response
1	Delayed response
2	Normal response
	Nociception
0	No deep nociception
1	Intact deep nociception, no superficial nociception
2	Nociception present

Table 9.6 Recommended parameters for IVDD.

Area	Dose (J/cm²)	Power (W)	Power density (W/cm²)
Spinal post-op	4-8	2-4	0.1-0.8
Acute	6-10	4-8	0.5-1.5
Chronic	8-20	8-15	1-3

deliver that dose and over what area. The power density that is used depends on the particular patient and condition: in the immediate postoperative period of spinal surgery, hypersensitivity and allodynia can be present; some patients show discomfort even with the regular wound parameters being applied at a distance. In such cases you will have to decrease power density to 0.1–0.8 W/cm² (compared to the 1–3 W/cm² you would use in a chronic condition) by defocusing at a longer distance, or by decreasing the wattage, move the hand faster, etc. This is the reason why you see such broad ranges in Table 9.6; again, this is just a framework, and for lower-sized or very sensitive patients you will need to start on the (lower) conservative side.

For acute cases, give a daily treatment for 3 days, then try to maintain a q48h schedule until there is some improvement. Chronic cases can start on a schedule of three times a week, until an improvement is noticed. In both cases, this should be noted in less than 2 weeks; otherwise reconsider the diagnosis and/or treatment plan. But don't wait that long to increase your stimulation if there is no obvious change; if after a couple of visits there is no improvement and the patient tolerates it, increase dose and/or power by about 20–30%.

9.8.2 Treating peripheral nerves

Peripheral nerve injuries can occur as a result of trauma, sustained compression, or inflammation. Together with brachial plexus injuries, the most commonly affected nerves are the facial, sciatic, and radial. Neurapraxia commonly resolves after a few weeks, but we can try to speed up this recovery with LT. An experimental model of sciatic lesion after crushing injury, in which rats were treated on a daily basis for 3 weeks, showed significantly better recovery in the laser group than in the control group; this was first noted 2 weeks after the beginning of treatment.[371] In a similar sciatic crushing injury model, transplantation

of mesenchymal stem cells acted synergistically with LT to enhance functional recovery.[372] One study reported a better effect on recovery when treatment was delayed 7 days from the injury than if it was started immediately after the injury, both functionally and in the morphology of myelinated fibers. [373] Different wavelengths have been used to achieve results, including 660 nm, 808 nm, and 905 nm, and one study found the combination of continuous (808 nm) and pulsed (905 nm) irradiation achieved the best outcome.[166][167]

Some clinical studies in humans affected with brachial plexus injuries, carpal tunnel syndrome, and other peripheral neuropathies report an improvement in nerve conductivity and functional recovery with LT.[374–376] It has been suggested that both the peripheral nerve area and the corresponding spinal segment are treated.[377]

Not all nerves are equally superficial, so the doses and power to be used may vary; if you are dealing with a facial nerve, it will be much easier to reach than a brachial plexus. Consider 4–12 J/cm² and 1–8 W, but keep your power density around 1–2 W/cm². In a rabbit model of sciatic nerve injury, different powers and power densities were tested, and penetration through the skin and biceps femoris muscle was measured. They found a dose of 8 J/cm² at the skin surface improved nerve recovery, with better functional outcomes 2 months after the injury. Comparing a superficial very high power density (7 W/cm², ouch!) with a moderate one (1.8 W/cm²), the very high values inhibited nerve regeneration, while the lower value, 1.8 W/cm², improved it.[378] So for a facial nerve, you would be using around 0.5–1 W/cm² (which is a 2.5–5 W output if your hand-piece gives you a spot size of 5 cm²), but about two to three times this power density for a radial or a sciatic nerve, since they are covered with more tissue – and as always, a good knowledge of the anatomy and nerve pathways is important.

9.8.3 Transcranial laser therapy

Applying LT through the skull to reach inside the brain represents a less common field in practice, but one with different potential clinical applications. But to have any effect, first we must carry the light through the skull – is that possible? Absolutely yes: in humans, about 5% of the applied energy gets into the brain at about 2 cm depth.[379] A study in research species showed how infrared light transmission through the skull changes with bone thickness, from 40% in the rat to about 11% in the rabbit.[380]

Since LT does penetrate the skull, it affects the blood flow in the brain (not just in a short-term, temperature-mediated reaction) via NO,[172] the metabolism of different cell types in the brain, and the inflammatory and apoptotic phenomena, transcranial laser therapy (TLT) may have a future role in the treatment of degenerative, traumatic, or vascular diseases of the brain[381]; hopefully clinical studies will develop following this research line. There are published results both *in vitro* and in animal **experimental models of different neurodegenerative diseases**, including the following.

- Familial amyotrophic lateral sclerosis: in a mouse model, motor function slightly improved in the early stage of disease with low-level LT, which correlated with immunohistochemical changes in the spinal cord, although survival and general motor performance did not change.[382]
- Alzheimer's disease: mouse models show LT ameliorates disease progression (in mice) because it decreases amyloid deposits.[383, 384] In cell cultures, it protects against amyloid-induced oxidative stress and inflammation[385] and mitigates amyloid-induced neuronal loss and dendritic atrophy by upregulating brain-derived neurotrophic factor (BDNF).[386]
- Parkinson's disease: mice treated with infrared light showed increased numbers of dopaminergic cells in the brain[387] – the progressive impairment of voluntary motor control is due to the loss of these cells.

Regarding **traumatic brain injury (TBI),** there are a few experimental reports with positive results in mice: LT in the 4 h following TBI reduces long-term neurological deficits and improves histological scores with a remarkable reduction in injury size.[388, 389] One of the

reported mechanisms is that LT improves BDNF, which enhances the formation of synapses.[390] Histologically, mice treated with LT have smaller lesion sizes, in time, which correlates with better cognitive and behavioral test results.[391]

Clinical reports in human medicine are scarce but do exist. Among these are two clinical cases in people with chronic TBI-associated cognitive dysfunction, in which transcranial LT with high dose (13.3 J/cm^2) but low power density (22 mW/cm^2) seemed to significantly help.[392]

By no means is this meant to encourage (nor to discourage) this clinical use, just to let you know some of what's been published. Clinical studies and reports are still anecdotal, and before LT is even considered for an acute case you would have to rule out any intracranial hemorrhage, or consider the risk of it, especially if the patient was under anticoagulant or fibrinolytic therapy.

The same would apply to stroke, but once the hemorrhagic type has been ruled out (by MRI/CT), if the problem is related to ischemia and cell death, could LT help? Animal models seem to point in that direction: acute cerebral ischemia was improved using LT, especially if the treatment was applied in the first 24 h after onset.[393, 394] But studies in humans have provided controversial (yet very interesting) results: a phase 1 trial with 130 patients with acute ischemic stroke found that TLT within 24 hours of onset was safe to use and seemed to improve clinical outcomes. [395] Then a larger trial was performed using 660 patients; this second trial found that patients treated with laser showed a more favorable trend in their clinical progression, but the difference between the TLT and placebo groups was not statistically significant.[396] Nevertheless, the results were meaningful enough to encourage additional research to find the treatment groups or types of patients that could be more consistently helped by the therapy. When patients were pooled with the previous similar study and the baseline characteristics and prognostic factors balanced between the two groups, it was found TLT patients had a statistically significant higher success rate.[397] Those results were not supported by the CT measurements: TLT did not decrease overall or cortical infarct volume. Neither did the results support the concept of a more likely effect on the cortex (due to the higher energy density that would penetrate there) compared with deeper structures.[398] The researchers kept an open door, saying that if MRI had been used, maybe small differences could have been detected, since it is a more sensitive and specific method for assessment of acute infarction. In the last phase of these trials, a double-blind, sham-controlled, randomized clinical study was performed, attempting to enroll 1000 patients with acute ischemic stroke treated in the first 24 hours. But after a futile analysis of 566 completed patients found no difference in clinical scores, it was cancelled.[399] Despite this, we hope more studies will be conducted along these lines, since there could be various explanations for these findings. For instance, the treatment parameters could have been non-optimal: a human skull is thicker than a murine one, they were using only 1 J/cm², and many other treatment details were not provided.

In a different field of application of TLT, a placebo-controlled clinical study in humans reported that TLT can have positive **cognitive and emotional** effects[400] related to frontal cortex stimulation. A previous study using a single dose provided clinically significant relief of depression symptoms[401]; in both cases, a very high dose but a relatively low power density was used – 60 J/cm² with 250 mW/cm².

Putting together the benefits of laser for blood flow in the brain, neuronal metabolism, and the described effects in animal models of neurodegenerative diseases, a potential field of application in small animal medicine that may show results in the future could be cognitive dysfunction syndrome, although there are no published trials. On the human side, TLT is also receiving attention as a potential tool for the treatment of cognitive dysfunction,[402] and hopefully more information in the form of placebo-controlled clinical studies will be available in the future.

Summary from a different perspective

Measuring the success (of laser or whatever) in musculoskeletal issues requires perhaps the most attention to detail, on the front end and the back. Proper diagnoses, pain scoring, range-of-motion measurement, and weight-bearing assessment all factor in. If you never implement a laser on musculoskeletal conditions ... you'd be missing out Presurgical and non-surgical cases alike are very likely to respond to laser because at the very core of these injuries, there are injured tissues that the body really does want to heal. Sometimes this requires your hands (or instruments) to help realign or affix or suture, but the vast majority of healing is done when your hands are no longer on the animal. And laser can help all those natural processes between visits, triggering cascades of events that lead to faster and stronger healing.

9.9 Case studies

The following are examples of the clinical use of LT in patients with a variety of conditions affecting the musculoskeletal system, whether these are fractures, osteoarthritis, trauma affecting muscle/tendons/bone, or other conditions. The same parameters, explanations, and reporting system that you can find in section 7.11 also applies here. Again, all treatments included **both CW and pulsed emission**, unless otherwise reported, with 20% of the energy being delivered in CW and the rest within a pulse (low to high) frequency range.

Case index

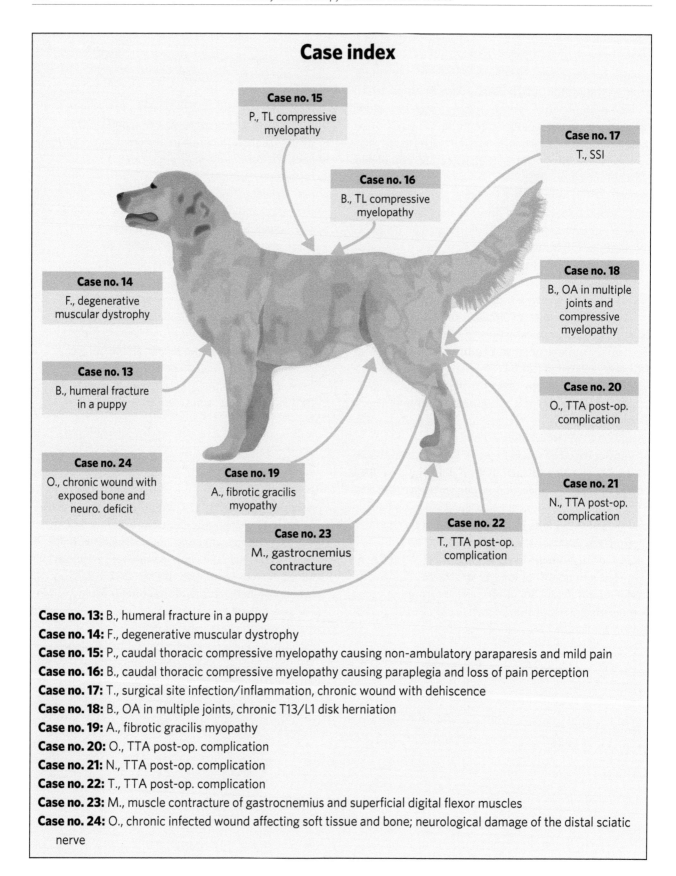

Case no. 15
P., TL compressive myelopathy

Case no. 16
B., TL compressive myelopathy

Case no. 17
T., SSI

Case no. 14
F., degenerative muscular dystrophy

Case no. 18
B., OA in multiple joints and compressive myelopathy

Case no. 13
B., humeral fracture in a puppy

Case no. 20
O., TTA post-op. complication

Case no. 24
O., chronic wound with exposed bone and neuro. deficit

Case no. 19
A., fibrotic gracilis myopathy

Case no. 21
N., TTA post-op. complication

Case no. 23
M., gastrocnemius contracture

Case no. 22
T., TTA post-op. complication

Case no. 13: B., humeral fracture in a puppy
Case no. 14: F., degenerative muscular dystrophy
Case no. 15: P., caudal thoracic compressive myelopathy causing non-ambulatory paraparesis and mild pain
Case no. 16: B., caudal thoracic compressive myelopathy causing paraplegia and loss of pain perception
Case no. 17: T., surgical site infection/inflammation, chronic wound with dehiscence
Case no. 18: B., OA in multiple joints, chronic T13/L1 disk herniation
Case no. 19: A., fibrotic gracilis myopathy
Case no. 20: O., TTA post-op. complication
Case no. 21: N., TTA post-op. complication
Case no. 22: T., TTA post-op. complication
Case no. 23: M., muscle contracture of gastrocnemius and superficial digital flexor muscles
Case no. 24: O., chronic infected wound affecting soft tissue and bone; neurological damage of the distal sciatic nerve

Case no. 13

B., canine, 3 months old, mixed breed, MNC, 7 kg

- **Complaint:** fracture.
- **History:** B. had been rescued after being hit by a car when he was 2 months old. He had a distal humeral fracture, which had been repaired 3 days before, i.e. a month after the accident, through a medial approach, using a clamp and rod internal fixation system and five screws. He was on cephalexin and carprofen.
- **Physical examination:** surgical wound over medial aspect of right humerus/elbow. Lameness score 4/5. Severe tension in the muscles over the scapula and biceps. Carpus carried in flexion and withdrawal reflex slightly delayed. VAS pain score 5/10.
- **Diagnosis:** postsurgical support for humeral fracture in a growing animal. Suspected radial neurapraxia.
- **Treatment:**
  - **Laser therapy:**
    - Treatment was started 3 days after surgery. Patient was treated twice a week initially and then once a week, including scapula, humerus, elbow, and antebrachium, down to the carpus.
    - A dose of 4–6 J/cm² was used (only 2–4 initially over the wound) over a total of 200 cm², with passive ROM during treatment.
  - **Other:**
    - Cephalexin and carprofen maintained for 5 days.
- **Outcome:** carpal movement and posture was normal after two sessions and VAS dropped to 2/10 during the second week. Two screws were removed in the fifth week after the initial surgery and the rest in the tenth week. Notice the open growth plates in the proximal radius and anconeal process even 10 weeks after surgery and after having been treated with LT (Fig. C13.4). At the moment of discharge, B. was able to run, even sprint to the right side.

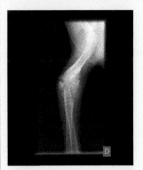
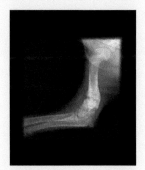

Figure C13.1 Fracture before surgery. (a) Craniocaudal and (b) mediolateral views.

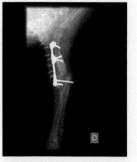
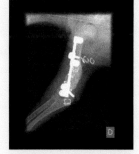

Figure C13.2 Immediately after surgical repair. (a) Craniocaudal and (b) mediolateral views.

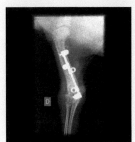
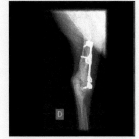

Figure C13.3 Week 5. (a) Craniocaudal and (b) mediolateral views.

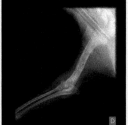

Figure C13.4 Week 10, mediolateral view. Note the open growth plates in the proximal radius and anconeal process.

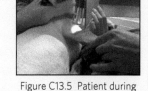

Figure C13.5 Patient during treatment with LT.

Pₐ (W)	Tx time	J/cm²	Total J/Tx	Spot (cm²)	W/cm²	Tx/week	No. Tx
4	250 s (4.1 min)	5	1000	5	0.8	2-1	8

Case no. 14

F., feline, 9 months old, Domestic Shorthair, MNC, 3.1 kg

- **Complaint:** severe generalized weakness.
- **History:** F. was found in the street as a kitten in a very poor condition. He had corneal ulcers and wore an E-collar for a month, while being kept inside a carrier. Since then his weakness had not improved, to the point he could barely move, had difficulties holding his head and the owners had to hand-feed him and help him to the sandbox. He lives on the sofa/bed without moving. The referring hospital performed radiographies, muscle (cranial tibial, quadriceps) and nerve (common peroneal) biopsy, and MRI. He is taking carnitine and a B-vitamin complex.
- **Radiographic findings:** generalized low bone density.
- **Pathology:** moderate primary non-inflammatory myopathy.
- **MRI:** no significant findings.
- **Physical examination:**
  - Body condition score 3/9.
  - Unable to walk. Plantigrade stance, with phalangeal and elbow flexion, and general spasticity.
  - Goniometry: the affected joints (the rest of the joints are normal).

| Joint | Range of motion (degrees) | |
	Right	Left
Knee	180	180
Elbow	90	92

- Limb circumference:
  - Forelimbs (20% of arm): right 9 cm; left 9.5 cm.
  - Hindlimbs (70% of thigh): right 21 cm; left 20 cm.
- Neurological exam: normal, except for some mild postural proprioceptive deficit in hind legs.
- Pain assessment: 6/10 NRS in elbows, shoulders, stifles, tarsi, thoracolumbar spine. Overload of supraspinatus, infraspinatus, and paravertebral muscles.
- **Diagnosis:** degenerative muscular dystrophy.
- **Treatment:**
  - **Laser therapy:**
    - Although the patient could only be seen once a week, LT was part of a broader treatment program.
    - Treatment area included the neck, elbows, and thoracolumbar spine.
    - Passive ROM and stretching were applied during the treatment.
  - **Other physical therapies:** twice a week for the first month, then once a week during the second month, then once every 2–3 weeks for 4 months.
    - Neuromuscular electrical stimulation (NMES): biphasic pulsed wave; 50 Hz, to stimulate lumbar muscles and triceps brachialis.
    - Transcutaneous electrical stimulation (TENS): electrodes are positioned bilateral to the spine (T13–L5) for 20 min.
    - Ultrasound: pulsing at 50%, 3.3 MHz, 5 cm probe, for 4 min over elbows and 4 min over biceps brachii during passive ROM and maintained stretching.
    - Pulsed magnetic therapy: initially 2–20 Hz over stifle and hip areas to treat pain, then 100 Hz for muscle stimulation.
  - **Exercise program:**
    - Assisted exercises: assisted stance, maintaining neck, elbow, and phalangeal extension. Balance and weight-shifting exercises while standing.
    - Active exercise: walking over soft non-slippery surface.
    - Manual intervention: stretching massage of forelimbs and spinal muscles. Passive ROM of all joints.
  - **Home exercise program:** all techniques were initially performed with the owners in the clinic to ensure proper delivery. Exercises were performed at home 3–4 times a week.

- Thermotherapy: local heat over elbows and thoracolumbar area.
- Passive exercises: joint mobilization, especially phalangeal extension of the four limbs, elbow extension, and knee flexion. Assisted standing. Soon joint manipulation was not tolerated at home and had to be discontinued.
- Active exercises: stimulating neck flexion to both sides, encouraging some walking over soft surfaces, using surfaces with some height difference. Stimulating movement with food.
- NMES: biphasic pulsed wave; 50 Hz, to stimulate hamstrings, quadriceps, triceps brachialis.
- **Owner education:** adapt the house so F. can use other places rather than just the sofa. Cover the floor with carpet or soft padding. Find a suitable cat scratcher to stimulate his desire to play and move, and a small sandbox he can enter without help. Avoid falls from sofa.
- **Outcome:**
  - Pain level was 4/10 after 1 week and 2/10 after 2 weeks. After the second week, F. was able to raise his head to look into your eyes and take a couple of steps.
  - During the next month he became more active and started to use the sandbox. On week 6, his elbow ROM had improved to 85°.
  - By the second month he was able to take small jumps, became more active, and engaged in playing. By the fourth month he was able to jump up onto and down from the sofa. Overall, he became more active, with less pain and more independence in his daily activities, which had a great impact in his quality of life.

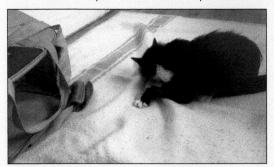

Figure C14.1 Patient unable to stand up.

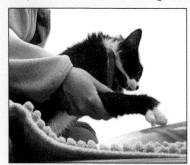

Figure C14.2 Patient unable to extend the neck.

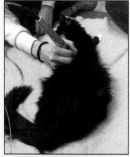

Figure C14.3 Laser therapy over the thoracic spinal muscles.

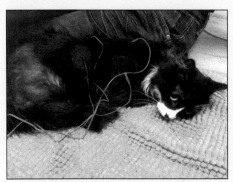

Figure C14.4 Treatment with TENS.

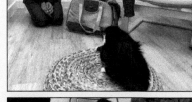
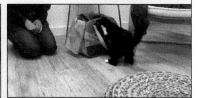
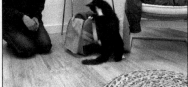
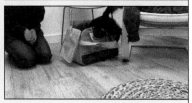

Figures C14.5 (a–d) Patient now able to take some steps and jump into his carrier.

Area	P_a (W)	Tx time	J/cm²	Total J/Tx	Spot (cm²)	W/cm²	Tx/week	No. Tx
Neck	5	2 min	8	600	5	1	1/week × 8 weeks, then 1/ month	12
TL spine	5	2 min	10	600	5	1		
Elbows	3	1.5 min	6	300	5	0.6		

Note: TL, thoracolumbar.

Case no. 15

P., canine, 10 years old, Pug, FNS, 6.7 kg

- **Complaint:** non-ambulatory paraparesis and difficult defecation.
- **History:** P. had started to show symptoms 6 months previously. She had initially been treated with steroids with little response, and she showed increased panting and restlessness. Two months previously a neurologist evaluated her and prescribed gabapentin, tramadol, firocoxib, and ozone therapy due to spinal pain, which improved with medical treatment. Nevertheless, a few days ago P. showed non-ambulatory paraparesis and MRI was recommended.
- **MRI:** arachnoid cyst causing severe compressive myelopathy at T12–T13. Hypoplastic vertebral facets at same location. Multifocal disk degeneration in other locations not causing spinal cord compression.
- **Physical examination:**
  - Body condition score 7/9.
  - Non-ambulatory paraparesis, dragged her weight on forelimbs, unable to support herself in standing position for more than a few seconds. Passive ROM not affected.
  - Symmetric hindlimb circumference (15 cm and 15.5 cm, measured at 70% of thigh).
  - Contracted forelimb muscles (triceps, biceps brachii, supraspinatus). Flaccid hypotrophic hindlimb muscles (quadriceps, gluteus, femoral biceps, semimembranosus, semitendinosus).
  - Increased sciatic and flexor patellar reflexes. Deep and superficial pain present. Severe proprioceptive deficit.
  - Absence of movement in the tail. Normal urinary and fecal continence.
  - Pain assessment: 2/10 NRS, mild discomfort in the caudal thoracic spine.
- **Diagnosis:** caudal thoracic compressive myelopathy causing non-ambulatory paraparesis and mild pain.
- **Treatment:**
  - **Laser therapy:**
    - Treatment area initially included T10–L1, with a dose of 8 J/cm^2, which after the second visit was increased to 10 J/cm^2 and extended to cover the whole T10–S1 area.
    - After treating twice a week for 2 weeks, a weekly treatment was performed for another month, and after that the patient was treated once a month. However, a much broader treatment plan was performed during those visits, and the owners committed to daily home exercise sessions.
  - **Medical treatment** with firocoxib and gabapentin was maintained for the first month.
  - **Acupuncture:** 20 min sessions once a week for 3 weeks, then once a month for 4 more months. Treatment included dry needle technique and electro-acupuncture with variable combinations of the following acupoints: GV20, BL-11, GV-6, GV-4, BL-23, *Shen shu, Shen peng*, ST-36, SP-3, KID-1, KID-3, BL-20, *Wei jie, Wei jian,* and *Liu feng*. Aqua-acupuncture was performed at *Hua-tuo-jia-ji* points from T10 to L2, BL-40, ST-36, and *Liu feng*, using diluted B12 vitamin. Herbal prescription of *Bu Yang Huang Wu* formula at 1 g/10 kg twice a day.
  - **Other physical therapies:** every 2 weeks initially, then once a month.
    - NMES: 40 Hz, biphasic, to stimulate hamstrings, quadriceps, and gluteus muscles; 10 min for each limb.
    - TENS: local treatment for 20 min. The electrodes were positioned bilateral to the spine (T11–L2).
    - Pulsed magnetic field (PMF) therapy: low frequency program 12–20 Hz.
  - **Exercise program:**
    - Assisted standing exercises, including weight-shifting, bicycling movement, assisted walking, and proprioceptive Physioroll exercises. Assisted treadmill was introduced after the second session and its duration progressively increased.
    - Manual intervention: massage of neck muscles (effleurage and petrissage). Passive ROM with bicycling movement of all limbs.
  - **Home exercise program:** all techniques were initially performed with the owners in the clinic to ensure proper delivery.

- Owners were advised to purchase an NMES device to perform stimulation at home, with electrodes on the hamstrings and gluteus muscles.
- Massage, standing exercises, slow assisted walking, passive ROM.
- **Owner education:** together with the exercises, a veterinary-formulated home-cooked diet was prescribed to control weight. Non-slippery surfaces were displayed at home, and owners were encouraged to walk her over different surfaces such as sand and grass.
- **Outcome:** pain disappeared after the second session, and after the third visit P. was able to stand by herself for several minutes and take some steps with assistance. By the fifth visit she was able to take a few steps without assistance (ambulatory paraparesis) and Cavaletti rails were introduced. By the seventh visit she was able to walk for 5 min without falling and had lost 1 kg and increased thigh circumference by 1 cm. A month later only a slight ataxia remained, which disappeared after two more visits. Owners were advised to perform a home exercise program on a regular (although less intense) basis.

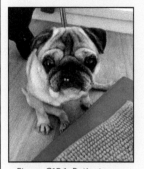

Figure C15.1 Patient, case no. 15.

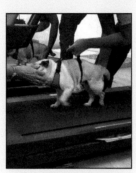

Figure C15.2 Assisted exercise on ground treadmill.

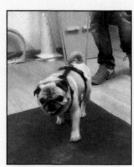

Figure C15.3 Sling-assisted walking.

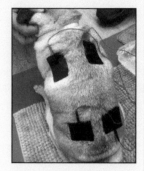

Figure C15.4 TENS over the thoracolumbar area.

P_a (W)	Tx time	J/cm²	Total J/Tx	Spot (cm²)	W/cm²	Tx/week	No. Tx
6	100–200 s (1.6–3.2 min)	8–10	600–1200	5	1.6	2/week, then 1 every 2 weeks, then 1/month	10

Case no. 16

B., canine, 9 years old, Dachshund, FS, 8.2 kg

- **Complaint:** non-ambulatory paraparesis and fecal/urinary incontinence.
- **History:** B. presented with acute paraplegia and loss of superficial pain perception 9 days ago; an MRI was performed, which diagnosed a caudal thoracic disk hernia. She underwent hemilaminectomy a week ago to decompress a T11–T12 disk hernia. She lost all pain perception after the procedure, so owners have been given a poor prognosis.
- **MRI:** T11–T12 hernia, with severe compressive myelopathy.
- **Physical examination:**
  - Body condition score 6/9.
  - There are no limitations in the ROM of the joints.
  - Limb circumference (70% of thigh): right 14.5 cm, left 13.5 cm.
  - Mild atrophy of paraspinal and hindlimb muscles.
  - Paraplegia, unable to support herself in standing position. Absence of movement in the tail.
  - No proprioception. Urinary and fecal incontinence. No superficial or deep pain perception in hindlimbs. Some pain perception at L3/L4 level.
  - Pain assessment: 0/10 NRS.

		Range of motion (degrees)		
		Hip	Knee	Tarsus
Right	Flexion	50	40	45
	Extension	150	170	170
Left	Flexion	40	35	35
	Extension	155	160	160

- **Diagnosis:** caudal thoracic compressive myelopathy causing paraplegia and loss of pain perception.
- **Treatment:**
  - **Laser therapy:**
    - Treatment area initially included T10–L2, with a dose of 8 J/cm^2, which after the second visit was increased to 10 J/cm^2 and extended to cover the whole T10–S1 area.
    - Daily treatments were performed for 4 days, then every other day for 3 weeks, twice a week for 2 more weeks and eventually a weekly treatment for 8 more weeks.
    - During some of the visits a much broader treatment plan was performed, and owners committed to home exercise sessions.
  - **Medical treatment:** she received meloxicam for the first 3 days but it was discontinued due to vomiting.
  - **Acupuncture:** 20 min sessions, initially three times a week for the first 2 weeks, then gradually decreasing the frequency of visits. Treatment included dry needle technique and electro-acupuncture with variable combinations of the following acupoints: GV-20, GV-14, GV-3, BL-18, BL-23, BL-24, BL-26, *Shen shu*, KID-1, LI-4, LIV-3, GB-34, ST-36 and *Hua-tuo-jia-ji*, as well as aqua-acupuncture at BL-40, ST-36, and *Liu feng*, using diluted B12 vitamin. Herbal prescription of Double P #2 and *Wu Bi Shan Yao* formula at 1 g/10 kg twice a day.
  - **Other physical therapies:** twice a week for the first month, then once a week.
    - NMES: biphasic, symmetric, and rectangular pulsed wave; 40 Hz, to stimulate hindlimb muscles (hamstrings and femoral quadriceps).
    - TENS: local treatment for 20 min, 5 Hz. The electrodes were positioned bilateral to the spine (T10–L2).
    - Cryotherapy at thoracolumbar incision site for 20 min (before laser therapy) during the first 2 weeks.

- **Exercise program:**
  - Assisted exercises: standing and weight-shifting using different surfaces, bicycling movement.
  - Hydrotherapy: started after the first month, with underwater treadmill and swimming pool twice a week, then once a week, once every 2 weeks, and later just once a month.
  - Manual intervention: gentle massage of hindlimb and forelimb musculature. Passive ROM of all joints of the pelvic limbs with bicycling movements.
- **Home exercise program:** all techniques were initially performed with the owners in the clinic to ensure proper delivery.
  - Passive exercises: gentle massage of hindlimb muscles two to three times/day, plus footpad friction massage and phalangeal stimulation. Passive ROM of all joints of pelvic limbs with bicycling movements.
  - Active exercises: assisted standing and weight-shifting on stable surfaces, then on a moderately unstable surface and on a bi-directional balance board. Slow supported leash walking was added after the first week, initially for 3–4 min, three times a day, then gradually increasing duration.
  - Other exercises were later performed as well, such as turning exercises during walking and sit-to-stand exercises; the schedule was adapted to the progress of the patient each week.
  - NMES: biphasic, symmetric, and rectangular pulsed wave; 40 Hz, to stimulate hindlimb muscles (hamstrings and femoral quadriceps).
  - TENS: local treatment for 20 min, 5 Hz. The electrodes were positioned bilateral to the spine (T10–L2).
- **Owner education:** exercise restriction, soft bedding to prevent ulcers. Bladder expression. Brief (later increased) assisted walking with a supporting harness and sling.
- **Outcome:**
  - On day 12, she was able to stand up by herself and had pain perception down to L5.
  - On day 15, she was able to take a few steps and recovered some urinary and fecal continence.
  - After 6 weeks, she recovered deep pain in the right hindlimb, and in the left limb after 10 weeks.
  - She was gradually able to take longer walks, up to 40 min by the fourth month.
  - She recovered continence by the sixth month.

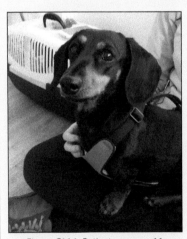

Figure C16.1 Patient, case no. 16.

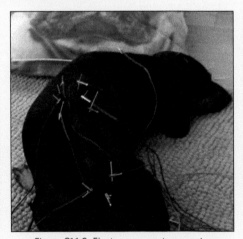

Figure C16.2 Electro-acupuncture session.

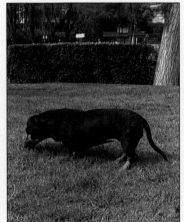

Figure C16.3 Ground exercises on different surfaces.

Area	P_a (W)	Tx time	J/cm²	Total J/Tx	Spot (cm²)	W/cm²	Tx/week	No. Tx
First week	6	1.5 min	8	400	6	1	4-3-2-1	25
Later	8	3 min	10	1200	5	1.6		

Case no. 17

T., canine, 4 years old, Portuguese Hound, FS, 20 kg

- **Complaint:** swelling of surgical sites.
- **History:**
  - T. had been hit by a bus a month before. As a consequence, she had an abdominal traumatic hernia (bladder and intestine), left hip fracture, and right sacroiliac luxation (Fig. C17.1a, b).
  - 48 h later she underwent hernia repair with a polypropylene mesh and fracture fixation with a dynamic compression plate and six screws (Fig. C17.2).
  - A week after surgery she was readmitted due to a large fluid collection and exudate from the hip wound, hindlimb edema, and pain.
  - She was put on ciprofloxacin, metronidazole, and cephalexin, but 2 weeks later she developed an infection and dehiscence in the abdominal wound and the hip area was inflamed.
  - She had lost 10 kg (about 30% of body weight) in a month. Blood culture was negative.
- **Physical examination:**
  - There was a 12 cm long dehiscence in the abdominal wound, which was inflamed. The subcutaneous tissue around it was severely inflamed (Fig. C17.3a).
  - The left gluteal area was moderately inflamed, although there was no open wound or discharge (Fig. C17.3b).
- **Diagnosis:** surgical site inflammation, chronic wound with dehiscence.
- **Treatment:**
  - **Wound management:** regular antiseptic lavage.
  - **Laser therapy:**
    - Treatment of the abdominal wound included a 5 cm margin around it, with a total area of 175–200 cm². Dose was 4 J/cm² for the first two treatments, and then increased to 10 J/cm². There was a fast clinical improvement (Figs C17.4a, C17.5a, C17.6a, C17.7a, C17.8a) and a week later the inflammation was so decreased (Fig. C17.5a) that stretch marks were evident.
    - The gluteal/hip area covered 200 cm² and was treated with higher power (5 W) and power density (1 W/cm²). Note how the area shows a concavity after five treatments (Fig.17.6b), even though it does not seem very inflamed in the initial pictures. Since the treatment was focused around the incision line, the hair grew faster here (Figs C17.6b, C17.7b, C17.8b).
  - **Others:** carprofen, tramadol, ciprofloxacin, metronidazole, and cephalexin were used for a week into the laser treatment, and then discontinued.
- **Outcome:** complete resolution of the inflammation. The patient was able to jump on the bed (not advised) a week after starting LT. No recurrence of inflammation or wound discharge.

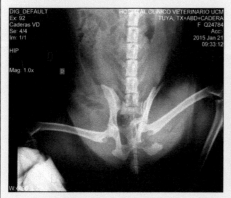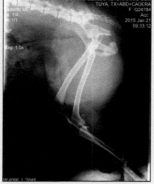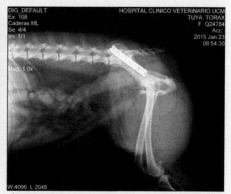

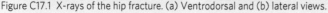

Figure C17.1 X-rays of the hip fracture. (a) Ventrodorsal and (b) lateral views.   Figure C17.2 Hip after surgery, lateral view.

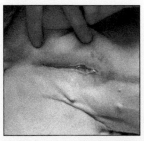
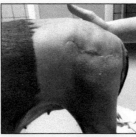
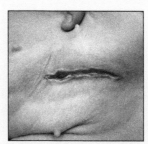
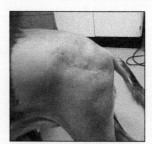

Figure C17.3 Three weeks after surgery; beginning of LT. (a) Abdominal wound and (b) gluteal area.

Figure C17.4 (a, b) Two days after beginning LT.

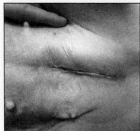
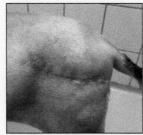
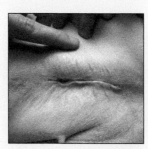
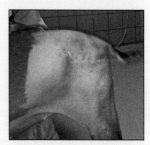

Figure C17.5 (a, b) One week after beginning LT.

Figure C17.6 (a, b) Day 9 of LT.

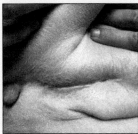
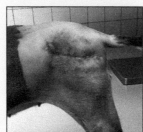
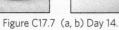
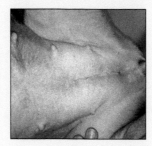
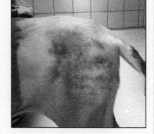

Figure C17.7 (a, b) Day 14.

Figure C17.8 (a, b) Patient is discharged.

Area	P_a (W)	Tx time	J/cm²	Total J/Tx	Spot (cm²)	W/cm²	Tx/week	No. Tx
Wound (175–200 cm²)	3	250 s (4.1 min)–500 s (8.3 min)	4–10	750–1500	6	0.5	4–3	7
Hip (200 cm²)	5	240 s (4 min)–320 s (5.3 min)	6–8	1200–1600	5	1	4–3	7

Case no. 18

B., canine, 8 years old, German Shepherd, MC, 39 kg

- **Complaint:** chronic right hindlimb lameness and weakness, occasional forelimb lameness.
- **History:** B. started to show symptoms 3 years ago, with hindlimb lameness and difficulty standing up. A few months ago forelimb lameness appeared. He gets chondroprotective nutraceuticals on a regular basis and NSAIDs when pain is worse (not at the moment). Lameness improves after exercise.
- **MRI:** T13–L1 disk protrusion with moderate spinal cord compression.
- **Radiographic findings**: severe bilateral hip OA, moderate left metatarsophalangeal OA.
- **Physical examination:**
  - Body condition score 6/9.
  - Decreased passive ROM.
  - Symmetric hindlimb circumference (right 35 cm and left 39 cm, measured at 70% of thigh) with mild atrophy of quadriceps, semitendinosus, and semimembranosus. Contracted triceps and infraspinatus muscles.
  - Mild synovial effusion in both stifles.
  - No neurological deficits.
  - Pain assessment: 2/10 NRS, mild discomfort at left metatarsophalangeal and T13/L1 area; difficulty standing up and sitting down; 4/10 pain on right knee flexion and right hip extension.

		Range of motion (degrees)		
		Hip	Knee	Tarsus
Right	**Flexion**	50	60	45
	Extension	155	170	165
Left	**Flexion**	55	45	45
	Extension	160	160	170

- **Diagnosis:** severe bilateral hip OA, bilateral knee arthritis, moderate left metatarsophalangeal OA, chronic T13/L1 disk herniation.
- **Treatment:**
  - **Laser therapy:**
    - Dose was 6–8 J/cm^2 over left metatarsophalangeal joints, 10–12 J/cm^2 over T10–L3 area and both hips, and 8–10 J/cm^2 over both stifles.
    - Treatment was performed every other day for the first week, then twice a week for 6 more weeks, once a week for 2 weeks, then every 2 weeks for maintenance.
  - **Other physical therapies:**
    - Twice a week for 3 weeks, once a week for 6 weeks, then every 2 weeks.
    - NMES: 40 Hz, biphasic, to stimulate hamstrings, quadriceps, and gluteus muscles; 10 min in each limb.
    - TENS: local treatment; 5 Hz, 30 min; electrodes are positioned bilateral to the spine (T13–L2), over right hip, right knee, and left metatarsophalangeal joint.
    - PMF therapy: low frequency (12–20 Hz), 90% intensity for 30 min, later increased to 100% for 40 min. Positioned over hip and shoulder areas.
    - Thermotherapy: infrared lamp during TENS treatment/PMF treatment.
    - Manual intervention: massage for 30 min with effleurage, petrissage, and longitudinal friction of all limbs, neck, and spine. Passive ROM exercises for all joints. Muscle stretching in right hindlimb.
  - **Home exercise program:** all techniques were performed with the owners in the clinic to ensure proper delivery. At home, owners performed them three times a week.

- TENS: T10–L3, right hip, right knee, and left metatarsophalangeal joints; 100 Hz for 30 min.
- NMES: right quadriceps and hamstrings; 40 Hz for 10 min.
- Massage, passive ROM.
- Slow ramp climbing, sit-to-stand exercises, Cavaletti.
- **Owner education:** as much controlled exercise as possible (walking on leash); rest is contraindicated. Avoid jumping and sleeping on cold hard surfaces. Avoid running up or down stairs or chasing rabbits. Weight control.
- **Outcome:**
  - Decreased pain on manipulation of affected areas after the second week; significant improvement in sitting/standing up after the third week. After 7 weeks right knee flexion improved to 55° and right hindlimb diameter increased from 35 to 37 cm (left 39 cm). Able to walk for 2 hours after 2 months.
  - A maintenance regime of LT and physiotherapy treatments every 2 weeks had to be maintained during the colder seasons, otherwise pain would reappear.

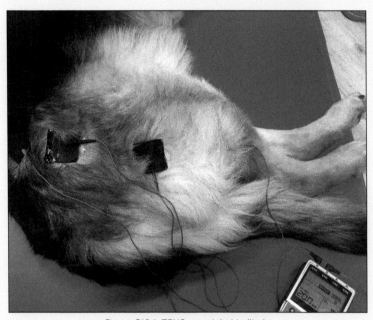

Figure C18.1 TENS over right hindlimb.

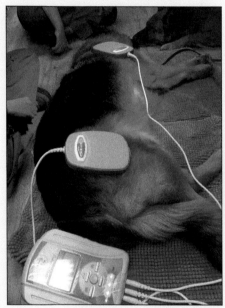

Figure C18.2 Thermotherapy during PMF session.

Area	P_a (W)	Tx time	J/cm²	Total J/Tx	Spot (cm²)	W/cm²	Tx/week	No. Tx
TL spine	**6–12**	4 min	12	2400		2.4		
Hip (each)	**6–12**	5 min	12	3600	5	2.4	3-2-1 then every 2 weeks	24
Stifle (each)	**8**	4.6 min	10	2250		1.6		
Left MTP	**6**	3.5 min	8	1280		1.2		

Note: MTP, metatarsophalangeal joints; TL, thoracolumbar.

Case no. 19

A., canine, 7 years old, German Shepherd, MC, 38 kg

- **Complaint:** pain and hindlimb lameness.
- **History:** he was diagnosed with gracilis muscle contracture in the left hindlimb 5 months ago. A month ago the right hindlimb seemed to start developing similar changes. He does not want to walk or play.
- **Physical examination:**
  - Abnormal gait with shortened stride and elastic, rapid medial rotation of the paw, external rotation of the calcaneus, and internal rotation of the stifle, typical of gracilis muscle myopathy (Fig. C19.1a, b).
  - Left hindlimb: severe gracilis fibrosis. The semitendinosus and semimembranosus muscles were very contracted and there was an abnormal fibrosis in the common calcaneal tendon. The extension of both the hock and stifle were very limited.
  - Right hindlimb: mild fibrosis of gracilis; contracture of the semitendinosus muscle was not as severe as in the contralateral limb, and neither was the limitation in ROM of the stifle and hock.
- **Diagnosis:** fibrotic gracilis myopathy, progressing to bilateral involvement.
- **Treatment:**
  - **Laser therapy:**
    - An area of 600 cm² was covered in each limb, from the calcaneus to the ischium.
    - With a dose of 8 J/cm², a total of 4800 J per limb was used in each session.
    - A. received LT three times a week during the first 2 weeks, then twice a week for 3 more weeks, then once a week for 6 more weeks.
  - **Others:** treadmill exercises, therapeutic massage and stretching techniques, dry needle.
- **Outcome:** after the second session, A. was eager to play again. Also after the second session, the right side contracture started to improve, with eventual resolution. ROM of the left stifle improved after four treatments. The left semitendinosus contracture progressively improved and the calcaneal tendon fibrosis disappeared. The left gracilis fibrosis did not disappear.

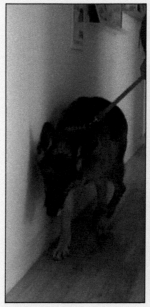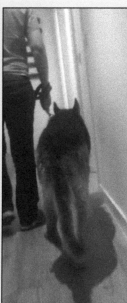

Figure C19.1 (a, b) Typical gait of gracilis muscle myopathy.

P$_a$ (W)	Tx time	J/cm²	Total J/Tx	Spot (cm²)	W/cm²	Tx/week	No. Tx
6	1600 s (26.7 min, 13.3 min each limb)	8	9600 (4800 each limb)	5	1	3-2-1	20

Case no. 20

O., canine, 3 years old, Greyhound, FS, 21 kg

- **Complaint:** open TTA wound.
- **History:** she underwent TTA surgery for right CCLR 8 days ago. She had an allergic reaction during surgery preparation, potentially to intravenous cephazolin, although the epidural morphine and bupivacaine were also considered. Wound is open and moist. She has been licking the bandage. She was on ciprofloxacin and also received tramadol for 4 days postoperatively. Last night she started to lick the wound. Orthopedic surgeon referred her for LT.
- **Physical examination:** surgical wound inflammation, with dehiscence in the distal half and partial exposure of metal plate. Mildly exudative and with some necrotic tissue.
- **Diagnosis:** surgical wound dehiscence and potential surgical site infection.
- **Treatment:**
  - **Wound management:** 0.05% chlorhexidine lavage and protective bandages. Keeping the E-collar on and preventing self-trauma was quite a challenge in this case, and some degree of dermatitis was present until wound closure.

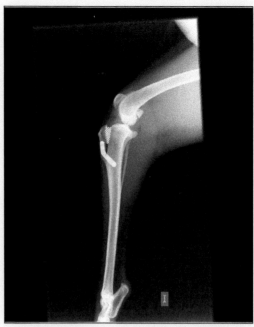

Figure C20.1 X-ray on the day of the surgery.

  - **Laser therapy:**
    - 5 J/cm^2 over the wound, increased to 10 J/cm^2 once the plate was covered, maintaining an average power of 1.5–3 W.
    - 6 J/cm^2 around the rest of the stifle and proximal tibia, with an average power of 5 W.
- **Outcome:** wound closure after 11 treatments over 5 weeks.

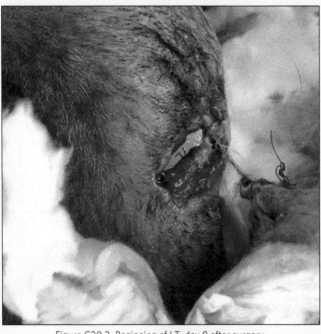

Figure C20.2 Beginning of LT, day 8 after surgery.

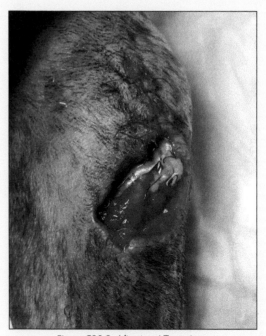

Figure C20.3 After two LT sessions.

Case no. 20 (cont.)

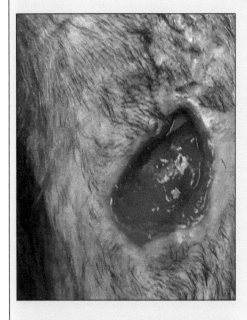

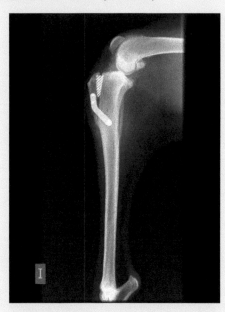

Figure C20.4 (a) Second week of treatment, 3 weeks after surgery. (b) X-ray shows correct evolution.

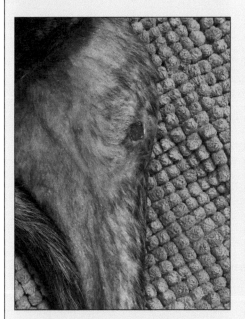

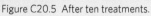

Figure C20.5 After ten treatments.

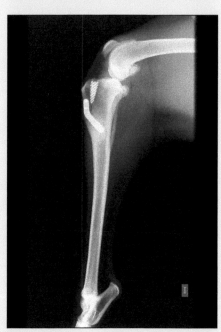

Figure C20.6 Four and a half months after surgery. X-ray shows full integration of plate.

Area	P_a (W)	Tx time	J/cm²	Total J/Tx	Spot (cm²)	W/cm²	Tx/week	No. Tx
Wound (50 cm²)	1.5–3	166s (2.7 min)–83s(1.4 min)	5	250	8	0.18–0.37	4-3-2-1	11
Stifle/prox. Tibia (150 cm²)	5	180s (3 min)	6	900	5	1	4-3-2-1	11

Case no. 21

N., canine, 4 years old, Boxer, MC, 36 kg

- **Complaint:** lameness and inflammation of the stifle.
- **History:**
  - N. underwent TTA surgery for partial left CCLR a week ago. Before surgery, his lameness was minimal. He has been on cephalexin since then.
  - Everything seemed to be going well until yesterday, when he started to be very lame in the same limb, so he came for a second opinion. No trauma after surgery.
  - Tramadol does not seem to be helping and owners want to avoid NSAIDs because he has chronic leishmaniasis and IRIS stage I renal disease.
- **Physical examination:** 4–5/5 left hindlimb lameness (Fig. C21.1a, b). Pain score 7/10. Severe inflammation of the stifle, with marked edema and tumefaction. Inflammation of the surgical incision (Fig. C21.1c).
- **Diagnosis:** surgical site inflammation.
- **Treatment:**
  - **Laser therapy:**
    - To treat the incision site plus its margin (total 50 cm²), a low power density was used (0.2 W/cm²), while slightly higher values can be reached around the rest of the joint. Power was kept low to moderate due to the severe inflammation.
    - The patient was treated on 2 consecutive days, then twice more at 48 h intervals, and once more another 72 h later.
- **Outcome:** in 9 days and with LT as the sole treatment, the inflammation was resolved (Fig. 21.2); lameness score was reduced to 1/5 and pain score to 1/10.

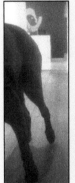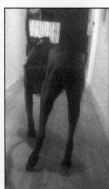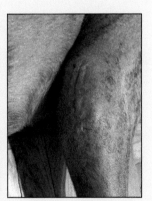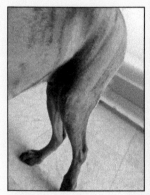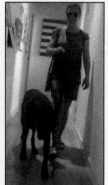

Figure C21.1 (a, b) Severe left hindlimb lameness and (c) severe inflammation of the stifle a week after surgery.

Figure C21.2 (a) Stifle and (b) patient walking 9 days later.

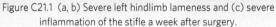

Area	P_a (W)	Tx time	J/cm²	Total J/Tx	Spot (cm²)	W/cm²	Tx/week	No. Tx
Wound (50 cm²)	**1.6**	125 s (2.1 min)	4	200	8	0.2	4-2	6
Stifle/prox. tibia (150 cm²)	**4**	262 s (4.4 min)	7	1050	5	0.8	4-2	6

Case no. 22

T., canine, 6 years old, Boxer, MC, 37 kg

- **Complaint:** discharge from surgical wound.
- **History:** T. had undergone TTA for CCLR 11 days before (Fig. C22.1). His orthopedic surgeon had just rechecked him and found there was discharge from the wound. He was worried about the patient, the procedure, and how this complication could affect implant integration, and referred T. for LT.
- **Physical examination:** moderate inflammation in the dorsal half of the surgical wound, with serohemorrhagic exudate (Fig. C22.2).
- **Diagnosis:** inflammation of the surgical site.
- **Treatment:**
  - **Wound management:** regular cleaning with chlorhexidine. Self-trauma prevention.
  - **Laser therapy:**
    - Two different treatments were performed in each session: one just above the incision, with lower dose and power, and another around the rest of the stifle and proximal tibia, with higher dose and power. In this way we could reach the osteotomy site without using excessive power over the wound and also avoid the metal plate, that would not allow the light to reach the tissues beneath it.
    - The patient came in 48 h later for a second laser session; the wound was no longer inflamed and had very minimal discharge (Fig. C22.3). A week later the problem seemed to be completely resolved (Fig. C22.4). A fourth treatment was performed on day 9 (Fig. C22.5), both over the wound and the proximal tibia.
- **Outcome:** resolution of the inflammation and discharge. Satisfactory clinical progression and bone healing, as the radiographic rechecks demonstrated (Figs C22.6 and C22.7).

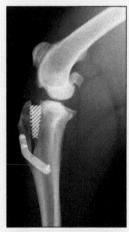

Figure C22.1 Radiography from the day of the surgery.

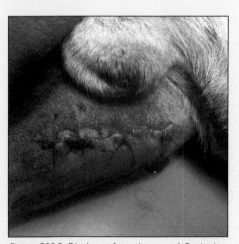

Figure C22.2 Discharge from the wound. Beginning of LT.

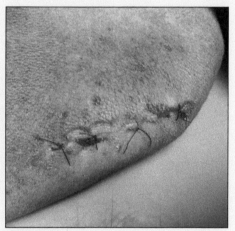

Figure C22.3 After 48 h, before second treatment.

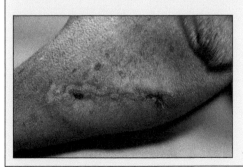

Figure C22.4 Day 7, third treatment.

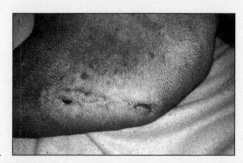

Figure C22.5 Day 9, last treatment.

Case no. 22 (cont.)

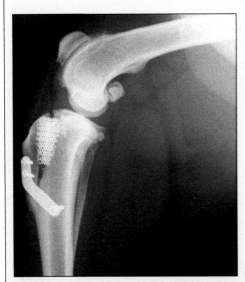

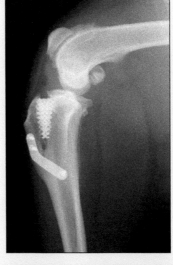

Figure C22.6 One month after surgery.

Figure C22.7 Two months after surgery.

Area	P_a (W)	Tx time	J/cm²	Total J/Tx	Spot (cm²)	W/cm²	Tx/week	No. Tx
Wound (40 cm²)	2	40 s	2	80	5	0.4	3-1	4
Stifle/prox. tibia (150 cm²)	5	180 s (3 min)	6	900	5	1	3-1	4

Case no. 23

M., canine, 8 years old, Border Collie, MNC, 20 kg

- **Complaint:** chronic right hindlimb lameness and weakness, occasional forelimb lameness.
- **History:** M. is a very active sports dog who is trained for obedience and has run four World Cups. Four months ago he presented with 5/5 acute lameness after running over frozen ground. He has improved since then but still shows abnormal gait. His referring veterinarian has performed ultrasound (no significant findings, apart from some inflammation in the gastrocnemius) and X-rays, and has diagnosed him with mild right hip OA and muscle contracture of gastrocnemius and superficial digital flexor muscles. He has recommended a month of NSAIDs and absolute rest.
- **Radiographic findings:** right femoral neck thickening, mild change in right coxofemoral angle. No radiographic changes in stifle and tarsus.
- **Physical examination:**
  - Body condition score 5/9.
  - 4/5 right hindlimb lameness, with shortened support phase and internal rotation of the tarsus of the affected limb during walking. Weight-bearing was significantly decreased during stance.
  - Goniometry: mild decrease in the right hindlimb passive ROM.
  - Asymmetric hindlimb circumference (right 24 cm and left 27 cm, measured at 70% of thigh).
  - No neurological deficits.
  - Pain assessment: 5/10 NRS, moderate pain during tarsus and hip manipulation.
- **Diagnosis:** mild right hip OA and muscle contracture of gastrocnemius and superficial digital flexor muscles.
- **Treatment:**
  - **Laser therapy:**
    - 6–8 J/cm^2 over gastrocnemius, superficial digital flexor, and tarsus; 10 J/cm^2 over right hip.
    - Three times a week for 3 weeks, then twice a week.
  - **Other physical therapies:**
    - Three times a week for 3 weeks, then twice a week.
    - Ultrasound: pulsed mode 50%, frequency 3.3 MHz, 5 cm probe over gastrocnemius and superficial digital flexor muscles.
    - Manual intervention: massage for 30 min with effleurage, petrissage, and longitudinal friction of affected limb, passive ROM exercises.
    - PMF therapy: 12–20 Hz over the hip area, 100% intensity for 40 min.
  - **Home exercise program:** all techniques were performed with the owners in the clinic to ensure proper delivery. At home, owners performed them twice a day.
    - Local heat for 15 min on gastrocnemius and right hip.
    - Massage, passive ROM.
  - **Owner education:** avoid intense or explosive exercise, just walking on leash. Do not train for the moment.
- **Outcome:**
  - Decreased pain on manipulation and improved weight-bearing after 1 week; almost normal after 2 weeks (1/5 lameness) but some pain persisted at the hip.

		Range of motion (degrees)		
		Hip	Knee	Tarsus
Right	**Flexion**	55	45	30
	Extension	157	170	170
Left	**Flexion**	50	42	35
	Extension	165	165	170

- Owners insisted he perform at championship after 2 weeks despite contraindication, which worsened pain. After another 2 weeks of rest and therapy, M. seemed back to normal and showed no lameness or pain, although it was still recommended that he avoid intense explosive exercise for the moment and wait for the next season to compete.

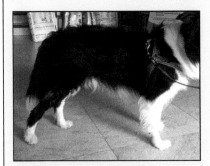

Figure C23.1 Decreased weight-bearing on right hindlimb.

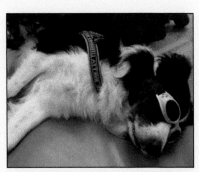

Figure C23.2 Patient M. during laser treatment.

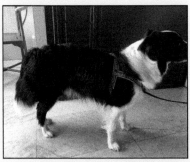

Figure C23.3 Improved weight-bearing.

Area	P_a (W)	Tx time	J/cm²	Total J/Tx	Spot (cm²)	W/cm²	Tx/week	No. Tx
Hip	**10**	3.3 min	10	2000		2		
Gastrocnemius	**6**	1.7 min	8	600	5	1.3	3-2	11
Tarsus	**6**	1.3 min	6	480		1.2		

Case no. 24

O., canine, 5 years old, Spanish Mastiff, MC, 75 kg

- **Complaint:** limb dragging and open wound.
- **History:** O. was hit by a car 6 months ago. He had a hip (left acetabulum) fracture and suspected sciatic damage but did not receive surgery. He has been dragging the leg since then. A month ago he received an orthosis, but it seems too small for him. The owners manage the wound with chlorhexidine and antibiotic ointment, but it has not improved. The referring veterinarian took a culture.
- **Physical examination:** open wound affecting the lateral half of the left foot, with exposure of the bones of the fifth digit (Fig. C24.1a, b). The left popliteal node is enlarged. No superficial or deep pain perception in the foot and up to the knee. Sciatic and patellar reflexes are present but not the flexor reflex.
- **Diagnosis:** chronic infected wound affecting soft tissue and bone. Neurological damage of the distal sciatic nerve.
- **Treatment:**
  - **Wound management:** lavaged with 0.05% chlorhexidine. Alginate dressing as a primary layer.
  - **Laser therapy:**
    - 5 J/cm^2 covering all the area up to the tarsus, and then increasing up to 10 J/cm^2.
    - The wound was initially very exudative, so treatments were performed 5 days a week in the first week (Figs C24.2 and C24.3); frequency of treatment then gradually decreased to just twice a week in the last week.
  - **Others:**
    - The initial antibiotic treatment was cephalexin and metronidazole. The culture results showed infection with *Proteus mirabilis* that was resistant to beta-lactamics, clindamycin, and doxycycline, and sensitive to quinolones, so treatment was changed to enrofloxacin for 2 weeks.
    - Support with a custom-made fiberglass splint.
- **Outcome:**
  - Closure of the wound in 40 days (Figs C24.4 to C24.7).
  - Recovery of pain perception from the stifle down to the tarsus and improvement of foot posture correction when he was re-evaluated in week 8; this was related to recovery of function in the sciatic nerve (but not the fibular or tibial nerves).

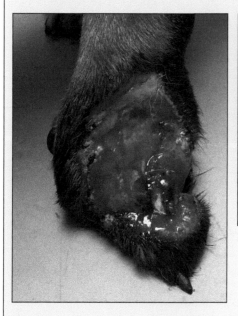
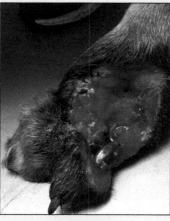
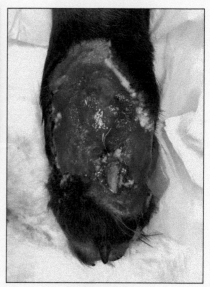

Figure C24.1 (a, b) Open wound before LT.

Figure C24.2 Day 1.

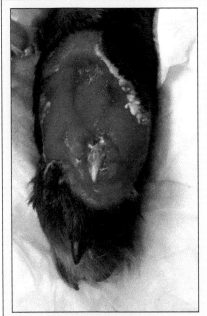

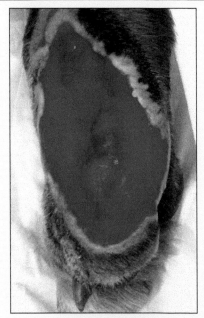

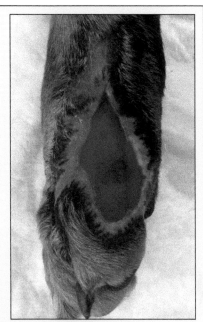

Figure C24.3 Day 3, after two treatments.

Figure C24.4 Day 8.

Figure C24.5 Day 22.

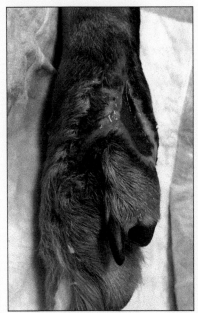

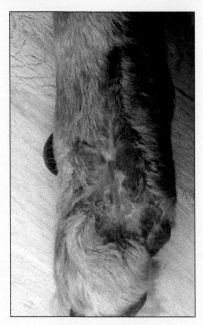

Figure C24.6 Day 30.

Figure C24.7 Day 40.

P$_a$ (W)	Tx time	J/cm^2	Total J/Tx	Spot (cm^2)	W/cm^2	Tx/week	No. Tx
3	333 s (5.4 min)–666 s (11 min)	5-10	1000–2000	5	0.4	5-2	20

PART 3

Using light in your practice

As you've seen, both of us have been collaborating throughout to give you a balanced view of both the scientific rigor and clinical intricacies of laser therapy. In this third part of the book, we have literally co-authored each section. This may seem strange to you since one of us (as admitted several times) is the geek with much less clinical experience. And the sections on integrating laser into your clinical routine would seem to be best explained by a clinician. But this geek has also developed the strategy, marketing, and client education for two separate laser companies and in three different markets: the early adopting US market back in 2010 where only about 10–15% of clinics had even heard of a laser, the earliest adopting European market in 2012 where virtually no therapy lasers were used in small animal practice, and again in 2018 in the US where laser has become more mainstream. So just as in the rest of this book, take in all the ideas we throw around, and discover which are the best for your particular environment.

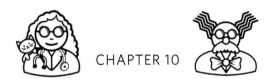

CHAPTER 10

Considering laser therapy for your practice

Nothing in life is to be feared, it is only to be understood. Now is the time to understand more, so that we may fear less.

— Marie Curie

We often purchase pieces of equipment for our practices and hospitals that allow us to work better as clinicians but that are not always an easy choice in financial terms. A new ultrasound machine, the latest toy for surgery, a computed tomography scanner … We hope the clinical benefits of laser therapy (LT) have been clarified in previous pages. But what about the financial side? The truth is that if the device is well chosen and used, implementing LT in your practice can help you pay for the ultrasound machine much faster. The versatility allows you to treat a wide variety of cases, whether you are in a general practice or in a sports medicine center. About 30–40% of US practices offer LT among their services, and hundreds of them do so in Europe.

10.1 Make an educated choice

At every veterinary conference you attend these days you will find many LT options. This market is sprouting; we hope that after reading this book you will know how to distinguish between a poor laser and a high-quality one. Their technical differences (diodes and wavelengths, power, pulsing, fiber durability, variety of spot sizes, either adjustable or with different treatment heads, etc.) do matter, and will not just influence their price, but also the efficacy of your treatments. The box on the next page lists the seven key points to look for.

The prices of LT devices are as varied as their characteristics. A well-powered device is commonly in the range of 17,000–32,000 USD, but return on investment is usually high and fast with the right device, proper use, and an implementation plan. There are good plans, and there are better plans, but the only bad plan is having no plan. The following are necessary questions and will help you make your calculations.

- How many patients per day/week do you treat that could benefit from LT? Remember LT is extremely versatile; unless you only see oncology and epileptic patients, many of your cases are going to benefit from it: in general practice, probably 50–70%. Think of all the post-ops, otitis, bite wounds, and degenerative joint disease (DJD) patients you treat, to mention just a few. Some of your past and current cases probably came to your mind while you were reading other sections of this book.

- How many of their owners would be willing to pay for it? You should expect at least 50%, but this will increase to about 80%. As with any other treatment, this depends in part on how, how much, and how fluently you and your staff talk to them about LT. A good implementation plan considers this. This is also related to how long you have been using LT and how familiar you are with seeing its effects and predicting how much and how fast it will help a patient. There will come a point when you will not hesitate to choose LT for a patient, in the same way you now have no doubt that a certain animal needs an non-steroidal anti-inflammatory drug (NSAID) or a particular surgical procedure.

- How much would you charge for a session? Remember that it does not take the same amount

Do need

1. Power output of at least 7 W (average, not just peak!), preferably 12–15 W: to improve penetration and shorten treatment times, especially in the case of deep tissues and broad areas.
2. Quality diodes with long manufacturer warranties. Diodes should produce light in the infrared spectrum and cover at least 800–920 nm, plus a red aiming/therapeutic beam, and ideally be able to work with multiple wavelengths simultaneously.
3. Interchangeable treatment heads and/or a built-in way to change the beam cross-section to modify power density, cover different areas, and treat from a distance without losing power density.
4. Easy and light to carry around, and battery-operated. A bigger device does NOT mean it is more powerful, and older, lower-power, primitive lasers were actually huge. Size doesn't mean quality.
5. Clear, intuitive software that is easy to update (best if it auto-updates via WiFi) and easy to customize to meet your patients' (and your clinic's) individual needs.
6. Ability to work both in continuous wave and pulsed mode, and able to pulse over a broad range of frequencies (at least greater than 10,000 Hz).
7. Reliable and accessible support. Although this book (we hope) helps you in a substantial way, it is important to have training, and clinical and technical support, from either the manufacturing/distributing company or other professionals. Dependable technical support is always necessary at some point; even the best laser will need check-ups/repairs throughout its lifetime.

Don't need

1. A tablet with fancy graphics as a giveaway: yes it is fancy, yes it may have some value in initially educating your clients, but don't let it change your focus of attention away from what's important in the laser.
2. A sales rep telling you a well-powered laser is dangerous because you will burn your patient. This scare tactic is the most common argument among people selling low-power devices and does drive me mad, because after thousands of treatments I have never ever been in that situation. You just need to understand the kind of tool you have in your hands (and you'd better after reading this book!).
3. A treatment menu with hundreds of options making you think you are choosing very specific settings for your patients, when actually half of them lead you to the same parameters. What is important is to understand why you are choosing what you choose. Do the thinking, don't just let the machine tell you what to do, because you should know better. If you do not want to do any thinking, you've wasted your time reading this book.

of time to treat a small laparotomy incision as the spine and hips of a Labrador. Consider also who is going to perform treatments, i.e. vets vs. technicians/nurses. Although the diagnosis and treatment plan should always be carried out by a veterinarian, a well-trained nurse can apply the laser treatment, once you decide the treatment parameters, area, and frequency of treatment.

So you can estimate the weekly laser revenue by multiplying the number of wound/DJD/otitis/acute trauma/post-op cases you see by the price you would charge for those and the percentage of owners who would agree to try this modality once you tell them about it. An Excel worksheet is very useful and easy to program to simulate different scenarios. Your monthly laser revenue will be about four times the weekly revenue, and if you subtract your lease/monthly payment for the device, you will estimate the monthly profit. A good laser should have a long working life and, if your plan is properly implemented, give you a substantial profit each year.

10.2 Laser safety and contraindications

Oddly enough, one of the most appropriate tenets of laser safety can be stated in terms of firearms: "Don't pull the trigger until you know what you're shooting at." (I currently live in the great southern state of Tennessee, so picture me saying that in a hillbilly, tobacco-spitting, moonshine-sipping, overall-wearing twang.) But seriously ...

Safety concerns have been thoroughly evaluated by governing bodies (Food and Drug Administration [FDA], Health Canada, Conformité Européen [CE] Marking, etc.) and international organizations (WALT, NAALT, etc.) via thermal tests, histology reports, and other worst-case scenario experiments. They all reach the same conclusions: LT is one of the safest in the world and undesired effects can be avoided if the therapist is educated. Reported side effects, (e.g. tiredness, nausea, headache, and increased pain) are always described as mild and actually have a prevalence similar to those in the placebo group when studied in humans. [100] Thousands of treatments are performed worldwide each day in human and veterinary patients. Safety is one of the reasons why LT is growing so fast. Having said this, every practice should be strict in their adherence to safety procedures when using laser. And knowing about safety is important even before you acquire a device.

Each country may have their own specific regulations for the safe use of laser devices, but all of them include eye protection, warning signs, and staff/pet owner education, among others. Being an educated laser user you will know why safety is important, but also how to erase any superstition related to this type of infrared electromagnetic radiation.

Basic facts

- Red and infrared lasers are non-ionizing, just like your infrared lamp in the intensive care unit, or the fluorescent bulb over your head.
- You are using a very special type of lamp, but a kind of a lamp nevertheless; when you turn it off, there is no radiation floating around or remaining in the room or in objects.
- In LT, we do not vaporize cells, or cut or burn the patient. That is done with other types of laser, coagulation devices, and laser sabers. Therefore, there is no toxic plume to be evacuated.

There is no universally endorsed contraindication list, however, and some of the conditions laser companies and training organizations include do not come from negative data points from any studies. Instead, this list is created mostly from theoretical possibilities

of danger and medical legal precautions. While it is absolutely necessary to disclose this list to your patients (and staff), it is useful to understand the actual dangers in each situation. Our version of the contraindications of LT is as follows:

- exposure to the eyes (main and absolute contraindication)
- known malignancies (although this paradigm may change in the future)
- gravid uterus
- the thyroid (relative)
- in local combination with steroid/NSAID injection.

Other situations, such as active growing epiphyses or epilepsy, are not contraindications per se, but precautions need to be taken and discussed with the owner. Let's explain in more detail, since knowing why the limits are in place and where their boundaries are enables you to extend the range of your applications safely and effectively.

10.2.1 Eye exposure

The eyes contain the most photosensitive cells in your body. This fact alone should throw up some red flags when dealing with high-powered light sources like lasers. But the most crucial feature of the eye relevant to safety is the lens and its focusing power. Briefly, whatever light that is not absorbed or reflected by the cornea passes through the lens and gets focused onto the retina, and in particular a central spot known as the fovea centralis, which then connects to the brain, where the light gets processed and interpreted as an image.

For a given wavelength of light, the laser parameter that dictates the safe/dangerous limit is power density (W/cm^2; i.e. the amount of energy delivered per second per unit area). Note: power alone says nothing about safety, since light from a 100 W lamp spread over an entire room is perfectly safe but light from a 0.5 W laser delivered through a 0.001 cm fiber can do surgery.

Once an external power density of 1 W/cm^2 (one that is perfectly safe for any tissue in your body) is focused by the lens, the retina is exposed to a power density of over 80 W/cm^2. This amount of focused energy can cause irreversible damage to the eye and can lead to partial or total blindness. You can see that even scattered light from high-powered sources poses

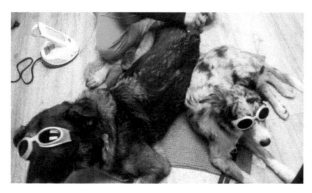

Figure 10.1 Both the patient and dog companion are using doggles.

a potential risk, which is why wavelength-specific eye protection must be used: everybody in the room has to wear the specific protective glasses (Fig. 10.1). These should be provided by the laser manufacturer and follow international regulations; they should indicate the wavelengths they block and the optical density for each of them. These glasses offer limited protection, though, and they are intended to protect you from indirect radiation, or from an accidental momentarily direct exposure; you are still not supposed to point the laser inside anyone's eyeball.

As for the patients, it is necessary to avoid their eye contact with the beam. So for safety, use the doggles (Fig. 10.2), a towel, or your hands every time you work around the head (Fig. 10.3) and forelimbs, but doggles are not that important if you are treating the lumbar area and you are blocking the view of the beam with your hand. For some head treatments, the straps of the doggles will be in your way to the treatment area. In such cases, cover the eyes with your assistant's or the owner's hands (Fig. 10.4), and avoid pointing the beam into the eye. Consider this too when dealing with the (really) very few patients who are reluctant to wear doggles – seriously, you will be surprised at how well they accept them.

A side note on doggles: one of the theories about why most patients seem to be quite relaxed with the doggles on is that because our animals can see at night (at least better than we can), this means they can see a little of the near-infrared spectrum. Well, laser safety goggles

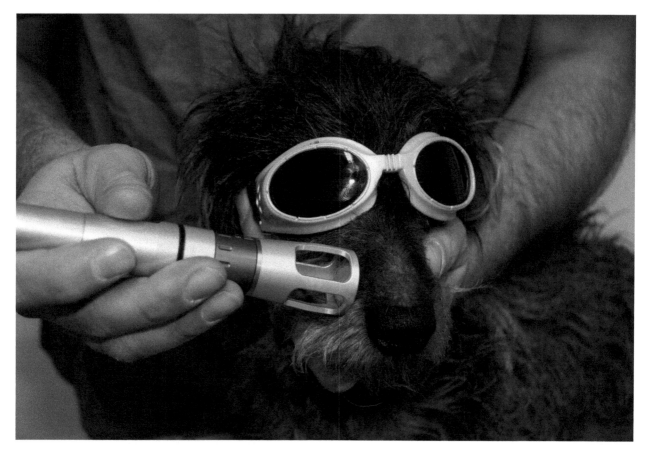

Figure 10.2 Patient wearing doggles for a sinus treatment.

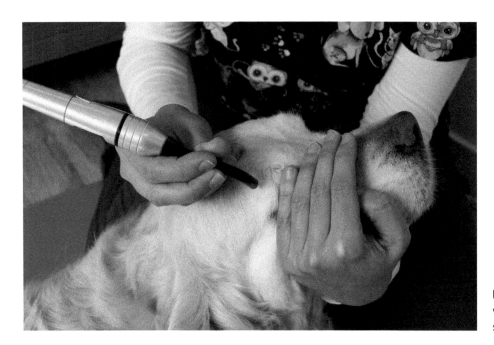

Figure 10.3 Eye protection with the hand while treating the supraciliary area.

(whether human-sized or animal-sized) block a large percentage of the near-infrared spectrum. So putting doggles on them makes the room that much dimmer for them (darker than night, in fact). That would put me to sleep too.

An important point, though, is that this lens magnification is the true source of danger, not the exposure of the retina to light. If the light does not pass through the lens and get magnified, then its power density is

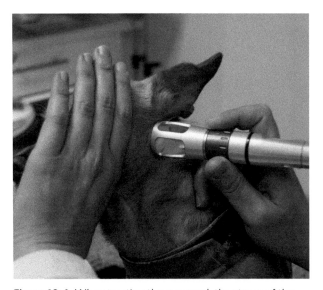

Figure 10.4 When treating the ear canal, the straps of the doggles are in the way, so one option is to protect the eye with the hand.

reduced at greater depths in the body, and so the same benefits you experience with laser on other related conditions of the body can be exploited safely around the eyes.

10.2.2 Neoplastic growths

Cancer cells proliferate faster than healthy ones and often "do things" they are not supposed to. The reason to avoid LT over a neoplastic growth or its surroundings is that we do not want to stimulate an already overstimulated cell line that is having a negative biological effect. Light does not distinguish between healthy or cancerous cells. Plus you would be having a pro-angiogenic effect and potentially facilitating cell dissemination, although a link between LT and an increased rate of metastasis has never been proven. Benign growths should also be avoided, since the increased metabolism could also have unwanted effects.

As happens with non-cancerous cells, the whole truth may be more complex; the net effect probably depends on both the type of cancer (cell line) and the parameters used (wavelength and dose, at least), plus other factors we may still ignore. For instance, using an *in vivo* model of squamous cell carcinoma, Myakishev-Rempel et al. found no effect on tumor growth after irradiating tumor-bearing mice with 5 J/cm^2 of red light.[403] Using a higher dose over squamous cell carcinoma tumors in hamsters, however, another study found an increase in progression and severity of the disease.[404] *In vitro* irradiation of the malignant osteosarcoma MG63 cell line stimulates growth with certain wavelengths but not others,[405] independently of the dose, while dose-dependent growth/inhibition was reported in different cancer cell lines (EMT-6 and RIF-1)[406] under red light stimulation. Neoplastic cells could be more responsive to laser stimulation than normal ones, according to the *in vitro* experiment published by Werneck et al., which also showed a significant influence of wavelength and irradiation time[407] (more irradiation time also means more cumulative dose). Neoplasias could also be more resistant to cell inhibition with very high dosages, and some authors relate this to cancer stem cells and their potentially increased capacity to overcome overproduction of reactive oxygen species.[408]

There are at least two scenarios where laser may not be such a bad idea. However, in each of these as well as virtually any scenario that involves a malignancy, there is always the risk that laser will stimulate the cancer and so written letters of disclosure and consent are highly recommended. The first is to prevent or treat surgical site complications after resection of a tumor where the pathology report makes you feel comfortable about the margins. You may think: "how far do I have to be from a tumor site, or from a previous tumor site, to consider LT to be safe?" There is no straight answer. Some types of neoplasia have a confined *in situ* growth, others can have relatively distant satellite nodules and even skip metastasis, as is seen in osteosarcomas or synovial sarcomas. An increase in tumor growth or recurrence has never been reported in the following clinical studies in human patients, but some of them are very recent and/or do not specifically evaluate the risk of recurrence or metastasis after LT.

- Head and neck cancer and chemotherapy- and radiotherapy-induced mucositis: although some studies show better results than others, no negative effects have been described. A growing body of evidence is accumulating regarding the benefits of LT for these patients, and guidelines and protocols have been published.[64, 65, 238, 409]
- In women who undergo mammary lumpectomy and develop radiation-induced dermatitis: initial studies with light emitting diode (LED) treatment did not find a therapeutic effect[410], but recently a study was published using LT with good results (not placebo-controlled).[411]

- Post-lymphadenectomy lymphedema: LT has been used for some years now to treat secondary lymphedema of the arm. Systematic reviews seem to conclude LT does help significantly.[412]

The second scenario is as palliative care at the end of a patient's life. If the patient's condition is severe and you're certain that he is nearing his end, but want to provide some heightened quality of life, LT may be an option. It can help to treat the inflammation and pain associated with certain types of cancer.

Solid tumors are also characterized by a certain degree of hypoxia, extracellular acidosis, and lack of cell nutrients.[413] This situation is similar to wounds to some extent, since they both trigger the same inflammatory mediators, which in this case can be released by tumor cells, by the stroma, or by other cells attracted to the site. The shared inflammatory mechanisms and the effect of LT on their control could explain the results obtained by Ottaviani and her team in 2016 when they found that laser irradiation of cultured melanoma cells increased their growth, but once implanted in live mice, laser irradiation of the mice decreased tumor progression.[414] This is not meant to encourage you to treat your oncological patients; the aim is to show that a lot more research is needed in this field, which could change our black-and-white traditional paradigm.

10.2.3   Pregnant uterus

There has never been a single report of a miscarriage or any deformity that can be linked to LT, but this is on everyone's list of no-no's. For pregnant veterinarians and technicians, the combination of clothing and the arm's length treatment distance mitigates any risk. Laser can affect muscle tone and blood flow, so although it is theoretically unlikely to have any effect, avoid performing laser treatments around the abdominal area of pregnant patients for medical legal reasons.

10.2.4   Recent infiltration of joints with steroids/ NSAIDs

LT directly over the site of a recent intramuscular or intra-articular injection can cause tenderness, swelling, and pain. The main reason is that the local drug concentration is very high, some of these drugs are photosensitive (others heat-sensitive), and this combination can lead to a flare-up. A standard recommendation is to wait the biological half-life of the drug (usually about 7–10 days) after the injection to treat over the site. Treating before an injection has no contraindication since the light is absorbed within nanoseconds of treatment, so if you want to inject, do the laser treatment first.

10.2.5   Thyroid

It has been advised to avoid laser over the thyroid gland. This organ is delicate, already very metabolically active, and the number of people being diagnosed with thyroid nodules is growing, so there are some concerns about potential uncontrolled stimulation of thyroid function both in medical and veterinary practice.

Could you send a patient into a thyroid storm? We are not aware of any single such report. There are a few animal studies on the effect of LT on thyroid activity, though. A dose of 4 J/cm^2 over the thyroid of mice increased their thyroid hormone production, without morphological changes,[415] but higher doses had previously been reported to potentially increase vessel diameter and numerical density of pinocytotic vesicles.[416] On the other hand, a study in 6-month-old rabbits found after repeated treatments that the effect was a decrease in total T3 and T4 serum concentrations, and an increase in serum TSH.[417] Another study showed a variable effect of infrared laser irradiation depending on age: laser increased the size of the thyroid capillaries in very young Wistar rats and had the opposite effect in older ones.[418]

One of the most interesting reports in this field was a study in people with chronic autoimmune thyroiditis. In a randomized, placebo-controlled clinical study, LT was able to dramatically decrease the need for thyroid replacement therapy and decreased some of the auto-immunity markers.[419] The potential for this use had been previously pointed out in the chronic autoimmune thyroiditis pilot study.[420] The same authors also found LT increased the levels of transforming growth factor (TGF)[421] and improved thyroid parenchyma vascularization.[422]

LT may have an impact on thyroid function even if laser is not directly applied over the thyroid area. Researchers have found some protocols applied to the mandible have no effect on thyroid activity,[423] while others demonstrated an effect on serum levels of T3 and calcium – which nevertheless remained within the normal range.[424]

The take-home message is: try not to aim at the thyroid area or focus a high dose specifically over the gland, and don't treat the neck of hyperthyroid patients, but otherwise treat cervical conditions whenever laser is indicated.

10.2.6   Other extra precautions

- As obvious as it may seem, do not laser over active bleeding: laser will stimulate blood flow into the area, which will increase the bleeding. If the bleeding is minimal, this may not have consequences, for example right after closing a spay incision, but to improve the situation you should apply some cold and light pressure to the wound first, then consider LT after bleeding has completely stopped.

- Be extra cautious in epileptic patients: it is known that pulsing visible red light as an aiming beam can trigger epileptic seizures in humans (make sure the pet owner and other people in the room are not epileptic themselves), and although most of the energy will be delivered using invisible light (infrared), LT devices generally use a visible pulsing red light. Laser can be considered in some epileptic patients provided the patient does not see the flashing red light at all, we are not working around the head, and the matter has been discussed with the owner. Why the head? When treating over the temporal, frontal, parietal, and occipital areas (brain projection areas), be aware of the fact that the skull is relatively transparent to the laser. It has been proposed that a power density of 1.6 W/cm^2 applied transcranially is equivalent to 1.1 W/cm^2 applied directly to an exposed cortex.[172] I had two personal communications from colleagues describing epileptic episodes after laser treatments for two wounds over the skull, in patients who had not previously been diagnosed as epileptics. So it is possible that the changes in cerebral blood flow unmask a cryptogenic/secondary epilepsy. I would also be especially cautious if I had to treat the neck of an epileptic patient with high power, since it can also affect cerebral blood flow.

- Refer to section 9.2.1, "Laser therapy in growing animals"; again, it is not an absolute contraindication, just a particular type of patient that can benefit a great deal from LT but already has a higher metabolic rate, so dosing and frequency of treatment should be adjusted.

• LT has often been avoided as a precaution in patients on photosensitizing medications. This is because, at least in theory, those patients could overreact to a certain amount of light (mainly ultraviolet) and develop a rash or another type of skin reaction. The list of potentially photosensitizing agents includes antihistaminics, sulfonamides, some essential oils, and tetracyclines, among others. Some herbal supplements such as *Hypericum perforatum* have also been described as potentially photosensitizing. Photosensitivity has also been described in lupus and secondary to severe liver disease. However, there is no reported case of laser having adverse effects in photosensitive patients, or in those on photosensitive medication. Current advice is to create a list of photosensitive medication and the peak wavelength of radiation required to activate the drug.[425] It is always advisable to wash off any topicals, such as antiseptics and massage oils/creams, before applying LT.

• Concerning the contraindication to using LT over the gonads: considering masculine gonads are more superficial and accessible, and how heat-sensitive they are, we would avoid treating the scrotal area with a high power, but that would be the only precaution. Navratil and Kymplova considered it more of a doubtful contraindication than a real danger.[426] Nevertheless, their article was published in 2004, before class IV therapy lasers were in use.

• When treating areas with reduced or absent sensitivity, keep that fact in mind, since you won't get any feedback from the patient. Just keep a hand in contact with the treatment surface to be fully aware of the temperature, or in the case of a wound, treat it as you would other wounds, but never slower.

• Although they are not very frequent nowadays, it is still possible to find ID tattoos on some patients; avoid that area, since the ink can absorb the light and cause pain (Fig. 10.5).

10.2.7 Compliance and regulatory considerations

We are not going to bore you with the paperwork involved in making sure your clinic complies with whatever state/province/country agency governs the use of laser-emitting medical devices. About half of that responsibility falls on the manufacturer/distributor of the laser, to provide the appropriate information

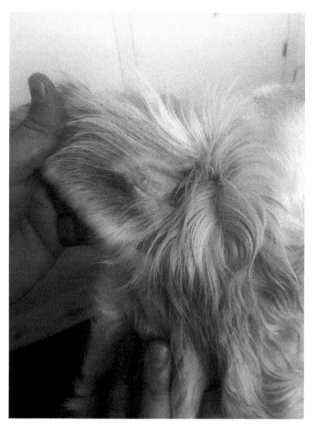

Figure 10.5 Ear ID tattoo in a patient with ear canal inflammation. Direct laser over the tattoo should be avoided, for example by covering it with your finger.

about their device as well as which safety categories it falls under. The other half of that responsibility falls on you to research the local laws and points of contact at the appropriate agencies.

That said, here is a (by no means comprehensive) list of topics you'll need to address in order to stay compliant and safe.

• Appointing a Laser Safety Officer, and the responsibilities of the person in that role.
• Training your staff on laser safety.
• Training your staff on the basic usage of the device.
• Laser warning signage: what it needs to look like and where it needs to be hung.
• Calculating the Nominal Ocular Hazard Zone (NOHZ).
• How to handle windows into the laser therapy room.
• Whether/how to handle inflammable gases (e.g. oxygen) around the laser.
• Setting up a door interlock circuit (which shuts

off the laser if the therapy room door is opened), if required.

10.3 How to charge for therapy and when

Part of your implementation plan should be how much and when to charge for LT. Without a pricing structure, you risk performing treatments as freebies, and this will be setting very low expectations if you want to increase the price later on. Do not devalue your clinical services, and consider that sometimes several visits are necessary to get an improvement; you may regret not charging anything for that time and effort.

The answer to the question about whether it is OK to do any free laser treatments is very personal. These are examples of particular situations in which you may want to consider it.

- During the first week or 2 weeks that you are trying LT. Some manufacturers will allow you to have this trial period, during which you may want to call in some friends, treat your staff's pets, or invite some clients to try this new modality you are considering.
- You want to try treating a condition for which you have not found any literature, and you are kind of thinking, "I know it will not hurt, but can LT really help here?" Most cases will need a few sessions to respond. Again, remember the time you will spend on this case.

Here are some of the factors you will want to consider when setting your prices.

- Will LT be an adjunct treatment in the visit or will the patient come just for the laser session?
- How much time will the session take? Note that it can range from 90 seconds to 20–30 minutes.
- Will the treatments be performed by the vets or the nurses?
- How many treatments do I expect the patient will need?

The following is a guide to help you formulate a plan; it includes average pricing for the US, UK, and Spain, but you may change it according to your business model and demographics.

POSTSURGICAL INCISIONS: £10, $8–15, AND €5–10

Unless you are using very low-cost business models, this is an almost invisible extra charge on a surgery bill in case you decide to make it non-elective, but with enough surgeries per week this is a very solid revenue stream. Yes, non-elective LT is an option: is bipolar coagulation elective to the owner because you just purchased it? The same applies here to a certain extent. Again, as a good surgeon, most of your incisions don't have trouble healing, but if you could improve it even more, isn't that valuable? Not convinced? Next time you have a long wound/incision, laser just the cranial (or caudal) half. You'll almost certainly notice a difference in healing in as little as a few days.

ORAL TREATMENTS: £10, $8–15, AND €5–15

A post-extraction or gingivectomy treatment takes less than 2 minutes and makes a difference in terms of swelling and pain. Some of these will be a one-time treatment, and others can benefit from a second treatment at the recheck. A full mouth gingivitis treatment may take up to 5 minutes.

WOUNDS: £10–30, $15–35, AND €12–30

Not all wounds are the same size and severity/extension, so the range of charges varies. Laser wound treatment can be as short as 1 minute or as long as 15 minutes. If you are managing the wound with bandages, or if it is a wound that requires surgical or extensive treatment in this phase, consider the costs of it. You can charge a package price, including bandage changes and laser as part of routine wound management – this way you will not overwhelm the client.

ORTHOPEDIC PROCEDURES: £20–30, $25–35, AND €15–20

You can consider starting to treat these patients even before surgery; in some cases this has been shown to decrease recovery time and improve quality of repair. This prep treatment would be the night before or the morning of the surgery, and then often the charging structure mirrors the number of interactions with the patient in his surgical journey: one treatment postsurgically (day of surgery, before you put on any bandage if that is the case), one or two follow-up treatments (on already scheduled follow-up visits) and ideally eventually blending into a rehabilitation plan that would include laser therapy.

ACUTE TRAUMAS: £25–30, $25–35, AND €15–25

Sprains, strains, fractures, roadside accidents, and other acute traumas can be treated immediately with LT (once stabilized) to decrease inflammation and pain. The treatment protocol depends on the severity of the trauma, tissues involved, etc., but often 3–6 treatments will be enough and can make a big difference.

CHRONIC PAIN CONDITIONS: £25–30, $25–35, AND €15–30

The price range is wide, since it does not take the same amount of time to treat the tarsus of a Poodle as the spine, hips, and knees of a Labrador. Also, if this is part of a rehabilitation plan, you may want to pack different modalities into the session price.

People comply more when they feel that they are getting a discount. Since LT is most often not a one-and-done modality, you may want to offer a bundle discount, generally 15–20% or a "buy five and get the sixth free." For more long-term treatments, you can bundle in 10 or 12 visits. This will increase compliance with the treatments, and has two further advantages: 1) payment upfront and 2) you are more likely to get to see that patient for the full treatment prescription and so your predicted efficacy will be higher. Also, every time your clients see you, you have the opportunity to solidify your relationship with them, find out more about the patients' progress in daily activities and behavior, and educate them on the variety of other services you offer for their best friend's benefit.

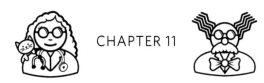

CHAPTER 11

Implementation of laser therapy in practice

Medicine is not only a science; it is also an art. It does not consist of compounding pills and plasters; it deals with the very processes of life, which must be understood before they may be guided.

— Paracelsus

11.1   Early implementation

There is no standard way for practices to integrate laser therapy (LT) into their workflow, but a plan has to be made to make the most of your new laser. The only truly bad plan is no plan. Pricing plans were discussed in Chapter 10, because they should be formulated even before purchasing a laser. All good plans share some foundations, so keep these in mind as a general framework.

1. **Prepare yourself:** get trained and do your studying. You got to this section of the book so you probably have step one checked. You don't need a PhD in lasers, but for starters you need a good core knowledge of which patients LT can help, why, and to what extent. Then you should learn about the important parameters, treatment regimes, how to adapt your treatments to each patient, and so on. Combine external resources with those provided by manufacturers, and try to stay updated in the field; yes, a lot will be coming in the next years! You must **have a pricing plan** from the beginning, before you actually start offering the service, although it's not uncommon to reformulate it later based on what you learn about your demographics in the early stages of implementation.

2. **Get your staff on board:** integrating LT in your patient care requires them to know the clinical benefits. Not just from the theory side, because they may also experience laser treatment with their own pets, or participate in sessions with the patients. Having your staff on board with LT can be more important than any external marketing, even if they are not the ones to perform the treatments.

    Of course, LT is not just about holding a magic light on top of the patient. All people using LT should be properly trained, for both the efficacy and the safety of the treatment. But the learning curve is quite fast, modern technology makes most devices easy to use, and a growing number of learning resources are available. If new staff join the practice, make sure they also get quality training. Encourage continuing education. You could even program case presentations and discussions.

    Also, everybody should know how to explain LT to clients. The person on the front desk does not need to use the same language or depth of detail as the clinical staff, but they absolutely need to know enough to help spread the word. Consider composing a script for a more homogenous explanation of the benefits and the top ten conditions to treat, for instance, so that when owners of pets with those conditions call in to schedule appointments, they can set the stage for this new (laser) technology.

3. **Make sure the laser is present:** the more visible and easy to reach, the more frequently it will be used. Have the laser device placed in a safe but accessible location (locked mode if not in use, for safety reasons), not inside a box in the darkest room.

4. **Let people know** you have a new, safe treatment to offer. Prepare and display information (boards, leaflets, testimonial binders, on digital screens, etc.). Use pictures of real cases, with before/after images if appropriate. Make videos about LT that you can use online but also on the computer or the waiting room screen if you have one. Manufacturing or distributing companies often have display material or information that can help get you started.

    Update your website, email your clients, and use social media. Who does not love pictures of patients in their doggles? Testimonials of successful cases will also help and add credibility, whether you include them on boards, videos, or emails, etc. If some good clients are willing to share information about LT in their social media, this can attract extra attention. Local press and magazines can be an option and reach a different target audience with less intense use of social media. And if you get the attention of the TV or radio, your audience will surely increase.

    Also, let your colleagues know about your new therapy; some of them will refer cases to you for laser treatment if they know about its uses, so consider gathering some information for them in the format you prefer, whether it's a newsletter, a professional journal, or a lecture, for example.

5. **Your laser session should be enjoyable for the patient, the therapist, and the owner.** This is actually easy to achieve, since the patient is going to experience pain relief and endorphin release; go with it. Come on: it is one of the occasions when we do something to our patients they actually like (Fig. 11.1).

    Try to work in a patient-friendly and fear-free way, at least as much as you can in that particular environment (Fig. 11.2). Really, decreasing your patient's fear and anxiety is ALWAYS worth it. Most canine and some feline patients will feel less stressed if treated and handled on the floor, rather than on a table, so please consider that. Some will like to be lying straight on the floor (Fig. 11.3), and

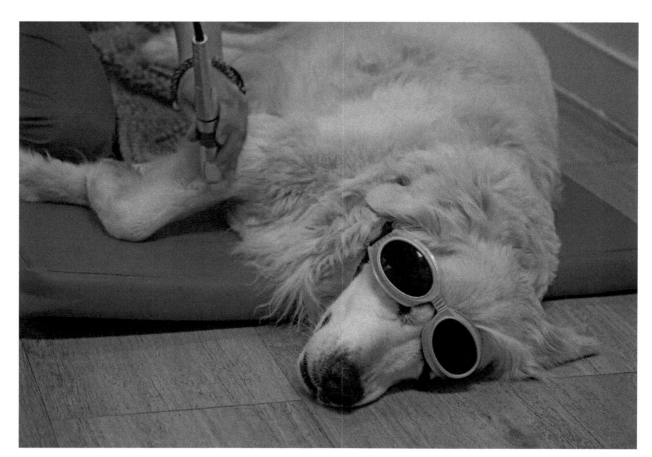

Figure 11.1 Patient relaxing during laser therapy.

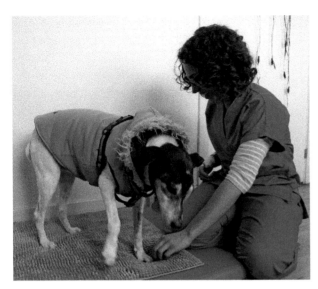

Figure 11.2 A warm, soft, quiet place has been prepared for this senior dog.

others will prefer to lie on a mattress or similar surface. Of course, many cats will prefer to be treated inside their carrier (removing the top) and that is an option for head/mouth and spine treatments, but usually not for limb problems. Some of your patients will require longer or multiple treatments, so make sure you and the owner take comfortable positions. Of course, most owners will love to see their pets in doggles.

6. The place where treatments take place has to be **safe, in terms of optical hazards**: if there are windows, consider blocking the view to avoid people or patients outside being accidentally pointed at with the laser beam. Avoid mirrors or highly reflecting surfaces; for instance, put an anti-slip mattress or a blanket over the steel table. At least, be aware of where those reflecting surfaces are, to avoid pointing the beam in that direction.

7. **Keeping treatment records is a must.** Just as with your other treatments, it is the only way we can reflect on what to change if we do not see the expected improvement, or keep track of the parameters that give the best results. Evolution since the last treatment, pain assessment, and treatment parameters should be recorded at every session. The treatment parameters should include dose, which also means the treatment area that has been calculated.

   Keeping track of treatments can also help you monitor what percentage of patients receive LT, whether the use is increasing or not, and who is using it more.

Next, we will propose several examples of implementation strategies, and help you decide how to answer the questions, "who do I start treating?" or "which should be my first patients?" Some strategies may be

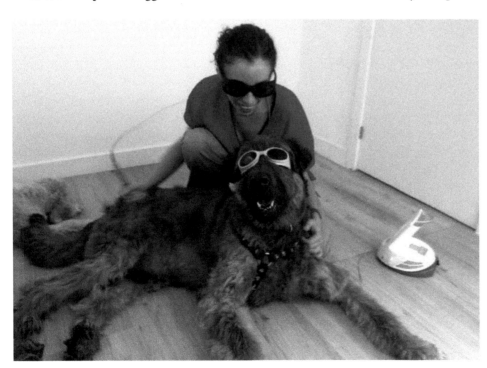

Figure 11.3 Other cool-seeking patients prefer to be straight on the floor.

used together, and others are incompatible. Choose and customize for your particular situation from the following list of ideas.

- **Patients with chronic pain conditions.** For instance, about 20% of our patients over 1 year of age suffer from osteoarthritis (OA) – this is not the only condition needing chronic pain management but probably the most common one. Chronic pain requires a multimodal approach and now you will be offering an option that will likely reduce the need for drugs, which are not free of side effects.

  NOTE: There are a couple of ways to look at combination treatments, especially when it comes to pharmaceuticals, since pet owners (and you, for that matter) are so used to a given result. If you keep the patient on the drugs and add laser, you will likely see an increased response. At that point you (and the owner) can decide if that heightened activity is desired (especially for show or competition animals). But you may decide to wean the patient off the drugs (once an improvement has been noted with LT) to see where they end up. Most likely by the time you get them off the drugs completely, you'll find that their activity (and pain and quality of life) measurements level off pretty close to where they were while on the drugs. This would NOT be a tie. This would be a BIG WIN, to be able to have pharmaceutical-level response without the drugs and their long list of potential side effects.

- **Conditions with the greatest clinical response.** The more confident you become about the clinical results you achieve with LT, the better you will convey that to your clients and the more they will accept laser treatments. If you are the kind of person who gets discouraged unless you see strong and fast results – someone who says, "how am I going to charge for a treatment if I do not have a high likelihood of success?" – then wounds (especially chronic and complicated ones) are probably your best chance of growing in confidence. Otitis, acute trauma, and chronic back pain are also on the top ten list of successfully treated conditions, although not all of them will need the same time to respond or achieve a similar degree of improvement. And from there, you and your staff will start to broaden the recommendations as you feel more confident.

- **A reduced price package for (almost) all post-ops.** Not only will your rate of postsurgical complications decrease (even more), but even the uncomplicated wounds will heal faster and better, and the hair will regrow faster as well. Sad as it is, many pet owners will judge the surgical procedure by the clipping (very sad) and how pretty the incision looks (not that sad: usually the prettiest incisions feel more comfortable and heal better). So improving all of these can go a long way with everyone. Adding a small amount (it will take little time to treat an incision) to the price of your surgeries will be unnoticeable for your clients, but at a certain volume of surgeries it really adds up. The exception, as you know, would be the oncological procedures, at least as a general rule.

- **Everything that walks through the door at low cost.** While you need to be aware of the few contraindications, your infrared laser is absolutely safe, and many patients respond favorably after a single treatment. For this reason, many practices now include LT as a part of their standard visit. This way, every owner gets not just information about the service, but also an initial experience. If you just slightly increase the price of the visit, revenue can become very significant. If you don't want to do this for every standard visit, consider doing it for certain types: geriatric check-ups, dental visits, otitis, rehabilitation visits, and so on.

- **Making use of the waiting room:** you can take advantage of the short time pet owners spend there to inform them about laser therapy in the most direct way, by having your receptionist or a nurse trained in LT and using a small, dedicated exam/treatment room. While the patient and owner are waiting, the receptionist offers this "complimentary" service in the treatment room after asking a few preliminary questions (i.e. "is there a known malignancy?" etc.). And while they treat, the pet owner is watching a short iPad video on laser, or the receptionist or nurse is just talking them through what the laser is and what it may help with. This way, the pet owner is already aware of the service and is likely to ask the vet if laser is right for their pet. If the answer is "yes," then the vet has already given one treatment free and so can create a bundled "package" price with an already-perceived discount. If not, no problem, it didn't cost any real money, just 5 minutes of the receptionist/nurse's time.

The clinician of us has a slight problem with this last strategy, thinking it carries the risk of an improper diagnosis (from a non-veterinarian receptionist), where a squamous cell carcinoma is mistaken for a simple wound, for instance. Plus there is the possibility of devaluing the therapy. Both are valid points, but I'll still emphasize that the waiting room is a VERY valuable place, confirmed by the amount of money big food and pharma companies spend on their marketing in that room. Either way, proceed with caution, and choose what's best for your clinic and its personnel.

11.2 How to integrate laser therapy with your current treatments

With LT, you are incorporating a new resource into your tool box. It is certainly one you will use often and in a variety of conditions, but it is not a magic wand. You are still going to prescribe drugs, perform surgeries, and use other modalities to help your patients. Yes, you will probably use less medication (or none in some conditions), a few surgeries will even be avoided, and recovery after injuries may need less rehab visits, but let's talk about how these coexist and integrate with laser.

11.2.1 Medications

As for compatibility, LT can be performed in patients under any oral medication; the only theoretical precaution would be with photosensitizing drugs, but as already mentioned, there are no reports of side effects nor a list of which drugs are activated at which wavelengths. Local drugs can be a different story: they can absorb the light and produce a local inflammatory reaction; that is why we absolutely avoid LT over joints that have been infiltrated with steroids or non-steroidal anti-inflammatory drugs (NSAIDs) in the last 1–2 weeks, and why it is recommended to clean topical products from a wound or from an ear canal before applying laser treatment.

One of the most common questions asked when clinicians start to work with LT is about how much and how fast it actually decreases the need for drugs. "When do I taper off painkillers?" "Is this patient going to need antibiotics or is LT enough?" Because this, together with how much improvement the patient can

achieve and how fast, is what REALLY matters to us as clinicians! And of course, part of the answer is that it depends on the case, but there are some guidelines.

My recommendation is that before you change your protocols (i.e. before you stop doing anything you were doing before you had the laser), just add it to your treatments. Give yourself some time to grow confident in the clinical results. If discontinuing an antibiotic course makes you uneasy, just don't do it (if justified). Keep treating the patients the same way, just adding the laser. After a few weeks or months you will feel confident to try some of the following changes.

- Antibiotics: first of all, whenever possible, please DO perform cultures and antibiograms as part of your routine to diagnose an infection. Overuse of antibiotics and resistance expansion is a very serious and growing problem, and a risk not just for our patients: there is resistance transfer from companion animals to their human companions (and vets!).[427]
- If there is a local superficial infection with mild signs, you may avoid antibiotics, especially if you can monitor the patient in upcoming sessions, which is usually the case with LT. You can still use antiseptics. If signs are severe or seem to be progressing, consider the antibiotic. An acute mild sacculitis or a hot spot can often be managed without antibiotics, but if the patient is hyperthermic and deteriorating it is probably time to think about other things as well.
- Keep using your (topical and/or systemic depending on the case) antibiotics for deep-seated infections such as bacterial cystitis, deep, purulent fistulae or otitis, osteomyelitis, etc. (please, please perform cultures).
- Analgesics: do not decrease the dose until the patient shows some significant improvement with LT. This can take very few days or several weeks, depending on the case, so too early a withdrawal could leave a gap of time between that and the effect of LT. Plus, it has been described how most of the effect of the NSAID often takes several weeks to be achieved. The exception, of course, would be a clinical contraindication to maintaining the use of those drugs (gastritis, renal conditions, and all those you know). In some cases you will be able to eliminate the need for analgesics, in others you will just decrease the dose or frequency, and in some you will maintain all

the prescriptions and add LT for better multimodal pain management.

11.2.2   Surgery

A few reconstructive surgeries will be avoided, and hopefully some ear canal ablations prevented ... but you still need to fixate your fractures, remove that infected tooth that is causing a sinus, decompress that spine that has lost pain perception today, and so on. The change is that the fracture and socket will heal faster and with less pain, and the spinal patient is likely to have an improved recovery. Some cases will not be that black-and-white, such as some partial cranial cruciate ligament tears.

Laser can be used before, during, and after surgeries. Treating beforehand improves the metabolic state of the tissue and this can manifest even as a significant difference in force plate peak vertical force 8 weeks after a TPLO.[284] During certain surgical procedures, such as after a non-oncological intestinal anastomosis or a cystotomy, laser can help you improve local oxygenation, reduce inflammation, and kick-start healing – and you know how important that is after an anastomosis. Most of your treatments will be postoperative, though, and you will be getting faster and better healing in general terms. You can review Chapters 7 and 9 for more details and treatment protocols.

11.2.3   Acupuncture

Acupuncture is one of the branches of Traditional Chinese Veterinary Medicine (TCVM). Some practitioners have a more traditional Chinese approach to acupuncture based on TCVM theory, diagnosis, and principles of treatment; others approach acupuncture from a more westernized perspective, since the effects can be explained (although not all, for the moment) in contemporary medical terms. Several endocrine, nervous, and immune mechanisms are involved, and a PubMed search will give you an idea of how extensive the research is concerning this topic. Having the best scientific basis whenever possible is actually compatible with a good knowledge of the traditional medical system that began thousands of years ago and led to the existence of the therapy we now try to explain in scientific terms. It is a fascinating medical approach that can broaden and change the way you work, and some excellent courses are available for veterinarians.

LT is compatible with your acupuncture treatments. Unlike acupuncture, LT is tolerated by all patients; if you want to combine both, LT can help your patient feel more relaxed before you do any needling; otherwise you can choose to do the laser before or after the acupuncture treatment.

Except in some severe cases, acupuncture treatments don't need as many initial visits as LT: while you may initially want to do 3–5 laser treatments in a week, you will probably needle the patient only 1–2 times; explain to the owner that some visits will be shorter than others and try to schedule both things for the same day.

Laser acupuncture

Acupuncture points can be stimulated in different ways. The traditional "dry needle" (Fig. 11.4) and moxibustion (Fig. 11.5) techniques were complemented in the 20th century by electric stimulation of the points, which facilitated a stronger stimulus and greater standardization in terms of time, intensity, and frequency of pulsing (Fig. 11.6). As the potential of laser therapy also spread in the last quarter of the 20th century, its use to stimulate such areas with different parameters

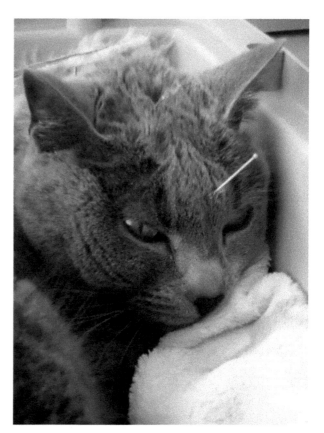

Figure 11.4 Dry needle acupuncture in a cat.

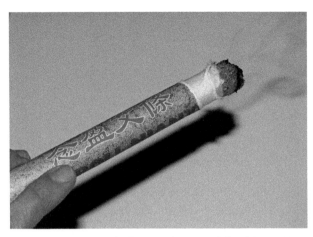

Figure 11.5 Moxa stick. A particular type of dried *Artemisia* leaves are rolled and burned next to the point to be stimulated.

of energy was gradually implemented among some acupuncture practitioners.

This should probably be caller laser acupoint stimulation rather than laser acupuncture. There is a literal laser acupuncture, mainly performed for research, in which real needles that are inserted several millimeters

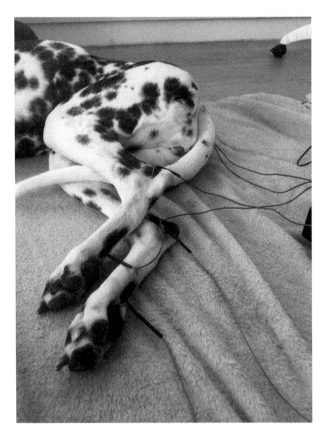

Figure 11.6 Electro-acupuncture in a canine patient.

into the body emit laser light.[428] What we are going to talk about, though, is holding the beam over the spot, at a given distance (0 to a few cm) and for a given time, with the aim of stimulating that particular acupoint. The first experiments were in the 1970s with very low-powered lasers. Nowadays, this can be performed with more powerful devices that offer more consistent penetration and shorter treatment times, although the power we use and need for laser acupuncture is much lower than the wattage (power) that is recommended to scan a whole area as in conventional LT. If acupuncture is the only use you want to give your laser, do not buy a class IV device: a good class III will be enough. If you have a class IV, and unless your probes or hand-pieces are very broad and unable to focus over a point, you can turn the power down to use it as a class III.

There is an obvious advantage when you use laser instead of needles: patient acceptance. If you are not an acupuncture practitioner, you would be surprised at how well most patients react during treatments, but there is still a percentage of them who find it difficult to tolerate needling and won't relax. And if they don't relax, the increase in cortisol levels inhibits the effects of acupuncture; in these cases, laser stimulation is an alternative, which all or almost all patients will accept. Even some owners who are very scared of needles themselves will like this option.

Effects

There are many objective ways in which the effects of laser acupuncture have been demonstrated, including measurements of physiological parameters, levels of biochemical mediators and markers,[429] and recently, advanced brain imaging, which shows how stimulation of acupoints activates certain areas of the brain, while stimulation of non-specific points does not.[430] It can also affect the blood flow velocity in cerebral arteries.[431]

The following are some of the reported effects; most of them, but not all, are related to analgesia. One common mechanism for laser- and acupuncture-induced analgesia is the release of endogenous opioids. The serotonergic system (5-HT1 and 5-HT2A receptors) is also involved.[432] Unfortunately, as we've seen with many papers on LT, not all parameters are always specified and they differ among studies, which makes it very difficult to compare them. Evidence supports some effects, and also the need for more quality research, however much of a cliché this sounds. The analgesic effect has been reported in experimental pain models, including neuropathic pain,[433] and clinical studies in people with musculoskeletal disorders, such as knee osteoarthritis,[434] subacromial impingement syndrome,[435] or rheumatoid polyarthritis,[436] to name a few. It's also been reported in the preoperative period; for instance, a recent report described improved analgesia in children after kidney biopsy[437]; and cats receiving laser acupuncture at ST-36 and SP-6 points (described in the section on "Acupoint selection") bilaterally prior to induction had lower analgesic requirements after spaying.[438] If you are curious, the study reports using 3 J/cm^2, 9 seconds/point, 904 nm, 124 Hz.

Laser acupuncture can also be anti-inflammatory, as described in experimental models and clinical studies. For example, 4 J/cm^2 of 830 nm light decreased carrageenan-induced paw edema in mice.[27] In human patients with arthritis, it increases antioxidant levels and decreases inflammatory biomarkers (4–6 J/cm^2), reduces periarticular swelling, and improves range of motion.[436, 439, 440]

Other reported effects in clinical studies are as follows.

- Improvement of symptoms (strength, ROM) in chronic post-stroke phase.[441]
- Decrease in morphine needs and hospital stay in newborns with neonatal abstinence syndrome.[442]
- Increase in salivary production in patients with Sjögren's syndrome[443] during treatment and several weeks after its cessation.
- Modulation of gastric motility.[444]
- It has an effectiveness similar to pharmacological treatment for nocturnal enuresis in children.[445]
- Decrease of postoperative vomiting in children – applied 15 min before induction and in the recovery room.[446]
- Improvement of asthma symptoms in children.[447]

A systematic review of randomized controlled trials that evaluated laser acupuncture vs. no treatment/sham procedure in people with different conditions concluded there was moderate positive evidence to support this use in the treatment of myofascial pain/musculoskeletal pain, postoperative nausea and vomiting, tension headache, and others.[448] A more recent systematic review with meta-analysis[449] included 49 randomized controlled studies on laser acupuncture and musculoskeletal disorders: two thirds of those reported a positive analgesic effect, and the remaining third, either no effect or inconclusive outcomes. The authors pointed out that these negative reports usually did not express parameters properly and/or used inadequate doses, and that half of them were actually of very low methodological quality, and they concluded that "the evidence is sufficiently robust to determine the effectiveness of laser acupuncture at long term for treating musculoskeletal conditions." According to the same review, its analgesic effects are not always immediately appreciated; the difference is more marked in long-term follow-ups. An idea to consider is to combine your laser acupuncture (distal points) with *regular* laser treatment of the affected area in musculoskeletal cases. Of course, the power used is very different, and as we have said, while you can turn down the power of your class IV laser to use it for acupuncture, you cannot make a class III laser (perfect for acupuncture) more powerful to allow you to treat a big area with a high enough dose using a scanning technique.

Laser acupuncture is more effective when the Traditional Chinese Medicine (TCM) pattern of disease is yang deficiency,[450] which makes sense since laser is energy/heat/yang. In TCM theory, yang represents heat, activity, movement (yes, in a very simplistic way). Yang deficiency patients show signs such as worsening in cold conditions. This means that your geriatric patients with low back pain and weakness or OA that worsens in cold weather will love your laser session even more – that works even if you do regular LT.

Parameters and technique

Wavelength: both red and infrared light have been used; infrared will have a deeper penetration, and longer infrared wavelengths will penetrate even more (with the outputs used in acupuncture, this means deeper as in a few mm). Some authors use the term laser moxibustion to refer to the use of infrared wavelengths similar to the infrared spectrum of moxibustion.[451]

Frequency: some of the published results have used continuous wave and others pulsed wave. I use the latter to help avoid a thermal effect. Some people hypothesize that each meridian/organ/location of disorder has its own frequency (for instance, 18,688 Hz for mental disorders, or 442 Hz to stimulate the Liver meridian) and therefore you should change it to be in tune with your target. The most popular series of frequencies are those from Nogier, Reininger, and Bahr.[452] Some practitioners have reported positive results, but this has not been scientifically proven.[453]

Dose: most studies use a dose of 1–50 J/cm². Some have proposed the use of low doses (0.5–2 J/cm²) to stimulate the acupoint, and higher ones (8–20 J/cm²) to sedate it, but this has not been proven, and some clinical studies use 20 J/cm² and more and still achieve stimulation. On the other hand, different doses/times of exposure can have different effects according to some studies. In He's paper on needle laser acupuncture,[428] red light from the needle had a physiological effect after 20 min of stimulation (total of 300 J, 600 J/cm²) but not after 10 or 30 min (both time and dose were different).

Now note that when we deal with acupoints or laser acupuncture, the treatment area, our target point, or the tip of the hand-piece/laser device can differ from 1 cm². So, for instance, if the tip of your laser is 0.5 cm² and you apply a total of 4 J to a point, you would be using 8 J/cm². If the tip is 0.25 cm², you would be applying 16 J/cm². The World Association of Photobiomodulation Therapy recommends a minimum dose of 1–6 J/point in its guidelines for class 3B lasers,[454, 455] which could mean a minimum of 2–12 J/cm². It makes sense to use a lower dose for more superficial acupoints, and a higher one for deeper points. For instance, the points *Tai-Yang* and SP-6 could be treated with 2–4 J/cm², while for the deeper points such as *Jian-jiao*, BL-23, or GB-21, I would use 10–20 J/cm².

Power: the authors recommend using 0.1 to 0.5 W, so 100–500 mW, although some studies achieve results with lower-powered devices, even 5 mW, but for a 5 mW device it would take more than half an hour to deliver 10 J. More power will reduce the treatment time and increase the density of photons that penetrate to the desired depth. Working at 0.2 W (200 mW) of average power (remember the difference between average and peak power!), applying 2 J takes 10 seconds. Applying 10 J would take 50 seconds at that same power, but by increasing it to 0.4 W the time would be cut in half. On the other hand, a very low-powered device working at 10 mW (0.01 W) would take more than 16 minutes to produce 10 J.

Also, power density can affect the biochemical response to laser acupuncture.[429] When selecting how high a power to use, consider very well the resulting power density. Laser acupuncture is usually performed with tips or probes that are narrow and concentrate the energy. If your tip is 0.5 cm² (on the broad side of tips for acupuncture), working at 1 W would give you 2 W/cm² of power density. Since the tip is not going to move during treatment (unlike scanning in LT) and the

distance from the skin is going to be very little or 0, it could be too much (especially in contact mode or with prolonged treatment time).

Whatever device you have, decide the dose you want (e.g. 10 J/cm²), check the area of the tip (e.g. 0.5 cm², which makes a dose of 5 J/point), decide the power you can and want to work with (probably lower if the animal is very sensitive; imagine 100 mW) and work out the treatment time this takes (5 J divided by 0.1 W is 50 s).

I usually work with 100–400 mW, at a distance of 0–10 mm from the point, for 10–50 seconds/point, to give a dose of 2 J/cm² (e.g. 100 mW for 10 s) to 20 J/cm² (e.g. 400 mW for 25 s).

Acupoint selection

The selection of points to stimulate can be the same as with conventional acupuncture, and laser also offers you the possibility of stimulating some points that because of their location are less commonly used, or very sensitive points that you feel the patient will not tolerate: you can combine needle stimulation of some points and laser for others.

Even at the risk of disappointing you, TCVM offers no cookbook of points, but these are some very commonly used ones that have also been proven, in a scientific way, to have an effect. Please note: these points are usually stimulated in combination with others. The described effects are just examples, and their use is much broader. I recommend *Xie's Veterinary Acupuncture*[456] and Schoen's *Veterinary Acupuncture*[457] if you want an acupuncture atlas (and more).

- LI-4 (*He-gu*): located in the forelimb, between the second and third metacarpal bones, in the middle of the length of this space (Fig. 11.7). It is reached from the dorsal surface toward the palmar, aiming at the third metacarpal. Very commonly used for immune regulation, nasal discharge, and general pain/inflammation – especially over the head and mouth.
- PC-6 (*Nei-guan*): in the medial side of the forelimb (Fig. 11.8). Find the distance from the transverse carpal crease to the elbow, and the point is one quarter of that distance from the carpus, over the interosseous space, between the flexor carpi radialis and the superficial digital flexor muscles. This point has an anti-nausea, anti-vomiting effect, reduces anxiety, and modulates cardiac rhythm, among others.

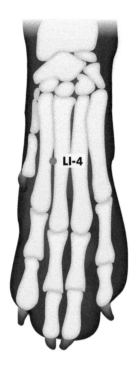

Medial   **Lateral**

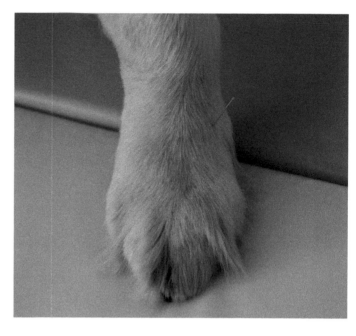

Figure 11.7 *Illustrator: Elaine Leggett.*

- ST-36 (*Hou-san-li*): this point lies on the cranio-lateral side of the tibia (Fig. 11.9). The needle with the red handle (ventral) shows point ST-36. The dorsal needle (blue handle) shows GB-34. It has a long, linear shape. As you palpate the tibial crest, go about 5–10 mm lateral to the cranial midline where the crest ends over the cranial tibial muscle. A very common point to regulate digestive problems and stimulate immunity, among others.
- SP-6 (*San-yin-jiao*): in the medial side of the

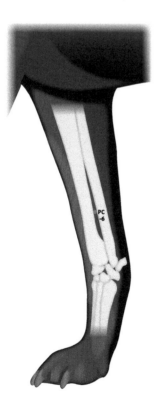

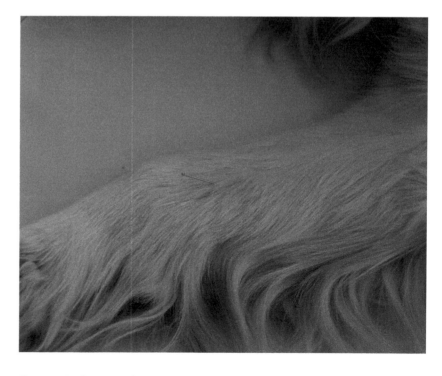

Figure 11.8 *Illustrator: Elaine Leggett.*

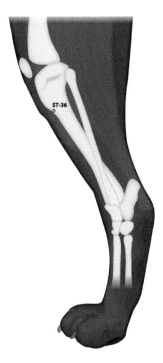

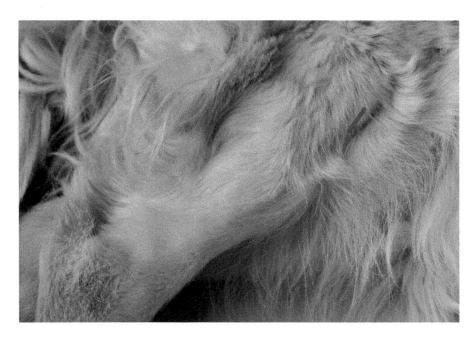

Figure 11.9 *Illustrator: Elaine Leggett.*

hindlimb (Fig. 11.10). Divide the distance from the tibial plateau to the tarsus into 13 parts; this point is approximately three parts from the tarsus, in a small depression you can palpate in the caudal side of the tibia, proximal to the medial malleolus. Very

commonly used for urogenital and caudal abdominal disorders and procedures.

- GB-34 (*Yang-ling-quan*): in the lateral side of the proximal tibia, in the depression felt just cranial and distal to the head of the fibula, over the fibular

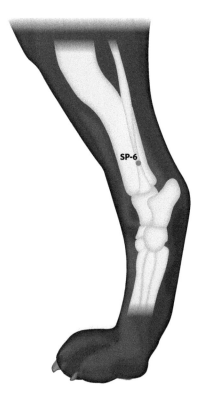

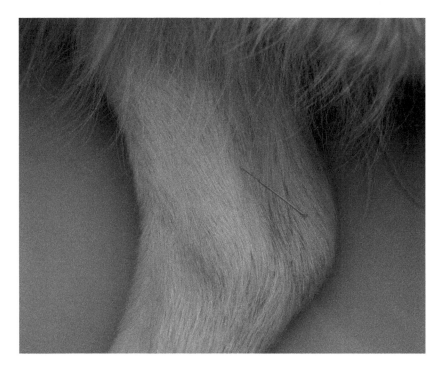

Figure 11.10 *Illustrator: Elaine Leggett.*

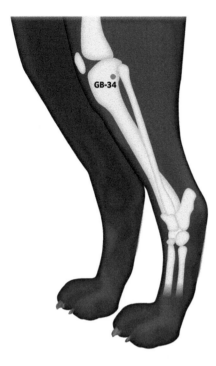

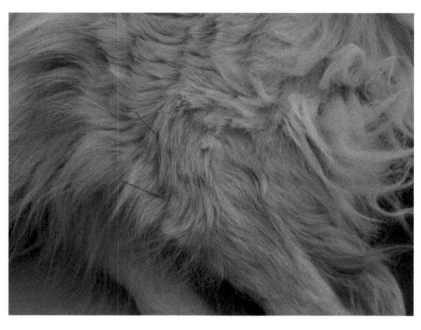

Figure 11.11 *Illustrator: Elaine Leggett.*

nerve (Fig. 11.11). The dorsal needle shows point GB-34. The ventral needle shows ST-36. Very commonly used for gastrointestinal disorders, especially vomiting, hindlimb weakness, and general pain management.

- *Bai-hui*: located in the dorsal midline, at the lumbosacral junction (L7–S1) – yes the same place you would put a lumbosacral epidural (Fig. 11.12). The cranial needle shows GV-4 (blue handle). The caudal needle (red handle) shows *Bai-hui*. It is used for hindlimb problems, including lumbosacral and coxofemoral conditions, among others.
- GV-4 (*Ming-men*): you can find this point on the

dorsal midline, between the spinous processes of L2–L3 vertebrae (Fig. 11.12). Used for lumbar disk problems and renal conditions, among others. Both this point and *Bai-hui* are the most efficacious points to warm up a patient – so those suffering from pain and weakness that worsen with cold will be especially happy to have these points/areas treated.

The time used to stimulate each point is very different from needle retention; an average acupuncture session takes about 20 minutes with the needles, but with laser we will stimulate each point for seconds, depending on

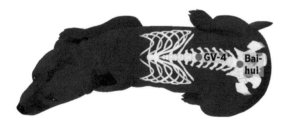

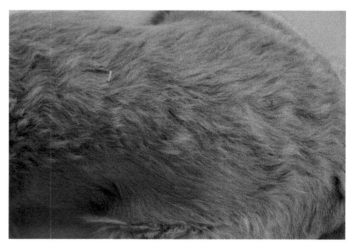

Figure 11.12 *Illustrator: Elaine Leggett.*

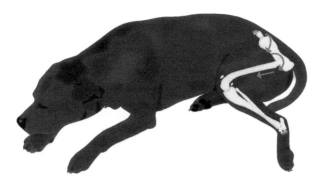

Figure 11.13 Suggested scanning of the hip and lateral femoral area.
Illustrator: Elaine Leggett.

the desired dose and output power (usually 10 to 60 s, although some studies take up to several minutes to achieve a certain dose if they use a low power device).

Another way to stimulate meridians in painful areas with the laser is the scanning technique, locally trailing a meridian pathway. This is preferably done in contact mode, using either your acupuncture hand-piece or a slightly wider one. For this method, a higher power can be used, since you will be moving the probe. Here are some examples of this technique.

- Scan the Gall Bladder meridian (Fig. 11.13). In the hip area, it covers the greater trochanter from cranial to caudal, and following the tract of the sciatic nerve distally, travels to the fourth digit of the pelvic limb.
- Scan the Large Intestine meridian in the elbow (Fig. 11.14). This meridian starts in the third digit and travels proximally to the nose. In the craniolateral aspect of the elbow, it runs between the extensor carpi radialis and the common digital extensor muscles, medial to the lateral epicondyle, and from there up to the acromion. We would treat from LI–8/9 (proximal radius) to LI–12/13 (distal third of humerus).
- Scan the Bladder meridian in a paravertebral treatment. This meridian starts at the eye, runs over the head and lateral to the spine and then travels down the lateral aspect of the hindlimb. The points will change depending on the spinal segments treated, but there are Bladder points lateral to each vertebral spinous process from T1 to L7 (also in the dorsolateral aspect of the neck).

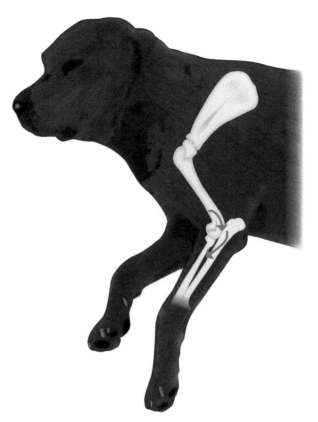

Figure 11.14 Suggested scanning of the lateral elbow area.
Illustrator: Elaine Leggett.

11.2.4 Other physical modalities

LT is synergistic with most physical therapies and modalities of regenerative medicine in its effects of stimulation of healing and decrease in inflammation and pain. LT is not a substitute for a full rehabilitation plan, but becomes an important part of almost all of them once you integrate LT into your practice. Experience will help you decide which modalities or combinations of them make more sense for each patient and each recovery phase.

Application of **cryotherapy** after LT is not recommended, since this would decrease blood flow after we have enhanced it. What about local cold prior to LT? That can actually be a great idea; recent studies show light penetration can be enhanced with prior cryotherapy.[458] This could be due to the reduction in skin and underlying tissue microcirculation (therefore less light is absorbed by hemoglobin and plasmatic water and more can travel through the tissue). Also, an experimental study showed cryotherapy followed by LT had a synergistic effect on the recovery of tendon injuries, improving both histological and biomechanical parameters.[459]

Therapeutic ultrasound (TU) is frequently used for the treatment of connective tissue such as tendon and ligament injuries or scar tissue. The transmission of the pressure of ultrasonic waves from the skin to deeper layers of tissue improves blood flow, muscle relaxation, collagen production, and tissue remodeling through thermal and non-thermal mechanisms. Some *in vitro* and clinical studies show LT can be superior to ultrasound in stimulating fibroblast activity,[136] but comparing different parameters necessarily produces different results; for instance, in the treatment of pain, LT is superior to TU in some studies,[460] but then in others (with low power and dose) TU has a more marked effect on anti-inflammatory biomarkers. The combination is possibly synergistic: a study on experimental tendon injury showed both TU and LT increased the amount of collagen production and the percentage of type I collagen, but the combination of both was even more effective, especially if LT was applied prior to TU.[138] A synergy in the analgesic effects was also described in a clinical trial using LT and TU for the treatment of hand osteoarthritis.[461]

Low-level electrical currents are often used in the form of transcutaneous electrical stimulation (TENS) and neuromuscular electrical stimulation (NMES). TENS provides analgesia by affecting the threshold and pathway of pain, while NMES use the electric impulse to stimulate muscle contraction (Fig. 11.15). Laser can be used with both in the same or separate sessions. LT before NMES can potentially help the patient make the most of the NMES, since according to animal models and human clinical studies it will improve the metabolism and contraction ability of the muscle and decrease muscle fatigue, exhaustion, and muscle stress indicators.[462]

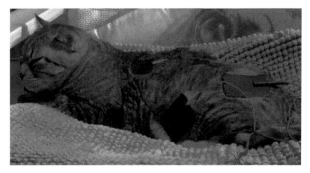

Figure 11.15 Feline patient receiving TENS therapy and simultaneous infrared heating.

Pulsed magnetic field therapy (PMF) uses magnetic fields to stimulate metabolism and healing processes. It is also used to decrease inflammation and pain, and can be combined with other modalities such as LT, TU, and others.[463] PMF therapy makes a great combination with LT, and can add to its physiological effects; the author has observed this effect in musculoskeletal pain and neurogenic bladder disorders.

Chiropractic and other manipulative techniques also combine very well with LT. In fact, chiropractors have been some of the first to incorporate LT into their practices, on both the human and the veterinary side. Myofascial pain, trigger points, and low back pain are some of the common conditions treated. LT prior to adjustments can help muscle relaxation and ease manipulation. A clinical study in human patients suffering from cervical pain due to vertebral facet dysfunction reported a potentiated efficacy when both chiropractic adjustments and LT were combined: patients improved their cervical mobility and reported less intense pain.[464]

11.2.5   Stem cells and platelet-rich plasma

Some of the most incredible advances in medicine are taking place in the fields of stem cell therapy, tissue engineering, and other areas of regenerative medicine. The aims of LT and other modalities of regenerative medicine are to increase tissue regeneration and modulate inflammation; therefore it makes sense to think there could be a potential synergy among them. That is why, among the ways to enhance cell viability and proliferation, researchers have investigated LT.

Stem cells are not just interesting because they can multiply once implanted to replenish a tissue; they also produce trophic factors with a paracrine action, i.e. they stimulate the growth of the host's own cells locally, increase vascularization, and modulate inflammation. Stem cells can be obtained from embryos, fetuses, or adults. Most clinical and preclinical studies use cells from adults, either from the same (autologous) or a different (heterologous) individual of the same species. Let's focus on adult stromal/mesenchymal stem cells (MSCs): these can be harvested from the bone marrow, adipose tissue, bone, dental pulp, periodontal ligament, and other locations. The stem cells we are starting to use in clinical practice are either from the bone marrow (BM-MSCs) or adipose tissue (AD-MSCs). So we either perform a bone marrow aspirate (easier than it sounds), usually from the wing of the ilium, or we take a piece of fat, generally from the inguinal area or falciform ligament.

When stem cells are cultivated, which usually takes about 20 days, one of the key questions is how to make them proliferate more; there is a critical number of cells that need to be implanted/administered to achieve an effect (several hundred thousand to several millions, depending on the case). After that, survival and success depend on the transplantation method – either in suspension or with different scaffolds, with or without growth factors – and recipient environment, both in terms of the microenvironment and considering the mechanical forces the area is subjected to.

Having said this, the following questions arise.

• Before the tissue is harvested, could LT improve local conditions for a more successful harvest?
• Can we encourage cells to survive and proliferate more while being cultured in vitro?
• Could preconditioning with LT improve local conditions in the area that will receive the stem cells?
• Would LT after implanting stem cells improve their viability and proliferation? Would that have a clinical effect?

In vitro experiments show LT increases human adipose stem cell viability and proliferation,[465] and the same results have been found in bone marrow mesenchymal stem cells: greater osteogenic potential after LT, plus an increase in extracellular levels of TGF-β, IGF-I, and ALP.[466] While growth factors increase, LT suppresses transcription factor NF-κB (via an increase in cAMP), and therefore the expression of IL-1β, IL-6, and IL-8; this also happens even when stem cells are previously challenged with lipopolysaccharide to experimentally induce inflammation.[467] These molecular changes lead to increased survival and proliferation. But stem cells don't just grow more and faster: they differentiate more into neurons and osteoblasts when treated with laser,[468] and all of these effects lead to improved tissue healing in experimental animals.[469] The optimal parameters to increase proliferation can be different from those to achieve maximal differentiation. A review of 73 publications concluded that both dose and power density influenced the results, and the maximum proliferation was achieved with 0.5 to 4 J/cm^2[470]. Power densities ranged from 2 to 125 mW/cm^2, with higher values in that range leading to more

proliferation. Also, irradiating cultures every day or every other day for a certain period gave better results than a single exposure.

Osteoarthritis and tendon and ligament injuries are the most common conditions in which stem cells are employed in clinical settings,[471, 472] but very promising results are being reported in inflammatory conditions of the nervous system,[473] spinal cord injuries,[474] inflammatory bowel disease,[475] and others. To answer the question about increased survival of stem cells and their clinical effect when combining them with applying LT to the animal, these are some of the fields in which the combination has been investigated with successful results in experimental models.

• Bone repair, and in particular in maxillofacial reconstruction: for example, LT has been used in the search for strategies to close large alveolar clefts in patients with cleft lips and palates. When dental pulp stem cells are treated in vitro with LT, they show enhanced osteogenic potential.[476]
• Myocardial infarction is a common cause of disease and death in humans, and stem cells are also being investigated in this field to help with recovery of the infarcted heart. In one particular study, treating stem cells with LT increased their survival, proliferation, and homing, which manifested as a decrease in the infarct size and cell death and therefore enhanced cardiac function.[477]
• Neurological injury: in a model of nerve crush injury, the combination of LT and stem cell implant provided better functional recovery than either therapy alone.[372]
• Hindlimb ischemia: treating the implanted stem cells with LT increased the angiogenesis, tissue regeneration, and functional recovery in a mouse model of hindlimb ischemia.[478]

Again, we know laser works. But these studies are actually *in vitro* and experimental. We can't just assume those laser-preconditioned cells that proliferate and work better in experimental animals will behave the same in clinical cases of a different species, and we still have questions about the best way to stimulate cells both in cultures and once implanted. The methodological heterogeneity of the studies does not help to determine which are the best parameters and the effect in clinical patients.[479] Clinical research will provide more answers to those key questions in the next years. My

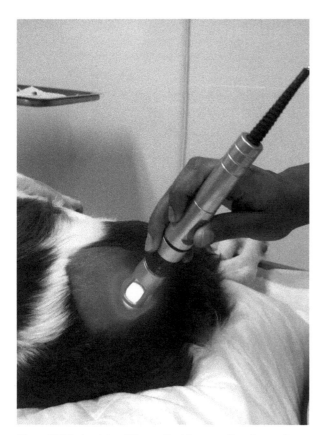

Figure 11.16 Applying LT over the hip area after stem cell infiltration of the joint in a case of severe hip OA.

several species: in a rabbit model where the Achilles tendon was damaged and treated with either therapy alone or in combination, both modalities by themselves led to a better repair when compared to no treatment (with no significant differences between them), but the combined treatment with PRP and LT was even more efficient.[143] The same was found in tenotomized rats, in which adding the two modalities enhanced type I collagen in the repaired tendon.[481] Similar results were seen in rat injured muscle: the combination of both therapies produced better histological scores than with either of them separately.[482] The same research group had previously found this combination also reduced the oxidative stress resulting from stretching injuries and modulated collagen production even better than the therapies did individually.[483] Although not all experiments conclude there is an additive effect,[484] at least there is no contraindication to trying this combination.

In fact, all three modalities can be combined. A clinical study (mentioned previously) reported good results with stem cells in combination with PRP to treat unilateral partial tears (≤ 50% as confirmed by arthroscopy) of cruciate ligaments. Those cases underwent a rehabilitation program after the intra-articular injection, which included LT and manual therapy once a week and a home exercise program for the first 8 weeks. Three months after treatment, a significant change was observed in functionality, pain, and arthroscopic parameters, including formation of new blood vessels and changes in fiber arrangement.[298]

guess is that the answers to most or all of them will be positive, but (again!) research has to demonstrate the optimal parameters, and clinical studies will take many years. Meanwhile, I suggest you treat those areas with moderate dose and power, according to the depth of the location and the state of the local tissue. That means for a wound/burn/superficial lesion you would use 1–4 J/cm², but about double for deeper-seated locations (Fig. 11.16).

The use of platelet-rich plasma (PRP) is also becoming more and more popular, as it is relatively easy to obtain and more affordable than stem cell therapy. Although experimental studies show positive results, not all clinical studies do. For instance, PRP did improve functionality and pain scores in dogs with OA,[479] but did not enhance osteotomy healing in dogs undergoing surgery for cruciate ligament rupture.[480] The combination of PRP and LT has been studied in

Like any new modality, we will continue to learn which treatments synergize with laser to best help our patients. And I'm sorry, but if you wait to see double-blinded studies with each possible permutation of treatments (control, laser + stem cells, stem cells + PRP, PRP + acupuncture, etc.), pull up a chair because it will be a while, especially with all the corporate interest (and conflicts of interest) out there between companies. But whether or not you expect to see a benefit from laser boils down to the question of whether whichever treatment you intend to enhance will benefit from better local circulation, tissue oxygenation, and cellular metabolism in the treatment area. If yes, then yes, laser will help.

The future light to be shed

The most fitting way we could think of to end this book is with a simple look forward. Though we clearly hope to be qualified enough to write this book and provide the insight we have given throughout, we also admit not to know everything. More than that, we as a community, both scientific and clinical, still have much to learn.

So as a tribute to the current limits of our knowledge, and in the hope of ever-so-slightly influencing the push to help us learn more, here is a quick list of questions/topics we collectively hope that people will spend time and resources to research.

FUNDAMENTAL SCIENCE

- Discover more specific resonant frequencies for a variety of tissue types.
- Uncover holographic techniques to better collimate light within tissue (https://www.ted.com/talks/mary_lou_jepsen_how_we_can_use_light_to_see_deep_inside_our_bodies_and_brains?language=en).
- Better understand the limits of pulse structure that can create photo-acoustic waves.

CLINICAL APPLICATIONS

- Light/brain interactions.
- Better understanding of the interaction of light with the immune system and its ability to help fight infection.
- Optimization of energy delivery to deeper tissues.
- Photodynamic therapy: using light to trigger tumor-specific drugs to kill cancer cells and bacteria.

Appendices

APPENDIX A

Pain assessment scales

A1 Glasgow Composite Pain Scale – short form

SHORT FORM OF THE GLASGOW COMPOSITE PAIN SCALE

Dog's name _____

Hospital Number _____ **Date** / / **Time**

Surgery Yes/No (delete as appropriate)

Procedure or Condition_____

_____

In the sections below please circle the appropriate score in each list and sum these to give the total score.

A. Look at dog in Kennel

Is the dog?

(i)

Quiet	0
Crying or whimpering	1
Groaning	2
Screaming	3

(ii)

Ignoring any wound or painful area	0
Looking at wound or painful area	1
Licking wound or painful area	2
Rubbing wound or painful area	3
Chewing wound or painful area	4

> In the case of spinal, pelvic or multiple limb fractures, or where assistance is required to aid locomotion do not carry out section **B** and proceed to **C**
> *Please tick if this is the case* ☐ then proceed to C.

B. Put lead on dog and lead out of the kennel.

When the dog rises/walks is it?

(iii)

Normal	0
Lame	1
Slow or reluctant	2
Stiff	3
It refuses to move	4

C. If it has a wound or painful area including abdomen, apply gentle pressure 2 inches round the site.

Does it?

(iv)

Do nothing	0
Look round	1
Flinch	2
Growl or guard area	3
Snap	4
Cry	5

D. Overall

Is the dog?

(v)

Happy and content or happy and bouncy	0
Quiet	1
Indifferent or non-responsive to surroundings	2
Nervous or anxious or fearful	3
Depressed or non-responsive to stimulation	4

Is the dog?

(vi)

Comfortable	0
Unsettled	1
Restless	2
Hunched or tense	3
Rigid	4

© University of Glasgow

Total Score (i+ii+iii+iv+v+vi) = _____

Glasgow Composite Measure Pain Scale: CMPS - Feline

Guidance for use

The Glasgow Feline Composite Measure Pain Scale (CMPS-Feline), which can be applied quickly and reliably in a clinical setting, has been designed as a clinical decision making tool for use in cats in acute pain. It includes 28 descriptor options within 7 behavioral categories. Within each category, the descriptors are ranked numerically according to their associated pain severity and the person carrying out the assessment chooses the descriptor within each category which best fits the cat's behavior/condition. It is important to carry out the assessment procedure as described on the questionnaire, following the protocol closely. The pain score is the sum of the rank scores. The maximum score for the 7 categories is 20. The total CMPS-Feline score has been shown to be a useful indicator of analgesic requirement and the recommended analgesic intervention level is 5/20.

Glasgow Feline Composite Measure Pain Scale: CMPS - Feline

Choose the most appropriate expression from each section and total the scores to calculate the pain score for the cat. If more than one expression applies choose the higher score

LOOK AT THE CAT IN ITS CAGE:

Is it?
Question 1

Silent/purring/meowing	0
Crying/growling/groaning	1

Question 2

Relaxed	0
Licking lips	1
Restless/cowering at back of cage	2
Tense/crouched	3
Rigid/hunched	4

Question 3

Ignoring any wound or painful area	0
Attention to wound	1

Question 4

    a)   Look at the following caricatures. Circle the drawing which best depicts the cat's ear position?

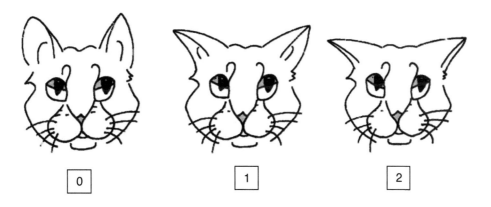

        0   1   2

    b) Look at the shape of the muzzle in the following caricatures. Circle the drawing which appears most like that of the cat?

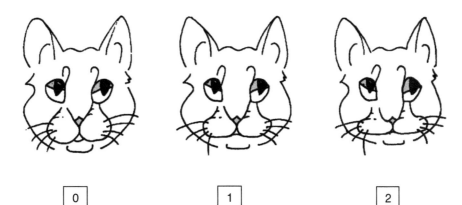

        0   1   2

APPROACH THE CAGE, CALL THE CAT BY NAME & STROKE ALONG ITS BACK FROM HEAD TO TAIL

Question 5
Does it?

Respond to stroking	0

Is it?

Unresponsive	1
Aggressive	2

IF IT HAS A WOUND OR PAINFUL AREA, APPLY GENTLE PRESSURE 5 CM AROUND THE SITE. IN THE ABSENCE OF ANY PAINFUL AREA APPLY SIMILAR PRESSURE AROUND THE HIND LEG ABOVE THE KNEE

Question 6
Does it?

Do nothing	0
Swish tail/flatten ears	1
Cry/hiss	2
Growl	3
Bite/lash out	4

Question 7
General impression
Is the cat?

Happy and content	0
Disinterested/quiet	1
Anxious/fearful	2
Dull	3
Depressed/grumpy	4

Pain Score ... /20

Canine Brief Pain Inventory

Description of pain:
Rate your dog's pain:

1. Fill in the oval next to the one number that best describes the pain at its **worst** in the last 7days.

   ○0   ○1   ○2   ○3   ○4   ○5   ○6   ○ 7   ○ 8   ○ 9   ○ 10

   No pain   Extreme pain

2. Fill in the oval next to the one number that best describes the pain at its **least** in the last 7 days.

   ○0   ○1   ○2   ○3   ○4   ○5   ○6   ○ 7   ○ 8   ○ 9   ○ 10

   No pain   Extreme pain

3. Fill in the oval next to the one number that best describes the pain at its **average** in the last 7 days.

   ○0   ○1   ○2   ○3   ○4   ○5   ○6   ○ 7   ○ 8   ○ 9   ○ 10

   No pain   Extreme pain

4. Fill in the oval next to the one number that best describes the pain as it is **right now**.

   ○0   ○1   ○2   ○3   ○4   ○5   ○6   ○ 7   ○ 8   ○ 9   ○ 10

   No pain   Extreme pain

Description of function:
Fill in the oval next to the one number that best describes how during the last 7 days **pain has interfered** with your dog's:

5. General Activity
   ○0   ○1   ○2   ○3   ○4   ○5   ○6   ○ 7   ○ 8   ○ 9   ○ 10

   Does not interfere   Completely interferes

6. Enjoyment of Life
   ○0   ○1   ○2   ○3   ○4   ○5   ○6   ○ 7   ○ 8   ○ 9   ○ 10

   Does not interfere   Completely interferes

7. Ability to Rise to Standing From Lying Down
   ○0   ○1   ○2   ○3   ○4   ○5   ○6   ○ 7   ○ 8   ○ 9   ○ 10

   Does not interfere   Completely interferes

Brief Pain Inventory, con't

8. Ability to Walk

    ○0   ○1   ○2   ○3   ○4   ○5   ○6   ○ 7   ○ 8   ○ 9   ○ 10

Does not interfere   Completely interferes

9. Ability to Run

    ○0   ○1   ○2   ○3   ○4   ○5   ○6   ○ 7   ○ 8   ○ 9   ○ 10

Does not interfere   Completely interferes

10. Ability to Climb Stairs, Curbs, Doorsteps, etc.

    ○0   ○1   ○2   ○3   ○4   ○5   ○6   ○ 7   ○ 8   ○ 9   ○ 10

Does not interfere   Completely interferes

Overall impression:

11. Fill in the oval next to the one number that best describes your dog's overall quality of life over the last 7 days.

○ Poor   ○ Fair   ○ Good   ○ Very Good   ○ Excellent

Texas A&M University College of Veterinary Medicine

Canine Lameness Assessment Questionnaire

Case Number _____   Owner's Name _____

Clinician _____   Dog's Name _____

Referring Veterinarian _____   Evaluator _____

Please **Read Instructions First:**

- Reply to the questions by **placing a vertical mark** on the corresponding line. This vertical mark corresponds to a place between the two extremes. The distance between your mark and the left end will be measured to quantify your response.

- Please **notice the labeling** on the left and right sides before marking it.

- When assessing your dog over the past week (or month), mark down his/her **usual condition.**

- **Thank you!**

1. How would you describe your overall assessment of your dog <u>in the last month</u>?

     poor   excellent

2. What kind of mood has your dog been <u>in the last month</u>?

     bad   good

3. How has your dog's attitude been <u>in the last month</u>?

     negative   positive

4. How frequently does your dog display comfort or "happy dog" postures (for example, lying on back with toy in mouth)? Not applicable: ☐

     rarely   frequently

5. Has your dog changed the <u>amount</u> of his/her daily activities?

            |_____|

            less   more

6. How willing is your dog to <u>play voluntarily</u>?

            |_____|

            not at all   very willingly

7. How often does your dog get exercise?

            |_____|

            less than once   all day
                                                               per day

8a. How stiff is your dog <u>when arising for the day</u>?

            |_____|

            not stiff   could not be
                                                         more stiff

8b. How stiff is your dog <u>at the end of the day</u> (post-activities)?

            |_____|

            not stiff   could not be
                                                         more stiff

9. Does your dog indicate any lameness at a walk?

            |_____|

            rarely   always

10. Does your dog indicate any pain when turning suddenly at a walk?

            |_____|

            rarely   always

Thank you for completing this questionnaire.

A5   Feline Musculoskeletal Pain Index (FMPI)

Veterinary Medicine
**Comparative Pain
Research Laboratory**

NOTES TO ACCOMPANY THE FMPI CLINICAL METROLOGY INSTRUMENT

Conditions of use:
- The FMPI is designed as a Clinical Metrology Instrument (Questionnaire) for the assessment of Feline Musculoskeletal Pain. It can be used in clinical research studies, and also by practitioners for individual case assessment.
- Use of this questionnaire in a commercial setting (e.g. company funded clinical trials) requires the permission for use of the FMPI under license from North Carolina State University.
- The FMPI will be acknowledged in any publication or report by citing the appropriate reference.
- The FMPI will be used only in the form presented here, and the format, wording and order of the questions and responses will not be changed.
- The FMPI must not be given to others.
- The FMPI must not be sold in any form.

The FMPI is a questionnaire with appropriate readability, reliability and proven discriminatory ability. *Full validity testing is continuing, and further versions of the FMPI may well take place in the future.*

Instructions:
1. The following instructions should be read to owners by the operator each time the FMPI is administered:
"This questionnaire asks you questions about your cat's ability to do various activities compared to what you think a normal adult cat without mobility impairment would be able to do.
Please read the questions carefully and place an 'X' in the appropriate box.
'Normal' is located here, and then there are various degrees of 'abnormal'. If the activity does not apply, such as if you do not have stairs in your home, check this box on the far right. <u>Owners should be encouraged to answer all questions at every evaluation, and only select 'Not applicable' if the question or activity truly does not apply for their cat.</u>

2. Upon completion of the questionnaire, the owner should return the questionnaire to the operator.

3. FMPI scores are calculated by assigning whole integer scores from 0 to 4, with 0 representing 'not at all', and 4 representing 'normal'.

4. The total FMPI score is the sum of scores for each question. Higher totals indicate less impairment with a possible range of (0-68). For analysis, total score or percent possible can be used. Calculation of percent possible is performed by taking the total score for the cat and dividing by the total possible points (the number of questions answered multiplied by 4).

FMPI%poss Score Q1-17 = (sum of Q1-17 scores) / (number of questions answered*4)

5. If repeat FMPI scores are acquired from an individual owner, they should not see their previous scores or responses prior to completing the questionnaire.

We welcome feedback on the FMPI. Please contact Dr. Duncan Lascelles using:
Duncan_Lascelles@ncsu.edu
The Comparative Pain Research Laboratory is very grateful to Morris Animal Foundation, Novartis Animal Health, and Boehringer Ingelheim Vetmedica Inc. for sponsoring the work that has led to the development and validation of the FMPI.

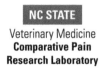

NC STATE
Veterinary Medicine
Comparative Pain
Research Laboratory

NAME: DATE:

FELINE MUSCULOSKELETAL PAIN INDEX

Please take some time to complete the following questions.

Please mark the circle that best describes your cat's ability to perform the following activities as compared to what you think a normal adult cat, without mobility impairment, would be able to do.

1. Walk and/or move easily?

○	○	○	○	○		○
Normal	Not quite normal	Moderately worse than normal	Barely, or with great effort	Not at all		Not applicable

2. Run?

○	○	○	○	○		○
Normal	Not quite normal	Moderately worse than normal	Barely, or with great effort	Not at all		Not applicable

3. Jump up (how well and how easily)?

○	○	○	○	○		○
Normal	Not quite normal	Moderately worse than normal	Barely, or with great effort	Not at all		Not applicable

4. Jump up to kitchen-counter height in one try?

○	○	○	○	○		○
Normal	Not quite normal	Moderately worse than normal	Barely, or with great effort	Not at all		Not applicable

Please rate your cat's ability to:

5. Jump down (how well and how easily)?					
O	O	O	O	O	O
Normal	Not quite normal	Moderately worse than normal	Barely, or with great effort	Not at all	Not applicable

6. Climb up stairs or steps?					
O	O	O	O	O	O
Normal	Not quite normal	Moderately worse than normal	Barely, or with great effort	Not at all	Not applicable

7. Go down stairs or steps?					
O	O	O	O	O	O
Normal	Not quite normal	Moderately worse than normal	Barely, or with great effort	Not at all	Not applicable

8. Play with toys and/or chase objects?					
O	O	O	O	O	O
Normal	Not quite normal	Moderately worse than normal	Barely, or with great effort	Not at all	Not applicable

9. Play and interact with other pets?					
O	O	O	O	O	O
Normal	Not quite normal	Moderately worse than normal	Barely, or with great effort	Not at all	Not applicable

Please rate your cat's ability to:

10. Get up from a resting position?						
O	O	O	O	O		O
Normal	Not quite normal	Moderately worse than normal	Barely, or with great effort	Not at all		Not applicable

11. Lie and/or sit down?						
O	O	O	O	O		O
Normal	Not quite normal	Moderately worse than normal	Barely, or with great effort	Not at all		Not applicable

12. Stretch?						
O	O	O	O	O		O
Normal	Not quite normal	Moderately worse than normal	Barely, or with great effort	Not at all		Not applicable

13. Groom himself or herself?						
O	O	O	O	O		O
Normal	Not quite normal	Moderately worse than normal	Barely, or with great effort	Not at all		Not applicable

14. Interact with you and family members?						
O	O	O	O	O		O
Normal	Not quite normal	Moderately worse than normal	Barely, or with great effort	Not at all		Not applicable

Please rate your cat's ability to:

15. Tolerate being touched and/or held?						
O	O	O	O	O		O
Normal	Not quite normal	Moderately worse than normal	Barely, or with great effort	Not at all		Not applicable

16. Eat?						
O	O	O	O	O		O
Normal	Not quite normal	Moderately worse than normal	Barely, or with great effort	Not at all		Not applicable

17. Use the litter box (get in and out, squat, cover waste?						
O	O	O	O	O		O
Normal	Not quite normal	Moderately worse than normal	Barely, or with great effort	Not at all		Not applicable

APPENDIX B

Goniometry

The purpose of this section is to facilitate your evaluation of the range of motion (ROM) of different joints when you assess patients and their progression. It describes anatomical landmarks, positioning of the patient, and the angle that is being measured. You can check the table at the end of Appendix B for measurements of each angle, according to different sources.

The authors would like to thank Dr. S. Salgado Sánchez DVM CCRP for her insight into this section and her help with the pictures.

B1 Forelimb

Bony landmarks

- Spine of the scapula.
- Humeral longitudinal axis: line from insertion of the infraspinatus muscle on the greater tubercle, in the proximal humerus, to lateral humeral epicondyle, in the distal humerus.
- Antebrachium longitudinal axis:
  - Lateral view: lateral humeral epicondyle to craniocaudal midpoint at the level of the ulnar styloid process.
  - Cranial view: line following medial aspect of the radius.
- Metacarpus:
  - Lateral view: longitudinal axis of metacarpals III and IV.
  - Cranial view: between longitudinal axes of metacarpals III and IV.

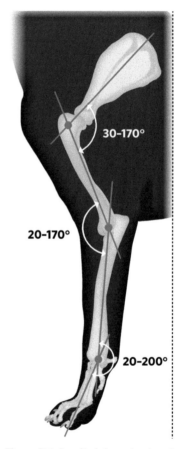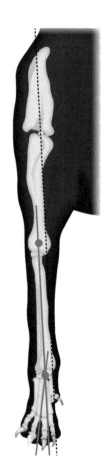

Figure B.1 Forelimb bony landmarks.
Illustrator: Elaine Leggett.

Shoulder

Shoulder flexion/extension

- Lateral recumbency.
- Humerus parallel to thoracic wall.

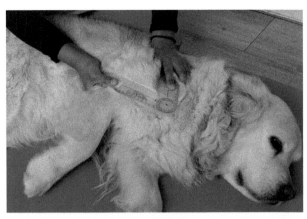

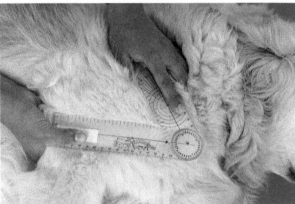

Figures B.2 and B.3 Shoulder flexion.

- The angle is determined by the line joining the scapular spine to the insertion of the infraspinatus muscle in the proximal humerus and the line following the humeral longitudinal axis.

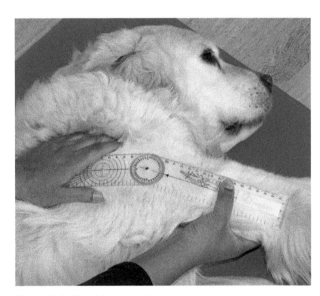

Figure B.4 Shoulder extension.

Shoulder abduction/adduction

- Cranial view.
- Standing position or lateral recumbency (preferred).
- Elbow and shoulder in extension.
- With scapula held against body wall, grasp the acromion with the thumb and forefinger of one hand or immobilize it with the back of the hand, and exert medial pressure on it to prevent movement of the scapula away from the body wall.
- One arm of the goniometer is parallel to the scapular spine, the other follows the humeral longitudinal axis. With the fulcrum over the shoulder joint, the outward (abaxial)/inward angle is measured from the zero position (parallel to the ground in recumbency, or perpendicular to it if standing).

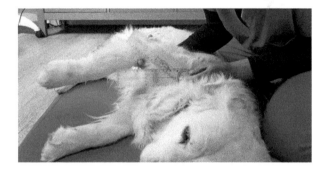

Figure B.5 Shoulder abduction.

Shoulder internal/external rotation

- Cranial view.
- Lateral recumbency (preferred).
- Elbow and shoulder in about 90° flexion.

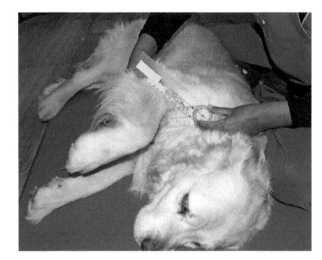

Figure B.6 Shoulder external rotation.

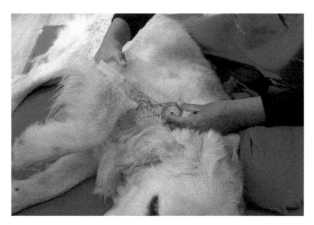

Figure B.7 Shoulder internal rotation.

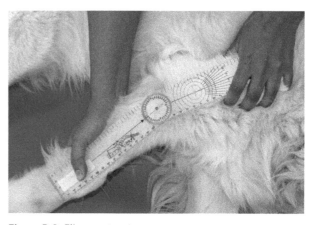

Figure B.9 Elbow extension.

- Prevent movement of the scapula away from the body wall.
- One arm of the goniometer is parallel to the ground, the other follows the humeral longitudinal axis. With the fulcrum over the shoulder joint, the external/internal rotation angle is measured by rotating the antebrachium inwards/outwards respectively (rotation of the antebrachium produces a rotation of the shoulder in the *opposite* direction).

Elbow

Elbow flexion/extension

- Lateral view.
- Humeral longitudinal axis to antebrachium longitudinal axis.

Radioulnar joints

Radioulnar pronation/supination

- Evertion/invertion of the paw from the head of the metacarpals.

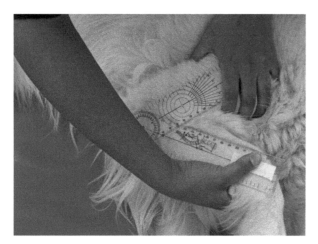

Figure B.8 Elbow flexion.

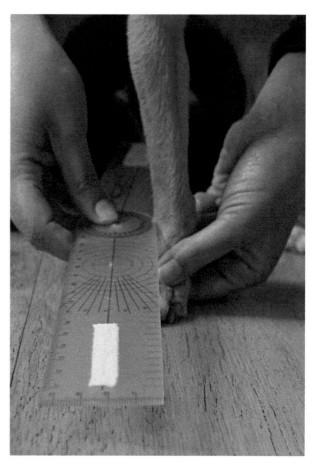

Figure B.10 Ready for pronation.

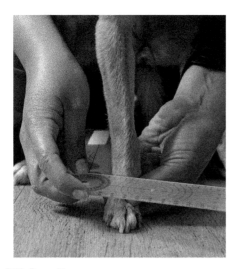

Figure B.11 Pronation.

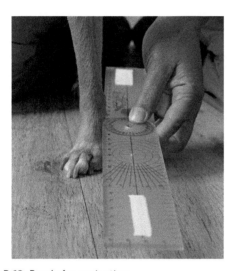

Figure B.12 Ready for supination.

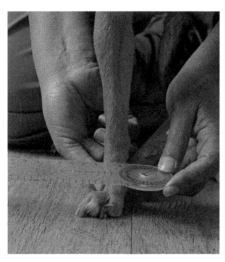

Figure B.13 Supination.

Carpus

Carpal flexion/extension

- Lateral view.
- Longitudinal axis of antebrachium to longitudinal axis of metacarpals (III/IV).

Carpus lateral/medial deviation

- Cranial view.
- Longitudinal axis of metacarpals (III/IV) to line parallel with medial border of the radius.

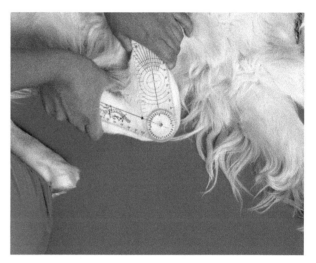

Figure B.14 Carpal flexion.

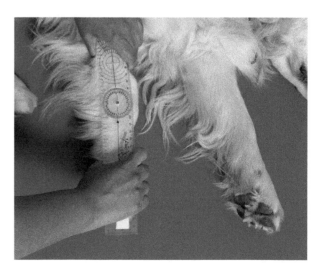

Figure B.15 Carpal extension.

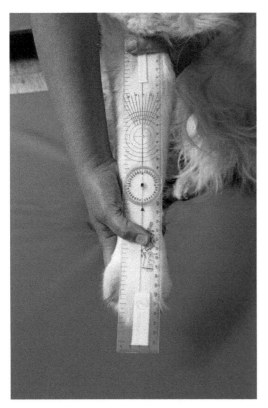

Figure B.16 Neutral position for lateral/medial deviation.

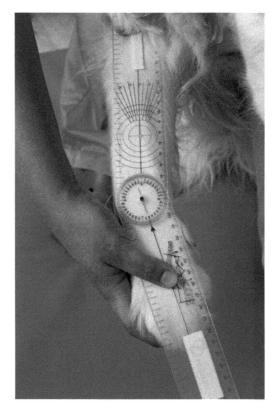

Figure B.18 Medial deviation.

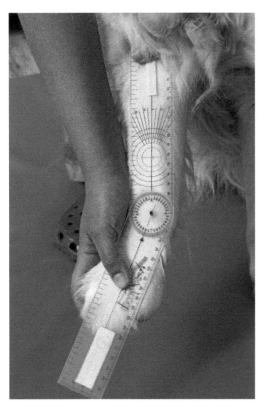

Figure B.17 Lateral deviation.

B2 Hindlimb

Bony landmarks

- Tuber sacrale, tuber coxae, and tuber ischiadicum.
- Femoral longitudinal axis: line from greater trochanter in the proximal femur, to lateral epicondyle in the distal femur.

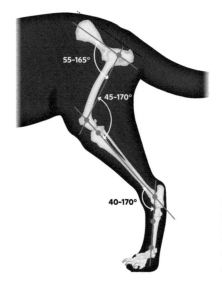

Figure B.19 Bony landmarks in the hindlimb.
Illustrator: Elaine Leggett.

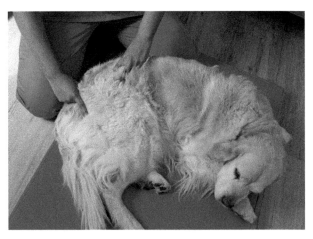

Figure B.20 Palpation of tuber ischiadicum, greater trochanter, tuber sacrale, and tuber coxae.

- Tibial longitudinal axis: line joining lateral epicondyle of femur, running over head of fibula, reaching lateral malleolus of fibula.
- Metatarsus: longitudinal axis of metatarsals III and IV.

Hip

Hip flexion/extension

- Lateral view.
- Angle between a line from the cranial iliac crest (midway between the tuber sacrale and tuber coxae) to the tuber ischiadicum, running over the greater trochanter, and the femoral longitudinal axis.

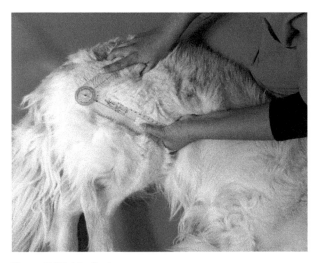

Figure B.21 Hip flexion.

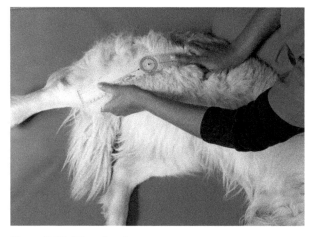

Figure B.22 Hip extension.

Hip abduction/adduction

- Lateral recumbency preferred to avoid pelvic tilting. Align both tuber ischii perpendicular to the ground.
- To measure the abduction angle, leave the fixed arm of the goniometer parallel to the ground, place the mobile arm following the femoral longitudinal axis and eventually the fulcrum over the coxofemoral joints. Open the angle as far as the patient allows, keeping the stifle and tarsus in extension.
- To measure the adduction angle, make sure the patient is close enough to the edge of the table to allow the movement. Place the fixed arm of the goniometer perpendicular to the ground, in line with both tuber ischii; the mobile arm follows the femoral longitudinal axis. The stifle and tarsus need to be extended.

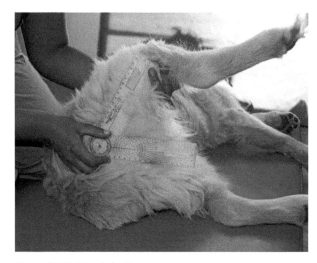

Figure B.23 Hip abduction.

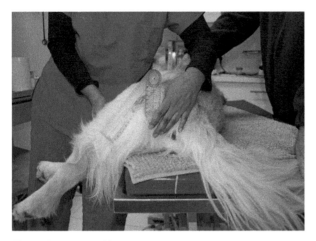

Figure B.24 Hip adduction.

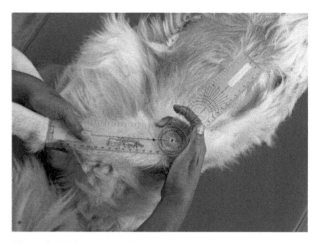

Figure B.26 Hip external rotation.

Hip external/internal rotation

- Dorsal recumbency with the tibia flexed at a right angle to the femoral shaft.
- Line up the patella and the coxofemoral joint perpendicular to the ground.
- The fixed arm of the goniometer is placed in line with the longitudinal axis of the body, the mobile arm is parallel to the tibia, and the fulcrum lies over the patella (Fig. B.25).
- The tibia is rotated *toward* the body to produce *external* rotation of the hip, and *away* from the body to rotate the hip *internally*.

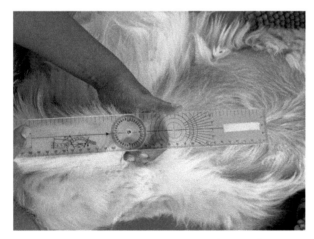

Figure B.25 Ready to measure hip external/internal rotation.

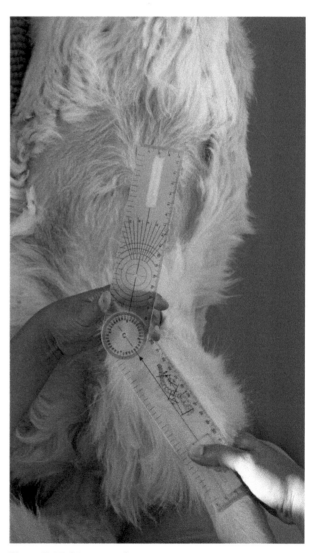

Figure B.27 Hip internal rotation.

- Lateral recumbency.
- Femoral longitudinal axis to tibial longitudinal axis.

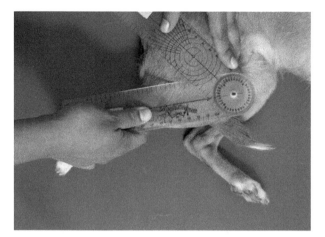

Figure B.28 Stifle flexion.

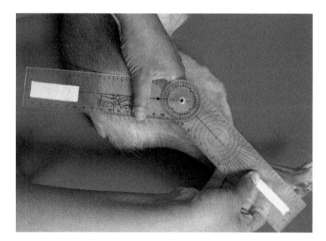

Figure B.29 Stifle extension.

- Lateral recumbency.
- Stifle must also be flexed to measure the flexion angle, due to limitation by the gastrocnemius muscle and common calcaneal tendon.
- Tibial longitudinal axis to metatarsus.

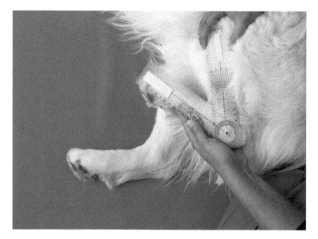

Figure B.30 Tibiotarsal flexion.

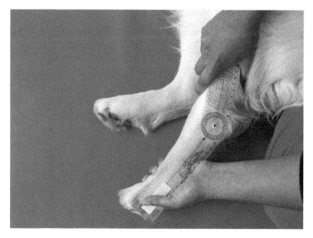

Figure B.31 Tibiotarsal extension.

Table 9.3 Range of motion (ROM).

Joint	Osteokinematic motion	Range of motion (degrees)					
		Millis and Levine[365]	Cook et al.[366]	Mann et al. (under general anesthesia)[363]	Jaegger et al. (Labradors) [361]	Thomovsky et al. (Dachshunds)[364]	Jaeger et al. (cats)[362]
Shoulder	Flexion	30–60			57		32
	Extension	160–170			165		163
	External rotation	40–50					
	Internal rotation	40–50					
	Abduction	40–50	32				
	Adduction	40–50					
Elbow	Flexion	20–40			36		22
	Extension	160–170			165		163
Radioulnar	Pronation	40–50					
	Supination	80–90					
Carpus	Flexion	20–35			32		22
	Extension	190–200			196		198
	Lateral (ulnar) deviation	10–20			12		10
	Medial (radial) deviation	5–15			7		7
Hip	Flexion	55		46	50	50	33
	Extension	160–165		164	162	155	164
	External rotation	50		50			
	Internal rotation	55		55			
	Abduction (flexed hip and 90° stifle)	120		118			
	Adduction (flexed hip and stifle at 90°)	63		64			
Stifle	Flexion	45		28	42	50	24
	Extension	160–170		172	162	160	164
Tarsus	Flexion	40		40	39	40	21
	Extension	170		175	164	167	167

Compilation of suggested treatment parameters

Table 4.1 Recommended parameters for pain management.

	Example	Dose (J/cm²)	Power (W)	Power density (W/cm²)
Acute superficial	Dog bite, acute tendinitis	2-5	1-4	0.2-1
Acute deep	Closed fracture	4-8	3-8	0.5-1.5
Chronic superficial	Non-healing ulcer, chronic tendinitis	4-15	2-5	0.5-1
Chronic deep	Spondylosis, hip dysplasia	8-20	6-15	1.5-3

Table 7.1 Recommended parameters for management of mucocutaneous conditions.

	Example	Dose (J/cm²)	Power (W)	Power density (W/cm²)
Acute superficial	Skin incision, hot spot	2-5	1-3	0.1-0.5
Acute deep	Acute sacculitis, penetrating wound	4-6	3-6	0.3-1
Chronic superficial	Non-healing ulcer	4-25	2-4	0.3-0.6
Chronic deep	Deep fistula	5-20	3-6	0.5-1.2

Table 7.2 Recommended parameters for lick granuloma.

Dose (J/cm²)	Power (W)	Power density (W/cm²)
4-30	2-4	0.5-0.8

Table 7.3 Recommended parameters for dermatitis.

	Example	Dose (J/cm²)	Power (W)	Power density (W/cm²)
Acute superficial	Hot spot	2-5	1-4	0.1-0.5
Chronic superficial	Chronic dermatitis	4-15	2-4	0.3-0.6

Table 7.4 Recommended parameters for otitis.

	Dose (J/cm²)	Power (W)	Power density (W/cm²)
Acute, pinna	2-4	1-3	0.2-0.6
Acute, canal	4-6	3-4	0.6-1
Chronic, pinna	4-6	2-3	0.2-0.6
Chronic, canal	6-12	4-8	0.8-1.2

Table 7.5 Recommended parameters for otohematoma.

Dose (J/cm²)	Power (W)	Power density (W/cm²)
4-6	1-3	0.2-0.5

Table 7.6 Recommended parameters for perineal treatments.

Dose (J/cm²)	Power (W)	Power density (W/cm²)
4-20	2-4	0.5-1

Table 7.7 Recommended parameters for oral treatments.

	Dose (J/cm²)	Power (W)	Power density (W/cm²)
Direct treatment	2-4	1-3	0.2-0.8
Through skin	6-10	4-6	0.6-1

Table 7.8 Recommended parameters for transabdominal treatments.

	Dose (J/cm²)	Power (W)	Power density (W/cm²)
Cat/small dog	4-10	3-6	1-2
Large dog	6-12	4-10	1-2

Table 7.9 Recommended parameters for transthoracic treatments.

	Dose (J/cm²)	Power (W)	Power density (W/cm²)
Cat/small dog	4-10	3-6	1-2
Large dog	6-12	4-10	1-2

Table 9.1 Recommended parameters for musculoskeletal conditions.

	Example	Dose (J/cm^2)	Power (W)	Power density (W/cm^2)
Acute superficial	Tendinitis	2-5	3-5	0.2-1
Acute deep	Closed fracture	4-8	4-8	0.5-1.5
Chronic superficial	Chronic tendinitis	4-15	4-6	0.5-1
Chronic deep	Spondylosis, hip dysplasia	8-20	6-15	1.5-3

Table 9.2 Examples of recommended parameters for chronic joint disorders.

Area	Patient	Dose (J/cm^2)	Power (W)	Power density (W/cm^2)
Carpus, tarsus	Cat, small dog	4-8	3-4	0.5-1
Elbow, stifle	Mid-sized dog	6-12	5-8	1-2
Spine, hip	Large dog	8-20	8-15	1.5-3

Table 9.6 Recommended parameters for IVDD.

Area	Dose (J/cm^2)	Power (W)	Power density (W/cm^2)
Spinal post-op	4-8	2-4	0.1-0.8
Acute	6-10	4-8	0.5-1.5
Chronic	8-20	8-15	1-3

Area Measurement Tool

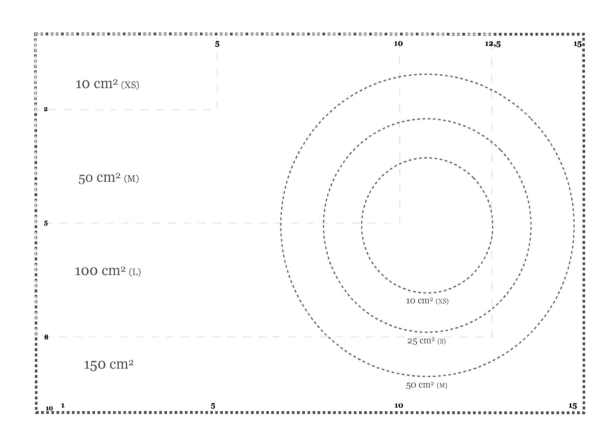

References

1. Suárez Redondo, M. Laser therapy approach to wound healing in dogs. *Veterinary Times*, 2015. **45**(37): pp. 25–7.

2. Fulop, A.M., et al. A meta-analysis of the efficacy of phototherapy in tissue repair. *Photomed Laser Surg*, 2009. **27**(5): pp. 695–702.

3. Usumez, A., et al. Effects of laser irradiation at different wavelengths (660, 810, 980, and 1,064 nm) on mucositis in an animal model of wound healing. *Lasers Med Sci*, 2014. **29**(6): pp. 1807–13.

4. Pereira, A.N., et al. Effect of low-power laser irradiation on cell growth and procollagen synthesis of cultured fibroblasts. *Lasers Surg Med*, 2002. **31**(4): pp. 263–7.

5. Rocha Júnior, A.M., et al. Modulation of fibroblast proliferation and inflammatory response by low intensity laser therapy in tissue repair process. *An Bras Dermatol*, 2006. **81**(2): pp. 150–6.

6. Martignago, C.C., et al. Effect of low-level laser therapy on the gene expression of collagen and vascular endothelial growth factor in a culture of fibroblast cells in mice. *Lasers Med Sci*, 2015. **30**(1): pp. 203–8.

7. Ayuk, S.M., N.N. Houreld, and H. Abrahamse. Collagen production in diabetic wounded fibroblasts in response to low-intensity laser irradiation at 660 nm. *Diabetes Technol Ther*, 2012. **14**(12): pp. 1110–7.

8. Alves, A.C., et al. Effect of low-level laser therapy on metalloproteinase MMP-2 and MMP-9 production and percentage of collagen types I and III in a papain cartilage injury model. *Lasers Med Sci*, 2014. **29**(3): pp. 911–9.

9. Zheng, J.M., et al. Surfaces and interfacial water: evidence that hydrophilic surfaces have long-range impact. *Adv Colloid Interface Sci*, 2006. **127**(1): pp. 19–27.

10. Chai, B., H. Yoo, and G.H. Pollack. Effect of radiant energy on near-surface water. *J Phys Chem B*, 2009. **113**(42): pp. 13953–8.

11. Santana-Blank, L., E. Rodrìguez-Santana, and K.E. Santana-Rodrìguez. Photobiomodulation of aqueous interfaces: finding evidence to support the exclusion zone in experimental and clinical studies. *Photomed Laser Surg*, 2013. **31**(9): pp. 461–2.

12. Kimura, K.W. and G.H. Pollack. Particle displacement in aqueous suspension arising from incident radiant energy. *Langmuir*, 2015. **31**(38): pp. 10370–6.

13. Gatsura, S.V., S.P. Gladkikh, and M.N. Titov. Effect of low-energy laser irradiation on the area of experimental myocardial infarction, lipid peroxidation, and hemoglobin affinity for oxygen. *Bull Exp Biol Med*, 2004. **137**(4): pp. 355–7.

14. Mittermayr, R., et al. Blue laser light increases perfusion of a skin flap via release of nitric oxide from hemoglobin. *Mol Med*, 2007. **13**(1–2): pp. 22–9.

15. Heu, F., et al. Effect of low-level laser therapy on blood flow and oxygen-hemoglobin saturation of the foot skin in healthy subjects: a pilot study. *Laser Ther*, 2013. **22**(1): pp. 21–30.

16. Karu, T.I., et al. Absorption measurements of cell monolayers relevant to mechanisms of laser phototherapy: reduction or oxidation of cytochrome c oxidase under laser radiation at 632.8 nm. *Photomed Laser Surg*, 2008. **26**(6): pp. 593–9.

17. Zhang, R., et al. Near infrared light protects cardiomyocytes from hypoxia and reoxygenation injury by a nitric oxide dependent mechanism. *J Mol Cell Cardiol*, 2009. **46**(1): pp. 4–14.

18. Lohr, N.L., et al. Enhancement of nitric oxide release from nitrosyl hemoglobin and nitrosyl myoglobin by red/near infrared radiation: potential role in cardioprotection. *J Mol Cell Cardiol*, 2009. **47**(2): pp. 256–63.

19. Kirkby, K.A., et al. The effects of low-level laser therapy in a rat model of intestinal ischemia-reperfusion injury. *Lasers Surg Med*, 2012. **44**(7): pp. 580–7.

20. Suami, H., et al. Lymphatic territories (lymphosomes) in a canine: an animal model for investigation of postoperative lymphatic alterations. *PLoS One*, 2013. **8**(7): pp. e69222.

21. Klabunde, R.E. *Cardiovascular Physiology Concepts*, 2nd edn. 2012, Lippincott Williams & Wilkins/Wolters Kluwer, Philadelphia, PA, pp. 60–123.

22. Honmura, A., et al. Analgesic effect of Ga-Al-As diode laser irradiation on hyperalgesia in carrageenin-induced inflammation. *Lasers Surg Med*, 1993. **13**(4): pp. 463–9.

23. Campana, V.R., et al. The relative effecs of He-Ne laser and meloxicam on experimentally induced inflammation. *Laser Ther*, 1999. **11**(1): pp. 36–42.

24. Albertini, R., et al. Effects of different protocol doses of low power gallium-aluminum-arsenate (Ga-Al-As) laser radiation (650 nm) on carrageenan induced rat paw ooedema. *J Photochem Photobiol B*, 2004. **74**(2–3): pp. 101–7.

25. Wu, Z.H., et al. Mitochondrial signaling for histamine releases in laser-irradiated RBL-2H3 mast cells. *Lasers Surg Med*, 2010. **42**(6): pp. 503–9.

26. Silveira, L.B., et al. Investigation of mast cells in human gingiva following low-intensity laser irradiation. *Photomed Laser Surg*, 2008. **26**(4): pp. 315–21.

27. Erthal, V., et al. Anti-inflammatory effect of laser acupuncture in ST36 (Zusanli) acupoint in mouse paw edema. *Lasers Med Sci*, 2016. **31**(2): pp. 315–22.

28. Ceylan, Y., S. Hizmetli, and Y. Silig. The effects of infrared laser and medical treatments on pain and serotonin degradation products in patients with myofascial pain syndrome. A controlled trial. *Rheumatol Int*, 2004. **24**(5): pp. 260–3.

29. Tomaz de Magalhães, M., et al. Light therapy modulates serotonin levels and blood flow in women with headache. A preliminary study. *Exp Biol Med (Maywood)*, 2016. **241**(1): pp. 40–5.

30. Campana, V., et al. He-Ne laser on microcrystalline arthropathies. *J Clin Laser Med Surg*, 2003. **21**(2): pp. 99–103.

31. Bortone, F., et al. Low level laser therapy modulates kinin receptors mRNA expression in the subplantar muscle of rat paw subjected to carrageenan-induced inflammation. *Int Immunopharmacol*, 2008. **8**(2): pp. 206–10.

32. Leal Junior, E.C., et al. Effects of low-level laser therapy (LLLT) in the development of exercise-induced skeletal muscle fatigue and changes in biochemical markers related to postexercise recovery. *J Orthop Sports Phys Ther*, 2010. **40**(8): pp. 524–32.

33. Sakurai, Y., M. Yamaguchi, and Y. Abiko. Inhibitory effect of low-level laser irradiation on LPS-stimulated prostaglandin E2 production and cyclooxygenase-2 in human gingival fibroblasts. *Eur J Oral Sci*, 2000. **108**(1): pp. 29–34.

34. Mizutani, K., et al. A clinical study on serum prostaglandin E2 with low-level laser therapy. *Photomed Laser Surg*, 2004. **22**(6): pp. 537–9.

35. Bjordal, J.M., et al. Low-level laser therapy in acute pain: a systematic review of possible mechanisms of action and clinical effects in randomized placebo-controlled trials. *Photomed Laser Surg*, 2006. **24**(2): pp. 158–68.

36. Prianti, A.C., Jr., et al. Low-level laser therapy (LLLT) reduces the COX-2 mRNA expression in both subplantar and total brain tissues in the model of peripheral inflammation induced by administration of carrageenan. *Lasers Med Sci*, 2014. **29**(4): pp. 1397–403.

37. Rodrigues, N.C., et al. Morphological aspects and Cox-2 expression after exposure to 780-nm laser therapy in injured skeletal muscle: an *in vivo* study. *Braz J Phys Ther*, 2014. **18**(5): pp. 395–401.

38. Sekhejane, P.R., N.N. Houreld, and H. Abrahamse. Irradiation at 636 nm positively affects diabetic wounded and hypoxic cells *in vitro*. *Photomed Laser Surg*, 2011. **29**(8): pp. 521–30.

39. Chen, Y.J., et al. Effect of low level laser therapy on chronic compression of the dorsal root ganglion. *PLoS One*, 2014. **9**(3): p. e89894.

40. Manchini, M.T., et al. Amelioration of cardiac function and activation of anti-inflammatory vasoactive peptides expression in the rat myocardium by low level laser therapy. *PLoS One*, 2014. **9**(7): p. e101270.

41. dos Santos, S.A., et al. Comparative analysis of two low-level laser doses on the expression of inflammatory mediators and on neutrophils and macrophages in acute joint inflammation. *Lasers Med Sci*, 2014. **29**(3): pp. 1051–8.

42. de Almeida, P., et al. What is the best treatment to decrease pro-inflammatory cytokine release in acute skeletal muscle injury induced by trauma in rats: low-level laser therapy, diclofenac, or cryotherapy? *Lasers Med Sci*, 2014. **29**(2): pp. 653–8.

43. Safavi, S.M., et al. Effects of low-level He-Ne laser irradiation on the gene expression of IL-1beta, TNF-alpha, IFN-gamma, TGF-beta, bFGF, and PDGF in rat's gingiva. *Lasers Med Sci*, 2008. **23**(3): pp. 331–5.

44. Boschi, E.S., et al. Anti-inflammatory effects of low-level laser therapy (660 nm) in the early phase in carrageenan-induced pleurisy in rat. *Lasers Surg Med*, 2008. **40**(7): pp. 500–8.

45. Wang, X.Y., et al. Effect of low-level laser therapy on allergic asthma in rats. *Lasers Med Sci*, 2014. **29**(3): pp. 1043–50.

46. Aimbire, F., et al. Low level laser therapy partially restores trachea muscle relaxation response in rats with tumor necrosis factor alpha-mediated smooth airway

muscle dysfunction. *Lasers Surg Med*, 2006. **38**(8): pp. 773–8.

47.   Xavier, M., et al. Low-level light-emitting diode therapy increases mRNA expressions of IL-10 and type I and III collagens on Achilles tendinitis in rats. *Lasers Med Sci*, 2014. **29**(1): pp. 85–90.

48.   Keshri, G.K., et al. Photobiomodulation with pulsed and continuous wave near-infrared laser (810 nm, Al-Ga-As) augments dermal wound healing in immunosuppressed rats. *PLoS One*, 2016. **11**(11): p. e0166705.

49.   Lavi, R., et al. Detailed analysis of reactive oxygen species induced by visible light in various cell types. *Lasers Surg Med*, 2010. **42**(6): pp. 473–80.

50.   Farivar, S., T. Malekshahabi, and R. Shiari. Biological effects of low level laser therapy. J *Lasers Med Sci*, 2014. **5**(2): pp. 58–62.

51.   Burger, E., et al. Low-level laser therapy to the mouse femur enhances the fungicidal response of neutrophils against *Paracoccidioides brasiliensis. PLoS Negl Trop Dis*, 2015. **9**(2): p. e0003541.

52.   Cerdeira, C.D., et al. Low-level laser therapy stimulates the oxidative burst in human neutrophils and increases their fungicidal capacity. *J Biophotonics*, 2016. **9**(11–12): pp. 1180–88.

53.   Ankri, R., et al. Visible light induces nitric oxide (NO) formation in sperm and endothelial cells. *Lasers Surg Med*, 2010. **42**(4): pp. 348–52.

54.   Mitchell, U.H. and G.L. Mack. Low-level laser treatment with near-infrared light increases venous nitric oxide levels acutely: a single-blind, randomized clinical trial of efficacy. *Am J Phys Med Rehabil*, 2013. **92**(2): pp. 151–6.

55.   Gal, D., et al. Percutaneous delivery of low-level laser energy reverses histamine-induced spasm in atherosclerotic Yucatan microswine. *Circulation*, 1992. **85**(2): pp. 756–68.

56.   Aimbire, F., et al. Effect of low level laser therapy on bronchial hyper-responsiveness. *Lasers Med Sci*, 2009. **24**(4): pp. 567–76.

57.   Nunez, S.C., et al. The influence of red laser irradiation timeline on burn healing in rats. *Lasers Med Sci*, 2013. **28**(2): pp. 633–41.

58.   Rabelo, S.B., et al. Comparison between wound healing in induced diabetic and nondiabetic rats after low-level laser therapy. *Photomed Laser Surg*, 2006. **24**(4): pp. 474–9.

59.   Ribeiro, M.A., et al. Immunohistochemical assessment of myofibroblasts and lymphoid cells during wound healing in rats subjected to laser photobiomodulation at 660 nm. *Photomed Laser Surg*, 2009. **27**(1): pp. 49–55.

60.   Gupta, A., et al. Superpulsed (Ga-As, 904 nm) low-level laser therapy (LLLT) attenuates inflammatory response and enhances healing of burn wounds. *J Biophotonics*, 2015. **8**(6): pp. 489–501.

61.   Vasheghani, M.M., et al. Effect of low-level laser therapy on mast cells in second-degree burns in rats. *Photomed Laser Surg*, 2008. **26**(1): pp. 1–5.

62.   Demir, H., H. Balay, and M. Kirnap. A comparative study of the effects of electrical stimulation and laser treatment on experimental wound healing in rats. *J Rehabil Res Dev*, 2004. **41**(2): pp. 147–54.

63.   Ottaviani, G., et al. Effect of class IV laser therapy on chemotherapy-induced oral mucositis: a clinical and experimental study. *Am J Pathol*, 2013. **183**(6): pp. 1747–57.

64.   Schubert, M.M., et al. A phase III randomized double-blind placebo-controlled clinical trial to determine the efficacy of low level laser therapy for the prevention of oral mucositis in patients undergoing hematopoietic cell transplantation. *Support Care Cancer*, 2007. **15**(10): pp. 1145–54.

65.   Kuhn, A., et al. Low-level infrared laser therapy in chemotherapy-induced oral mucositis: a randomized placebo-controlled trial in children. *J Pediatr Hematol Oncol*, 2009. **31**(1): pp. 33–7.

66.   Fekrazad, R. and N. Chiniforush. Oral mucositis prevention and management by therapeutic laser in head and neck cancers. *J Lasers Med Sci*, 2014. **5**(1): pp. 1–7.

67.   Gobbo, M., et al. Evaluation of nutritional status in head and neck radio-treated patients affected by oral mucositis: efficacy of class IV laser therapy. *Support Care Cancer*, 2014. **22**(7): pp. 1851–6.

68.   de Lima, F.M., et al. Low-level laser therapy attenuates the myeloperoxidase activity and inflammatory mediator generation in lung inflammation induced by gut ischemia and reperfusion: a dose-response study. *J Lasers Med Sci*, 2014. **5**(2): pp. 63–70.

69.   Silva, V.R., et al. Low-level laser therapy inhibits bronchoconstriction, Th2 inflammation and airway remodeling in allergic asthma. *Respir Physiol Neurobiol*, 2014. **194**: pp. 37–48.

70.   von Leden, R.E., et al. 808 nm wavelength light induces a dose-dependent alteration in microglial polarization and resultant microglial induced neurite growth. *Lasers Surg Med*, 2013. **45**(4): pp. 253–63.

71.   Oliveira, F.A., et al. Low-level laser therapy decreases renal interstitial fibrosis. *Photomed Laser Surg*, 2012. **30**(12): pp. 705–13.

72.   Yamato, M., A. Kaneda, and Y. Kataoka. Low-level laser therapy improves crescentic glomerulonephritis in rats. *Lasers Med Sci*, 2013. **28**(4): pp. 1189–96.

73.   Alves, A.C., et al. Effect of low-level laser therapy on the expression of inflammatory mediators and on neutrophils and macrophages in acute joint inflammation. *Arthritis Res Ther*, 2013. **15**(5): p. R116.

74.   Xavier, M., et al. Anti-inflammatory effects of low-level light emitting diode therapy on Achilles tendinitis in rats. *Lasers Surg Med*, 2010. **42**(6): pp. 553–8.

75.   Gavish, L., et al. Low-level laser irradiation inhibits abdominal aortic aneurysm progression in apolipoprotein E-deficient mice. *Cardiovasc Res*, 2009. **83**(4): pp. 785–92.

76.   Wang, Y., et al. Low-level laser therapy attenuates LPS-induced rats mastitis by inhibiting polymorphonuclear neutrophil adhesion. *J Vet Med Sci*, 2014. **76**(11): pp. 1443–50.

77.   Albertini, R., et al. Anti-inflammatory effects of low-level laser therapy (LLLT) with two different red wavelengths (660 nm and 684 nm) in carrageenan-induced rat paw edema. *J Photochem Photobiol B*, 2007. **89**(1): pp. 50–5.

78.   Hsieh, Y.L., et al. The fluence effects of low-level laser therapy on inflammation, fibroblast-like synoviocytes, and synovial apoptosis in rats with adjuvant-induced arthritis. *Photomed Laser Surg*, 2014. **32**(12): pp. 669–77.

79.   Knazovicky, D., et al. Widespread somatosensory sensitivity in naturally occurring canine model of osteoarthritis. *Pain*, 2016. **157**(6): pp. 1325–32.

80.   Hunt, J.R., et al. Electrophysiological characterisation of central sensitisation in canine spontaneous osteoarthritis. *Pain*, 2018. **159**(11): pp. 2318–30.

81.   Finnerup, N.B., et al. Pain and dysesthesia in patients with spinal cord injury: A postal survey. *Spinal Cord*, 2001. **39**(5): pp. 256–62.

82.   Wakabayashi, H., et al. Effect of irradiation by semiconductor laser on responses evoked in trigeminal caudal neurons by tooth pulp stimulation. *Lasers Surg Med*, 1993. **13**(6): pp. 605–10.

83.   Chow, R., et al. Inhibitory effects of laser irradiation on peripheral mammalian nerves and relevance to analgesic effects: a systematic review. *Photomed Laser Surg*, 2011. **29**(6): pp. 365–81.

84.   Yan, W., R. Chow, and P.J. Armati. Inhibitory effects of visible 650-nm and infrared 808-nm laser irradiation on somatosensory and compound muscle action potentials in rat sciatic nerve: implications for laser-induced analgesia. *J Peripher Nerv Syst*, 2011. **16**(2): pp. 130–5.

85.   Ohno, T. Pain suppressive effect of low power laser irradiation. A quantitative analysis of substance P in the rat spinal dorsal root ganglion [Article in Japanese]. *Nihon Ika Daigaku Zasshi*, 1997. **64**(5): pp. 395–400.

86.   Hsieh, Y.L., et al. Fluence-dependent effects of low-level laser therapy in myofascial trigger spots on modulation of biochemicals associated with pain in a rabbit model. *Lasers Med Sci*, 2015. **30**(1): pp. 209–16.

87.   Hsieh, Y.L., Y.C. Fan, and C.C. Yang. Low-level laser therapy alleviates mechanical and cold allodynia induced by oxaliplatin administration in rats. *Support Care Cancer*, 2016. **24**(1): pp. 233–42.

88.   Laakso, E. and P.J. Cabot. Nociceptive scores and endorphin-containing cells reduced by low-level laser therapy (LLLT) in inflamed paws of Wistar rat. *Photomed Laser Surg*, 2005. **23**(1): pp. 32–5.

89.   Hsieh, Y.L., et al. Low-level laser therapy alleviates neuropathic pain and promotes function recovery in rats with chronic constriction injury: possible involvements in hypoxia-inducible factor 1α (HIF-1α). J Comp Neurol, 2012. **520**(13): pp. 2903–16.

90.   Hagiwara, S., et al. GaAlAs (830 nm) low-level laser enhances peripheral endogenous opioid analgesia in rats. *Lasers Surg Med*, 2007. **39**(10): pp. 797–802.

91.   Meireles, A., et al. Avaliação do papel de opioides endógenos na analgesia do laser de baixa potência, 820 nm, em joelho de ratos. Wistar Rev Dor, 2012. **13**(2): pp. 152–5.

92.   Hochman, B., et al. Low-level laser therapy and light-emitting diode effects in the secretion of neuropeptides SP and CGRP in rat skin. *Lasers Med Sci*, 2014. **29**(3): pp. 1203–8.

93.   Mathews, K., et al. Guidelines for recognition, assessment and treatment of pain: WSAVA Global Pain Council members and co-authors of this document. *J Small Anim Pract*, 2014. **55**(6): pp. E10–68.

94.   Holton, L., et al. Development of a behaviour-based scale to measure acute pain in dogs. Vet Rec, 2001. **148**(17): pp. 525–31.

95.   Reid, S.M., et al. Development of a real-time reverse transcription polymerase chain reaction assay for detection of marine caliciviruses (genus *Vesivirus*). J Virol Methods, 2007. **140**(1–2): pp. 166–73.

96.   Calvo, G., et al. Development of a behaviour-based measurement tool with defined intervention level for assessing acute pain in cats. *J Small Anim Pract*, 2014. **55**(12): pp. 622–9.

97.   Brondani, J.T., S.P. Luna, and C.R. Padovani. Refinement and initial validation of a multidimensional composite scale for use in assessing acute postoperative pain in cats. *Am J Vet Res*, 2011. **72**(2): pp. 174–83.

98.   Brondani, J.T., et al. Validation of the English version of the UNESP-Botucatu multidimensional composite pain scale for assessing postoperative pain in cats. *BMC Vet Res*, 2013. **9**: p. 143.

99.   Robinson, N.G. Photomedicine, not opioids, for chronic pain. *Photomed Laser Surg*, 2016. **34**(10): pp. 433–4.

100.   Chow, R.T., et al. Efficacy of low-level laser therapy in the management of neck pain: a systematic review and meta-analysis of randomised placebo or active-treatment controlled trials. *Lancet*, 2009. **374**(9705): pp. 1897–908.

101.   Bjordal, J.M., et al. A systematic review with

procedural assessments and meta-analysis of low level laser therapy in lateral elbow tendinopathy (tennis elbow). *BMC Musculoskelet Disord*, 2008. **9**: p. 75.

102. Bjordal, J.M., et al. A systematic review of low level laser therapy with location-specific doses for pain from chronic joint disorders. *Aust J Physiother*, 2003. **49**(2): pp. 107–16.

103. Fulop, A.M., et al. A meta-analysis of the efficacy of laser phototherapy on pain relief. *Clin J Pain*, 2010. **26**(8): pp. 729–36.

104. Kreisler, M.B., et al. Efficacy of low level laser therapy in reducing postoperative pain after endodontic surgery–a randomized double blind clinical study. *Int J Oral Maxillofac Surg*, 2004. **33**(1): pp. 38–41.

105. Moore, K.C., et al. The effect of infra-red diode laser irradiation on the duration and severity of postoperative pain: a double blind trial. *Laser Ther*, 1992. **4**(4): pp. 145–9.

106. Ojea, A.R., et al. Beneficial effects of applying low-level laser therapy to surgical wounds after bariatric surgery. *Photomed Laser Surg*, 2016. **34**(11): pp. 580–4.

107. Nesioonpour, S., et al. Does low-level laser therapy enhance the efficacy of intravenous regional anesthesia? *Pain Res Manag*, 2014. **19**(6): pp. e154–8.

108. Ribas, E.S., et al. Use of low intensity laser treatment in neuropathic pain refractory to clinical treatment in amputation stumps. *Int J Gen Med*, 2012. **5**: pp. 739–42.

109. Falaki, F., A.H. Nejat, and Z. Dalirsani. The effect of low-level laser therapy on trigeminal neuralgia: A review of literature. *J Dent Res Dent Clin Dent Prospects*, 2014. **8**(1): pp. 1–5.

110. de Andrade, A.L., P.S. Bossini, and N.A. Parizotto. Use of low level laser therapy to control neuropathic pain: A systematic review. *J Photochem Photobiol B*, 2016. **164**: pp. 36–42.

111. Roberts, D.B., R.J. Kruse, and S.F. Stoll. The effectiveness of therapeutic class IV (10 W) laser treatment for epicondylitis. *Lasers Surg Med*, 2013. **45**(5): pp. 311–7.

112. Basso, F.G., et al. Biostimulatory effect of low-level laser therapy on keratinocytes *in vitro*. *Lasers Med Sci*, 2013. **28**(2): pp. 367–74.

113. Arany, P.R., et al. Activation of latent TGF-beta1 by low-power laser *in vitro* correlates with increased TGF-beta1 levels in laser-enhanced oral wound healing. *Wound Repair Regen*, 2007. **15**(6): pp. 866–74.

114. Saygun, I., et al. Effects of laser irradiation on the release of basic fibroblast growth factor (bFGF), insulin like growth factor-1 (IGF-1), and receptor of IGF-1 (IGFBP3) from gingival fibroblasts. *Lasers Med Sci*, 2008. **23**(2): pp. 211–5.

115. Houreld, N. and H. Abrahamse. Low-intensity laser irradiation stimulates wound healing in diabetic wounded fibroblast cells (WS1). *Diabetes Technol Ther*, 2010. **12**(12): pp. 971–8.

116. Jere, S.W., N.N. Houreld, and H. Abrahamse. Photobiomodulation at 660nm stimulates proliferation and migration of diabetic wounded cells via the expression of epidermal growth factor and the JAK/STAT pathway. *J Photochem Photobiol B*, 2018. **179**: pp. 74–83.

117. Hawkins, D.H. and H. Abrahamse. The role of laser fluence in cell viability, proliferation, and membrane integrity of wounded human skin fibroblasts following helium-neon laser irradiation. *Lasers Surg Med*, 2006. **38**(1): pp. 74–83.

118. Goncalves, W.L., et al. Influence of He-Ne laser therapy on the dynamics of wound healing in mice treated with anti-inflammatory drugs. *Braz J Med Biol Res*, 2007. **40**(6): pp. 877–84.

119. Meireles, G.C., et al. Effectiveness of laser photobiomodulation at 660 or 780 nanometers on the repair of third-degree burns in diabetic rats. *Photomed Laser Surg*, 2008. **26**(1): pp. 47–54.

120. Kayak, B.S., A. Maiya, and P. Kumar. Influence of helium-neon laser photostimulation on excision wound healing in Wistar rats. *OnLine J Biol Sci*, 7(2): pp. 89–92.

121. Novaes, R.D., et al. The energy density of laser light differentially modulates the skin morphological reorganization in a murine model of healing by secondary intention. *Int J Exp Pathol*, 2014. **95**(2): pp. 138–46.

122. Demidova-Rice, T.N., et al. Low-level light stimulates excisional wound healing in mice. *Lasers Surg Med*, 2007. **39**(9): pp. 706–15.

123. Gonzaga Ribeiro, M.A., et al. Morphological analysis of second-intention wound healing in rats submitted to 16 J/cm2 lambda 660-nm laser irradiation. *Indian J Dent Res*, 2009. **20**(3): p. 390.

124. Sperandio, F.F., et al. Low-level laser irradiation promotes the proliferation and maturation of keratinocytes during epithelial wound repair. *J Biophotonics*, 2015. **8**(10): pp. 795–803.

125. Gagnon, D., et al. An *in vitro* method to test the safety and efficacy of low-level laser therapy (LLLT) in the healing of a canine skin model. *BMC Vet Res*, 2016. **12**: p. 73.

126. Liao, X., et al. Helium-neon laser irradiation promotes the proliferation and migration of human epidermal stem cells *in vitro*: proposed mechanism for enhanced wound re-epithelialization. *Photomed Laser Surg*, 2014. **32**(4): pp. 219–25.

127. Stadler, I., et al. 830-nm irradiation increases the wound tensile strength in a diabetic murine model. *Lasers Surg Med*, 2001. **28**(3): pp. 220–6.

128. Peplow, P.V., T.Y. Chung, and G.D. Baxter. Laser

photobiomodulation of wound healing: a review of experimental studies in mouse and rat animal models. *Photomed Laser Surg*, 2010. **28**(3): pp. 291–325.

129.   Santos, N.R., et al. Influence of the combination of infrared and red laser light on the healing of cutaneous wounds infected by *Staphylococcus aureus*. *Photomed Laser Surg*, 2011. **29**(3): pp. 177–82.

130.   Yu, W., J.O. Naim, and R.J. Lanzafame. Effects of photostimulation on wound healing in diabetic mice. *Lasers Surg Med*, 1997. **20**(1): pp. 56–63.

131.   Al-Watban, F.A., X.Y. Zhang, and B.L. Andres. Low-level laser therapy enhances wound healing in diabetic rats: a comparison of different lasers. *Photomed Laser Surg*, 2007. **25**(2): pp. 72–7.

132.   Minatel, D.G., et al. Phototherapy promotes healing of chronic diabetic leg ulcers that failed to respond to other therapies. *Lasers Surg Med*, 2009. **41**(6): pp. 433–41.

133.   Kaviani, A., et al. A randomized clinical trial on the effect of low-level laser therapy on chronic diabetic foot wound healing: a preliminary report. *Photomed Laser Surg*, 2011. **29**(2): pp. 109–14.

134.   Houreld, N.N. Shedding light on a new treatment for diabetic wound healing: a review on phototherapy. *ScientificWorldJournal*, 2014. **2014**: p. 398412.

135.   Maltese, G., et al. A pilot study to evaluate the efficacy of class IV lasers on nonhealing neuroischemic diabetic foot ulcers in patients with type 2 diabetes. *Diabetes Care*, 2015. **38**(10): pp. e152–3.

136.   De Oliveira, R.F., et al. Comparison between the effect of low-level laser therapy and low-intensity pulsed ultrasonic irradiation *in vitro*. *Photomed Laser Surg*, 2008. **26**(1): pp. 6–9.

137.   Gal, P., et al. Effect of equal daily doses achieved by different power densities of low-level laser therapy at 635 nm on open skin wound healing in normal and corticosteroid-treated rats. *Lasers Med Sci*, 2009. **24**(4): pp. 539–47.

138.   Wood, V.T., et al. Collagen changes and realignment induced by low-level laser therapy and low-intensity ultrasound in the calcaneal tendon. *Lasers Surg Med*, 2010. **42**(6): pp. 559–65.

139.   Casalechi, H.L., et al. Analysis of the effect of phototherapy in model with traumatic Achilles tendon injury in rats. *Lasers Med Sci*, 2014. **29**(3): pp. 1075–81.

140.   Oliveira, F.S., et al. Effect of low level laser therapy (830 nm) with different therapy regimes on the process of tissue repair in partial lesion calcaneous tendon. *Lasers Surg Med*, 2009. **41**(4): pp. 271–6.

141.   Guerra Fda, R., et al. Pulsed LLLT improves tendon healing in rats: a biochemical, organizational, and functional evaluation. *Lasers Med Sci*, 2014. **29**(2): pp. 805–11.

142.   Guerra Fda, R., et al. LLLT improves tendon healing through increase of MMP activity and collagen synthesis. *Lasers Med Sci*, 2013. **28**(5): pp. 1281–8.

143.   Allahverdi, A., et al. Evaluation of low-level laser therapy, platelet-rich plasma, and their combination on the healing of Achilles tendon in rabbits. *Lasers Med Sci*, 2015. **30**(4): pp. 1305–13.

144.   Tsai, W.C., et al. Low-level laser irradiation stimulates tenocyte migration with up-regulation of dynamin II expression. *PLoS One*, 2012. **7**(5): p. e38235.

145.   Ozkan, N., et al. Investigation of the supplementary effect of GaAs laser therapy on the rehabilitation of human digital flexor tendons. *J Clin Laser Med Surg*, 2004. **22**(2): pp. 105–10.

146.   Ben-Dov, N., et al. Low-energy laser irradiation affects satellite cell proliferation and differentiation *in vitro*. *Biochim Biophys Acta*, 1999. **1448**(3): pp. 372–80.

147.   Shefer, G., et al. Low-energy laser irradiation promotes the survival and cell cycle entry of skeletal muscle satellite cells. *J Cell Sci*, 2002. **115**(Pt 7): pp. 1461–9.

148.   Nakano, J., et al. Low-level laser irradiation promotes the recovery of atrophied gastrocnemius skeletal muscle in rats. *Exp Physiol*, 2009. **94**(9): pp. 1005–15.

149.   Rochkind, S., S. Geuna, and A. Shainberg. Phototherapy and nerve injury: focus on muscle response. *Int Rev Neurobiol*, 2013. **109**: pp. 99–109.

150.   Albuquerque-Pontes, G.M., et al. Effect of pre-irradiation with different doses, wavelengths, and application intervals of low-level laser therapy on cytochrome c oxidase activity in intact skeletal muscle of rats. *Lasers Med Sci*, 2015. **30**(1): pp. 59–66.

151.   Shefer, G., et al. Primary myogenic cells see the light: improved survival of transplanted myogenic cells following low energy laser irradiation. *Lasers Surg Med*, 2008. **40**(1): pp. 38–45.

152.   Oron, U., et al. Attenuation of infarct size in rats and dogs after myocardial infarction by low-energy laser irradiation. *Lasers Surg Med*, 2001. **28**(3): pp. 204–11.

153.   Tuby, H., L. Maltz, and U. Oron. Implantation of low-level laser irradiated mesenchymal stem cells into the infarcted rat heart is associated with reduction in infarct size and enhanced angiogenesis. *Photomed Laser Surg*, 2009. **27**(2): pp. 227–33.

154.   Kazemi Khoo, N., et al. Application of low-level laser therapy following coronary artery bypass grafting (CABG) surgery. *J Lasers Med Sci*, 2014. **5**(2): pp. 86–91.

155.   Gavish, L., L. Perez, and S.D. Gertz. Low-level laser irradiation modulates matrix metalloproteinase activity and gene expression in porcine aortic smooth muscle cells. *Lasers Surg Med*, 2006. **38**(8): pp. 779–86.

156.   Stein, A., et al. Low-level laser irradiation promotes proliferation and differentiation of human osteoblasts *in vitro*. *Photomed Laser Surg*, 2005. **23**(2): pp. 161–6.

157. Favaro-Pipi, E., et al. Low-level laser therapy induces differential expression of osteogenic genes during bone repair in rats. *Photomed Laser Surg*, 2011. **29**(5): pp. 311–7.

158. Ueda, Y. and N. Shimizu. Effects of pulse frequency of low-level laser therapy (LLLT) on bone nodule formation in rat calvarial cells. *J Clin Laser Med Surg*, 2003. **21**(5): pp. 271–7.

159. Pinheiro, A.L. and M.E. Gerbi. Photoengineering of bone repair processes. *Photomed Laser Surg*, 2006. **24**(2): pp. 169–78.

160. Saracino, S., et al. Superpulsed laser irradiation increases osteoblast activity via modulation of bone morphogenetic factors. *Lasers Surg Med*, 2009. **41**(4): pp. 298–304.

161. Santiago, V.C., A. Piram, and A. Fuziy. Effect of soft laser in bone repair after expansion of the midpalatal suture in dogs. *Am J Orthod Dentofacial Orthop*, 2012. **142**(5): pp. 615–24.

162. Walter, C., A.M. Pabst, and T. Ziebart. Effects of a low-level diode laser on oral keratinocytes, oral fibroblasts, endothelial cells and osteoblasts incubated with bisphosphonates: An *in vitro* study. *Biomed Rep*, 2015. **3**(1): pp. 14–18.

163. de Vasconcellos, L.M., et al. Healing of normal and osteopenic bone with titanium implant and low-level laser therapy (GaAlAs): a histomorphometric study in rats. *Lasers Med Sci*, 2014. **29**(2): pp. 575–80.

164. Scalize, P.H., et al. Low-level laser therapy improves bone formation: stereology findings for osteoporosis in rat model. *Lasers Med Sci*, 2015. **30**(5): pp. 1599–607.

165. Shamir, M.H., et al. Double-blind randomized study evaluating regeneration of the rat transected sciatic nerve after suturing and postoperative low-power laser treatment. *J Reconstr Microsurg*, 2001. **17**(2): pp. 133–7; discussion 138.

166. Gigo-Benato, D., et al. Low-power laser biostimulation enhances nerve repair after end-to-side neurorrhaphy: a double-blind randomized study in the rat median nerve model. *Lasers Med Sci*, 2004. **19**(1): pp. 57–65.

167. Barbosa, R.I., et al. Comparative effects of wavelengths of low-power laser in regeneration of sciatic nerve in rats following crushing lesion. *Lasers Med Sci*, 2010. **25**(3): pp. 423–30.

168. Moges, H., et al. Effect of 810 nm light on nerve regeneration after autograft repair of severely injured rat median nerve. *Lasers Surg Med*, 2011. **43**(9): pp. 901–6.

169. Marcolino, A.M., et al. Assessment of functional recovery of sciatic nerve in rats submitted to low-level laser therapy with different fluences. An experimental study: laser in functional recovery in rats. *J Hand Microsurg*, 2013. **5**(2): pp. 49–53.

170. Wu, X., et al. 810 nm Wavelength light: an effective therapy for transected or contused rat spinal cord. *Lasers Surg Med*, 2009. **41**(1): pp. 36–41.

171. Byrnes, K.R., et al. Light promotes regeneration and functional recovery and alters the immune response after spinal cord injury. *Lasers Surg Med*, 2005. **36**(3): pp. 171–85.

172. Uozumi, Y., et al. Targeted increase in cerebral blood flow by transcranial near-infrared laser irradiation. *Lasers Surg Med*, 2010. **42**(6): pp. 566–76.

173. Lapchak, P.A. and L. De Taboada. Transcranial near infrared laser treatment (NILT) increases cortical adenosine-5'-triphosphate (ATP) content following embolic strokes in rabbits. *Brain Res*, 2010. **1306**: pp. 100–5.

174. Lapchak, P.A., J. Wei, and J.A. Zivin. Transcranial infrared laser therapy improves clinical rating scores after embolic strokes in rabbits. *Stroke*, 2004. **35**(8): pp. 1985–8.

175. Oron, A., et al. Low-level laser therapy applied transcranially to rats after induction of stroke significantly reduces long-term neurological deficits. *Stroke*, 2006. **37**(10): pp. 2620–4.

176. de Oliveira, R.F., et al. Benefits of laser phototherapy on nerve repair. *Lasers Med Sci*, 2015. **30**(4): pp. 1395–406.

177. Belda, F.J., et al. Supplemental perioperative oxygen and the risk of surgical wound infection: a randomized controlled trial. *JAMA*, 2005. **294**(16): pp. 2035–42.

178. Bornstein, E., et al. Near-infrared photoinactivation of bacteria and fungi at physiologic temperatures. *Photochem Photobiol*, 2009. **85**(6): pp. 1364–74.

179. Percival, S.L., I. Francolini, and G. Donelli. Low-level laser therapy as an antimicrobial and antibiofilm technology and its relevance to wound healing. *Future Microbiol*, 2015. **10**(2): pp. 255–72.

180. Jawhara, S. and S. Mordon. Monitoring of bactericidal action of laser by *in vivo* imaging of bioluminescent *E. coli* in a cutaneous wound infection. *Lasers Med Sci*, 2006. **21**(3): pp. 153–9.

181. Krespi, Y.P., V. Kizhner, and C.O. Kara. Laser-induced microbial reduction in acute bacterial rhinosinusitis. *Am J Rhinol Allergy*, 2009. **23**(6): pp. e29–32.

182. Karu, T., et al. Effects of near-infrared laser and superluminous diode irradiation on *Escherichia coli* division rate. *IEEE Journal of Quantum Electronics*, 1990. **26**(12): pp. 2162–5.

183. Nussbaum, E.L., L. Lilge, and T. Mazzulli. Effects of 630-, 660-, 810-, and 905-nm laser irradiation delivering radiant exposure of 1–50 J/cm2 on three species of bacteria *in vitro*. *J Clin Laser Med Surg*, 2002. **20**(6): pp. 325–33.

184. Chan, Y. and C.H. Lai. Bactericidal effects of different laser wavelengths on periodontopathic germs in

photodynamic therapy. *Lasers Med Sci*, 2003. **18**(1): pp. 51–5.

185. Nussbaum, E.L., L. Lilge, and T. Mazzulli. Effects of low-level laser therapy (LLLT) of 810 nm upon *in vitro* growth of bacteria: relevance of irradiance and radiant exposure. *J Clin Laser Med Surg*, 2003. **21**(5): pp. 283–90.

186. Pereira, P.R., et al. Effects of low intensity laser in *in vitro* bacterial culture and *in vivo* infected wounds. Rev Col Bras Cir, 2014. **41**(1): pp. 49–55.

187. Bayat, M., M.M. Vasheghani, and N. Razavi. Effect of low-level helium-neon laser therapy on the healing of third-degree burns in rats. *J Photochem Photobiol B*, 2006. **83**(2): pp. 87–93.

188. Kaya, G.S., et al. The use of 808-nm light therapy to treat experimental chronic osteomyelitis induced in rats by methicillin-resistant *Staphylococcus aureus*. *Photomed Laser Surg*, 2011. **29**(6): pp. 405–12.

189. Krespi, Y.P., et al. Laser disruption and killing of methicillin-resistant *Staphylococcus aureus* biofilms. *Am J Otolaryngol*, 2011. **32**(3): pp. 198–202.

190. Silva, D.C., et al. Low level laser therapy (AlGaInP) applied at 5J/cm2 reduces the proliferation of *Staphylococcus aureus* MRSA in infected wounds and intact skin of rats. *An Bras Dermatol*, 2013. **88**(1): pp. 50–5.

191. Manevitch, Z., et al. Direct antifungal effect of femtosecond laser on *Trichophyton rubrum* onychomycosis. *Photochem Photobiol*, 2010. **86**(2): pp. 476–9.

192. Araujo, B.F., et al. Effects of low-level laser therapy, 660 nm, in experimental septic arthritis. *ISRN Rheumatol*, 2013. **2013**: p. 341832.

193. Lipovsky, A., et al. Visible light-induced killing of bacteria as a function of wavelength: implication for wound healing. *Lasers Surg Med*, 2010. **42**(6): pp. 467–72.

194. Keijzer, M., et al. Light distributions in artery tissue: Monte Carlo simulations for finite-diameter laser beams. *Lasers Surg Med*, 1989. **9**(2): pp. 148–54.

195. Firbank, M., et al. Measurement of the optical properties of the skull in the wavelength range 650–950 nm. *Phys Med Biol*, 1993. **38**(4): pp. 503–10.

196. Beek, J.F., et al. The optical properties of lung as a function of respiration. *Phys Med Biol*, 1997. **42**(11): pp. 2263–72.

197. Ma, X., et al. Bulk optical parameters of porcine skin dermis at eight wavelengths from 325 to 1557 nm. *Opt Lett*, 2005. **30**(4): pp. 412–4.

198. Jacques, S.L. and B.W. Pogue. Tutorial on diffuse light transport. *J Biomed Opt*, 2008. **13**(4): p. 041302.

199. Hall, G., et al. Goniometric measurements of thick tissue using Monte Carlo simulations to obtain the single scattering anisotropy coefficient. *Biomed Opt Express*, 2012. **3**(11): pp. 2707–19.

200. Stephens, B.J. and L. Ramball Jones. Tissue optics. In: Hamblin, M., T. Agrawal, and M. de Sousa (eds) *Handbook of Low-Level Laser Therapy*. 2016, Pan Stanford Publishing, Singapore, pp. 67–86.

201. Hashmi, J.T., et al. Effect of pulsing in low-level light therapy. *Lasers Surg Med*, 2010. **42**(6): pp. 450–66.

202. Mbene, A.B., N.N. Houreld, and H. Abrahamse. DNA damage after phototherapy in wounded fibroblast cells irradiated with 16 J/cm(2). *J Photochem Photobiol B*, 2009. **94**(2): pp. 131–7.

203. Karu, T.I., L.V. Pyatibrat, and T.P. Ryabykh. Nonmonotonic behavior of the dose dependence of the radiation effect on cells *in vitro* exposed to pulsed laser radiation at lambda = 820 nm. *Lasers Surg Med*, 1997. **21**(5): pp. 485–92.

204. Prado, R.P., et al. Experimental model for low level laser therapy on ischemic random skin flap in rats. *Acta Cir Bras*, 2006. **21**(4): pp. 258–62.

205. Carvalho, R.L., et al. Effects of low-level laser therapy on pain and scar formation after inguinal herniation surgery: a randomized controlled single-blind study. *Photomed Laser Surg*, 2010. **28**(3): pp. 417–22.

206. Olivieri, L., et al. Efficacy of low-level laser therapy on hair regrowth in dogs with noninflammatory alopecia: a pilot study. *Vet Dermatol*, 2015. **26**(1): pp. 35–9, e11.

207. da Silva, E.B., et al. Macro and microscopic analysis of island skin grafts after low-level laser therapy. *Rev Col Bras Cir*, 2013. **40**(1): pp. 44–8.

208. Kubota, J. Effects of diode laser therapy on blood flow in axial pattern flaps in the rat model. *Lasers Med Sci*, 2002. **17**(3): pp. 146–53.

209. Pinfildi, C.E., et al. Effect of low-level laser therapy on mast cells in viability of the transverse rectus abdominis musculocutaneous flap. *Photomed Laser Surg*, 2009. **27**(2): pp. 337–43.

210. Pinfildi, C.E., et al. What is better in TRAM flap survival: LLLT single or multi-irradiation? *Lasers Med Sci*, 2013. **28**(3): pp. 755–61.

211. Kubota, J. Defocused diode laser therapy (830 nm) in the treatment of unresponsive skin ulcers: a preliminary trial. *J Cosmet Laser Ther*, 2004. **6**(2): pp. 96–102.

212. Dantas, M.D., et al. Improvement of dermal burn healing by combining sodium alginate/chitosan-based films and low level laser therapy. *J Photochem Photobiol B*, 2011. **105**(1): pp. 51–9.

213. Castro, B., et al. Development and preclinical evaluation of a new galactomannan-based dressing with antioxidant properties for wound healing. *Histol Histopathol*, 2015. **30**(12): pp. 1499–512.

214. Balasch, J., et al. Case report on the treatment of surgically debrided deep wounds with a new antioxidant wound dressing in two dogs. *Adv Anim Vet Sci*, 2016. **4**(7): pp. 389–393.

215. Lilge, L., K. Tierney, and E. Nussbaum. Low-level laser therapy for wound healing: feasibility of wound dressing transillumination. *J Clin Laser Med Surg*, 2000. **18**(5): pp. 235–40.

216. de Jesus Guirro, R.R., et al. Analysis of low-level laser radiation transmission in occlusive dressings. *Photomed Laser Surg*, 2010. **28**(4): pp. 459–63.

217. Franz, M.G., et al. Guidelines to aid healing of acute wounds by decreasing impediments of healing. *Wound Repair Regen*, 2008. **16**(6): pp. 723–48.

218. Perego, R., et al. Low-level laser therapy: Case-control study in dogs with sterile pyogranulomatous pododermatitis. *Vet World*, 2016. **9**(8): pp. 882–7.

219. Stich, A.N., W.S. Rosenkrantz, and C.E. Griffin. Clinical efficacy of low-level laser therapy on localized canine atopic dermatitis severity score and localized pruritic visual analog score in pedal pruritus due to canine atopic dermatitis. *Vet Dermatol*, 2014. **25**(5): pp. 464–e74.

220. Maleki, S., et al. Effect of local irradiation with 630 and 860 nm low-level lasers on tympanic membrane perforation repair in guinea pigs. *J Laryngol Otol*, 2013. **127**(3): pp. 260–4.

221. Rhee, C.K., et al. Effect of low-level laser therapy on cochlear hair cell recovery after gentamicin-induced ototoxicity. *Lasers Med Sci*, 2012. **27**(5): pp. 987–92.

222. Tamura, A., et al. Low-level laser therapy for prevention of noise-induced hearing loss in rats. *Neurosci Lett*, 2015. **595**: pp. 81–6.

223. Tauber, S., et al. Lightdosimetric quantitative analysis of the human petrous bone: experimental study for laser irradiation of the cochlea. *Lasers Surg Med*, 2001. **28**(1): pp. 18–26.

224. Ghibaudo, G. and G. Marchingiglio. Use of low level laser therapy (LLLT) for drug unresponsive perianal fistulas in German shepherd dogs. *Vet Dermatol*, 2016. **27**(Suppl 1): p. 27.

225. Kim, C.H., K.A. Cheong, and A.Y. Lee. 850nm light-emitting-diode phototherapy plus low-dose tacrolimus (FK-506) as combination therapy in the treatment of *Dermatophagoides farinae*-induced atopic dermatitis-like skin lesions in NC/Nga mice. *J Dermatol Sci*, 2013. **72**(2): pp. 142–8.

226. Nikou Khorsand, T., et al. Comparison between the effect of low level laser therapy and injection of botox in treatment of anal fissure (clinical trial, case control). Paper presented at the 7th International WALT Congress, 2008, Johannesburg, Sun City, South Africa. Available at: https://www.researchgate.net/publication/266675695_COMPARISON_BETWEEN_THE_EFFECT_OF_LOW_LEVEL_LASER_THERAPY_AND_INJECTION_OF_BOTOX_IN_TREATMENT_OF_ANAL_FISSURE_CLINICAL_TRIAL_CASE_CONTROL (accessed September 2018).

227. Aranha, A.C., L.A. Pimenta, and G.M. Marchi. Clinical evaluation of desensitizing treatments for cervical dentin hypersensitivity. *Braz Oral Res*, 2009. **23**(3): pp. 333–9.

228. Amorim, J.C., et al. Clinical study of the gingiva healing after gingivectomy and low-level laser therapy. *Photomed Laser Surg*, 2006. **24**(5): pp. 588–94.

229. Qadri, T., et al. The short-term effects of low-level lasers as adjunct therapy in the treatment of periodontal inflammation. *J Clin Periodontol*, 2005. **32**(7): pp. 714–9.

230. Pejcic, A., et al. The effects of low level laser irradiation on gingival inflammation. *Photomed Laser Surg*, 2010. **28**(1): pp. 69–74.

231. Igic, M., et al. Cytomorphometric and clinical investigation of the gingiva before and after low-level laser therapy of gingivitis in children. *Lasers Med Sci*, 2012. **27**(4): pp. 843–8.

232. Qadri, T., et al. Role of diode lasers (800–980 nm) as adjuncts to scaling and root planing in the treatment of chronic periodontitis: a systematic review. *Photomed Laser Surg*, 2015. **33**(11): pp. 568–75.

233. Doeuk, C., et al. Current indications for low level laser treatment in maxillofacial surgery: a review. *Br J Oral Maxillofac Surg*, 2015. **53**(4): pp. 309–15.

234. de Paula Eduardo, C., et al. Laser phototherapy in the treatment of periodontal disease. A review. *Lasers Med Sci*, 2010. **25**(6): pp. 781–92.

235. Khadra, M., et al. Determining optimal dose of laser therapy for attachment and proliferation of human oral fibroblasts cultured on titanium implant material. *J Biomed Mater Res A*, 2005. **73**(1): pp. 55–62.

236. Massotti, F.P., et al. Histomorphometric assessment of the influence of low-level laser therapy on peri-implant tissue healing in the rabbit mandible. *Photomed Laser Surg*, 2015. **33**(3): pp. 123–8.

237. Tang, E. and P. Arany. Photobiomodulation and implants: implications for dentistry. *J Periodontal Implant Sci*, 2013. **43**(6): pp. 262–8.

238. Cruz, L.B., et al. Influence of low-energy laser in the prevention of oral mucositis in children with cancer receiving chemotherapy. *Pediatr Blood Cancer*, 2007. **48**(4): pp. 435–40.

239. Correa, F., et al. Low-level laser therapy (GaAs lambda = 904 nm) reduces inflammatory cell migration in mice with lipopolysaccharide-induced peritonitis. *Photomed Laser Surg*, 2007. **25**(4): pp. 245–9.

240. Irani, S., et al. Effect of low-level laser irradiation on *in vitro* function of pancreatic islets. *Transplant Proc*, 2009. **41**(10): pp. 4313–5.

241. Huang, L., et al. Photoactivation of Akt1/GSK3beta isoform-specific signaling axis promotes pancreatic beta-cell regeneration. *J Cell Biochem*, 2015. **116**(8): pp. 1741–54.

242. Gutnova, S.K. The evaluation of exocrinous function of pancreas in patients with chronic pancreatitis [Article in Russian]. *Klin Lab Diagn*, 2011(12): pp. 44–5.

243. Lim, J., et al. Effects of low-level light therapy on streptozotocin-induced diabetic kidney. *J Photochem Photobiol B*, 2010. **99**(2): pp. 105–10.

244. Lim, J., et al. Effects of low-level light therapy on hepatic antioxidant defense in acute and chronic diabetic rats. *J Biochem Mol Toxicol*, 2009. **23**(1): pp. 1–8.

245. Zigmond, E., et al. Low-level light therapy induces mucosal healing in a murine model of dextran-sodium-sulfate induced colitis. *Photomed Laser Surg*, 2014. **32**(8): pp. 450–7.

246. Burduli, I.M. and S.K. Gutnova. Efficacy of different laser treatments in combined therapy of patients with gastroduodenal ulcer [Article in Russian].*Ter Arkh*, 2008. **80**(2): pp. 30–3.

247. Oron, U., et al. Enhanced liver regeneration following acute hepatectomy by low-level laser therapy. *Photomed Laser Surg*, 2010. **28**(5): pp. 675–8.

248. de Castro e Silva Junior, O., et al. Laser enhancement in hepatic regeneration for partially hepatectomized rats. *Lasers Surg Med*, 2001. **29**(1): pp. 73–7.

249. Araujo, T.G., et al. Low-power laser irradiation fails to improve liver regeneration in elderly rats at 48 h after 70% resection. *Lasers Med Sci*, 2015. **30**(7): pp. 2003–8.

250. Takhtfooladi, M.A., H.A. Takhtfooladi, and M. Khansari. The effects of low-intensity laser therapy on hepatic ischemia-reperfusion injury in a rat model. *Lasers Med Sci*, 2014. **29**(6): pp. 1887–93.

251. Oliveira-Junior, M.C., et al. Low-level laser therapy ameliorates CCl4-induced liver cirrhosis in rats. *Photochem Photobiol*, 2013. **89**(1): pp. 173–8.

252. Ucero, A.C., et al. Laser therapy in metabolic syndrome-related kidney injury. *Photochem Photobiol*, 2013. **89**(4): pp. 953–60.

253. Asghari, A., M.A. Takhtfooladi, and H.A. Hoseinzadeh. Effect of photobiomodulation on ischemia/reperfusion-induced renal damage in diabetic rats. *Lasers Med Sci*, 2016. **31**(9): pp. 1943–8.

254. Takhtfooladi, H.A., et al. Evaluation of low-level laser therapy on skeletal muscle ischemia-reperfusion in streptozotocin-induced diabetic rats by assaying biochemical markers and histological changes. *Lasers Med Sci*, 2016. **31**(6): pp. 1211–7.

255. de Lima, F.M., et al. Low-level laser therapy restores the oxidative stress balance in acute lung injury induced by gut ischemia and reperfusion. *Photochem Photobiol*, 2013. **89**(1): pp. 179–88.

256. Ashrafzadeh Takhtfooladi, M., et al. Effect of low-level laser therapy on lung injury induced by hindlimb ischemia/reperfusion in rats. *Lasers Med Sci*, 2015. **30**(6): pp. 1757–62.

257. Krespi, Y.P. and V. Kizhner. Laser-assisted nasal decolonization of *Staphylococcus aureus*, including methicillin-resistant *Staphylococcus aureus*. *Am J Otolaryngol*, 2012. **33**(5): pp. 572–5.

258. Naghdi, S., et al. A pilot study into the effect of low-level laser therapy in patients with chronic rhinosinusitis. *Physiother Theory Pract*, 2013. **29**(8): pp. 596–603.

259. Choi, B., et al. Effects of low level laser therapy on ovalbumin-induced mouse model of allergic rhinitis. *Evid Based Complement Alternat Med*, 2013. **2013**: p. 753829.

260. Lee, H.M., et al. A comparative pilot study of symptom improvement before and after phototherapy in Korean patients with perennial allergic rhinitis. *Photochem Photobiol*, 2013. **89**(3): pp. 751–7.

261. Aghamohammadi, D., et al. Effect of low level laser application at the end of surgery to reduce pain after tonsillectomy in adults. *J Lasers Med Sci*, 2013. **4**(2): pp. 79–85.

262. Marinho, R.R., et al. Potentiated anti-inflammatory effect of combined 780 nm and 660 nm low level laser therapy on the experimental laryngitis. *J Photochem Photobiol B*, 2013. **121**: pp. 86–93.

263. Lutai, A.V., L.A. Egorova, and E.A. Shutemova. Laser therapy of elderly patients with pneumonia [Article in Russian]. *Vopr Kurortol Fizioter Lech Fiz Kult*, 2001. **May-Jun**(3): pp. 15–18.

264. Amirov, N.B., et al. Serum concentrations of trace elements and microcirculation during laser therapy for pneumonia [Article in Russian]. *Probl Tuberk*, 2002(2): pp. 17–20.

265. Kochetov, A.M., et al. The use of low-energy laser radiation in the combined treatment of patients with acute pneumonia [Article in Russian]. *Vrach Delo*, 1990. **Feb**(2): pp. 70–1.

266. Tiukhin, N.S., M.V. Semynin, and N.A. Stogova. Laser therapy in patients with inflammatory pleural exudates [Article in Russian]. *Probl Tuberk*, 1997(4): pp. 38–40.

267. World Association of Laser Therapy (WALT). Consensus agreement on the design and conduct of clinical studies with low-level laser therapy and light therapy for musculoskeletal pain and disorders. *Photomed Laser Surg*, 2006. **24**(6): pp. 761–2.

268. Karu, T.I., L.V. Pyatibrat, and G.S. Kalendo. Studies into the action specifics of a pulsed GaIAs laser (λ=S20 nm) on a cell culture. *Lasers Life Sci*, 2001. **9**: pp. 211–7.

269. Karu, T.I. Low-power laser therapy. In: Vo-Dinh, T. (ed.) *Biomedical Photonics Handbook*. 2003, CRC Press, Boca Raton, Florida, Chapter 48.

270. Katz, U. Cellular water content and volume regulation in animal cells. *Cell Biochem Funct*, 1995. **13**(3): pp. 189–93.

271. Duthey, B. Background Paper 6.24: Low back pain. Update on 2004 Background Paper. In: WHO (ed.)

Priority Medicines for Europe and the World. 2013, WHO, Geneva.

272.   Wittenauer, R., L. Smith, and K. Aden. Background Paper 6.12: Osteoarthritis. Update on 2004 Background Paper. In: WHO (ed.) *Priority Medicines for Europe and the World*. 2013, WHO, Geneva.

273.   Merli, L.A., et al. Effect of low-intensity laser irradiation on the process of bone repair. *Photomed Laser Surg*, 2005. **23**(2): pp. 212–5.

274.   Liu, X., et al. Effect of lower-level laser therapy on rabbit tibial fracture. *Photomed Laser Surg*, 2007. **25**(6): pp. 487–94.

275.   Mayer, L., et al. Effects of low-level laser therapy on distraction osteogenesis: a histological analysis. *RFO, Passo Fundo*, 2012. **17**(3): pp. 326–31.

276.   Son, J., et al. Bone healing effects of diode laser (808 nm) on a rat tibial fracture model. *In Vivo*, 2012. **26**(4): pp. 703–9.

277.   Lirani-Galvao, A.P., V. Jorgetti, and O.L. da Silva. Comparative study of how low-level laser therapy and low-intensity pulsed ultrasound affect bone repair in rats. *Photomed Laser Surg*, 2006. **24**(6): pp. 735–40.

278.   Gerbi, M.E., et al. Infrared laser light further improves bone healing when associated with bone morphogenic proteins: an *in vivo* study in a rodent model. *Photomed Laser Surg*, 2008. **26**(1): pp. 55–60.

279.   Valiati, R., et al. Effect of low-level laser therapy on incorporation of block allografts. *Int J Med Sci*, 2012. **9**(10): pp. 853–61.

280.   Chang, W.D., et al. Therapeutic outcomes of low-level laser therapy for closed bone fracture in the human wrist and hand. *Photomed Laser Surg*, 2014. **32**(4): pp. 212–8.

281.   Cepera, F., et al. Effect of a low-level laser on bone regeneration after rapid maxillary expansion. *Am J Orthod Dentofacial Orthop*, 2012. **141**(4): pp. 444–50.

282.   Doshi-Mehta, G. and W.A. Bhad-Patil. Efficacy of low-intensity laser therapy in reducing treatment time and orthodontic pain: a clinical investigation. *Am J Orthod Dentofacial Orthop*, 2012. **141**(3): pp. 289–97.

283.   Kraus, K.H. and B.J. Bayer. Delayed unions, nonunions, and malunions. In: Tobias, K.M. and S.A. Johnston (eds) *Veterinary Surgery: Small Animal*. 2012, Elsevier Saunders, Canada, p. 647.

284.   Rogatko, C.P., W.I. Baltzer, and R. Tennant. Preoperative low level laser therapy in dogs undergoing tibial plateau levelling osteotomy: A blinded, prospective, randomized clinical trial. *Vet Comp Orthop Traumatol*, 2017. **30**(1): pp. 46–53.

285.   Renwick, S.M., et al. Influence of class IV laser therapy on the outcomes of tibial plateau leveling osteotomy in dogs. *Vet Surg*, 2018. **47**(4): pp. 507–15.

286.   Oliveira, S.P., et al. Low-level laser on femoral growth plate in rats. *Acta Cir Bras*, 2012. **27**(2): pp. 117–22.

287.   Cressoni, M.D., et al. Effect of GaAlAs laser irradiation on the epiphyseal cartilage of rats. *Photomed Laser Surg*, 2010. **28**(4): pp. 527–32.

288.   Cheetham, M.J., R.S. Young, and M. Dyson. Histological effects of 820 nm laser irradiation on the healthy growth plate of the rat. *Laser Ther*, 1992. **4**(2): pp. 59–64.

289.   de Andrade, A.R., et al. The effects of low-level laser therapy, 670 nm, on epiphyseal growth in rats. *ScientificWorldJournal*, 2012. **2012**: p. 231723.

290.   Peterson, H.A. and M.B. Wood. Physeal arrest due to laser beam damage in a growing child. *J Pediatr Orthop*, 2001. **21**(3): pp. 335–7.

291.   Boldrini, C., et al. Biomechanical effect of one session of low-level laser on the bone-titanium implant interface. *Lasers Med Sci*, 2013. **28**(1): pp. 349–52.

292.   Reddy, G.K., L. Stehno-Bittel, and C.S. Enwemeka. Laser photostimulation of collagen production in healing rabbit Achilles tendons. *Lasers Surg Med*, 1998. **22**(5): pp. 281–7.

293.   Fung, D.T., et al. Therapeutic low energy laser improves the mechanical strength of repairing medial collateral ligament. *Lasers Surg Med*, 2002. **31**(2): pp. 91–6.

294.   Pires, D., et al. Low-level laser therapy (LLLT; 780 nm) acts differently on mRNA expression of anti- and pro-inflammatory mediators in an experimental model of collagenase-induced tendinitis in rat. *Lasers Med Sci*, 2011. **26**(1): pp. 85–94.

295.   Bublitz, C., et al. Low-level laser therapy prevents degenerative morphological changes in an experimental model of anterior cruciate ligament transection in rats. *Lasers Med Sci*, 2014. **29**(5): pp. 1669–78.

296.   Wang, P., et al. Effects of low-level laser therapy on joint pain, synovitis, anabolic, and catabolic factors in a progressive osteoarthritis rabbit model. *Lasers Med Sci*, 2014. **29**(6): pp. 1875–85.

297.   Bjordal, J.M., R.A. Lopes-Martins, and V.V. Iversen. A randomised, placebo controlled trial of low level laser therapy for activated Achilles tendinitis with microdialysis measurement of peritendinous prostaglandin E2 concentrations. *Br J Sports Med*, 2006. **40**(1): pp. 76–80; discussion 76–80.

298.   Canapp, S.O., Jr., et al. Partial cranial cruciate ligament tears treated with stem cell and platelet-rich plasma combination therapy in 36 dogs: A retrospective study. *Front Vet Sci*, 2016. **3**: p. 112.

299.   Leal-Junior, E.C., et al. Superpulsed low-level laser therapy protects skeletal muscle of mdx mice against damage, inflammation and morphological changes delaying dystrophy progression. *PLoS One*, 2014. **9**(3): p. e89453.

300.   Carvalho, A.F., et al. The low-level laser on acute myositis in rats. *Acta Cir Bras*, 2015. **30**(12): pp. 806–11.

301. Pertille, A., A.B. Macedo, and C.P. Oliveira. Evaluation of muscle regeneration in aged animals after treatment with low-level laser therapy. *Rev Bras Fisioter*, 2012. **16**(6): pp. 495–501.

302. Leal Junior, E.C., et al. Effect of 830 nm low-level laser therapy applied before high-intensity exercises on skeletal muscle recovery in athletes. *Lasers Med Sci*, 2009. **24**(6): pp. 857–63.

303. Felismino, A.S., et al. Effect of low-level laser therapy (808 nm) on markers of muscle damage: a randomized double-blind placebo-controlled trial. *Lasers Med Sci*, 2014. **29**(3): pp. 933–8.

304. McPartland, J.M. Travell trigger points—molecular and osteopathic perspectives. *J Am Osteopath Assoc*, 2004. **104**(6): pp. 244–9.

305. Cummings, M. and P. Baldry. Regional myofascial pain: diagnosis and management. *Best Pract Res Clin Rheumatol*, 2007. **21**(2): pp. 367–87.

306. McPartland, J.M. and J.P. Goodridge. Counterstrain diagnostics and traditional osteopathic examination of the cervical spine compared. *J Bodyw Mov Ther*, 1997. **1**(3): pp. 173–8.

307. Janssens, L.A. Trigger point therapy. *Probl Vet Med*, 1992. **4**(1): pp. 117–24.

308. Janssens, L.A.A. Trigger points in 48 dogs with myofascial pain syndromes. *Vet Surg*, 1991. **20**(4): pp. 274–8.

309. Uemoto, L., et al. Laser therapy and needling in myofascial trigger point deactivation. *J Oral Sci*, 2013. **55**(2): pp. 175–81.

310. Gur, A., et al. Efficacy of 904 nm gallium arsenide low level laser therapy in the management of chronic myofascial pain in the neck: a double-blind and randomize-controlled trial. *Lasers Surg Med*, 2004. **35**(3): pp. 229–35.

311. Johnston, S.A. Osteoarthritis. Joint anatomy, physiology, and pathobiology. *Vet Clin North Am Small Anim Pract*, 1997. **27**(4): pp. 699–723.

312. Rialland, P., et al. Clinical validity of outcome pain measures in naturally occurring canine osteoarthritis. *BMC Vet Res*, 2012. **8**: p. 162.

313. Slingerland, L.I., et al. Cross-sectional study of the prevalence and clinical features of osteoarthritis in 100 cats. *Vet J*, 2011. **187**(3): pp. 304–9.

314. Lascelles, B.D., et al. Cross-sectional study of the prevalence of radiographic degenerative joint disease in domesticated cats. *Vet Surg*, 2010. **39**(5): pp. 535–44.

315. Schmidt, J. Even painkillers for dogs have serious risks. *USA Today*, 2005, 4 November.

316. Penumudi, A. Nexvet canine osteoarthritis drug meets main goal in study. 2015. Available at: https://www.reuters.com/article/us-nexvet-study/ nexvet-canine-osteoarthritis-drug-meets-main-goal-in-study-idUSKCN0T523520151116 (accessed September 2018).

317. Carmichael, S. Optimising efficacy and minimising toxicity of NSAIDs. 2016. *Proceedings of the 22nd FECAVA Eurocongress, Vienna, Austria*. Available at: http://www.fecava2016.org/programme (accessed September 2018).

318. Smith, G.K., et al. Lifelong diet restriction and radiographic evidence of osteoarthritis of the hip joint in dogs. *J Am Vet Med Assoc*, 2006. **229**(5): pp. 690–3.

319. Impellizeri, J.A., M.A. Tetrick, and P. Muir. Effect of weight reduction on clinical signs of lameness in dogs with hip osteoarthritis. *J Am Vet Med Assoc*, 2000. **216**(7): pp. 1089–91.

320. Salinardi, B.J., et al. Matrix metalloproteinase and tissue inhibitor of metalloproteinase in serum and synovial fluid of osteoarthritic dogs. *Vet Comp Orthop Traumatol*, 2006. **19**(1): pp. 49–55.

321. Alam, M.R., et al. Biomarkers for identifying the early phases of osteoarthritis secondary to medial patellar luxation in dogs. *J Vet Sci*, 2011. **12**(3): pp. 273–80.

322. Hurlbeck, C., et al. Evaluation of biomarkers for osteoarthritis caused by fragmented medial coronoid process in dogs. *Res Vet Sci*, 2014. **96**(3): pp. 429–35.

323. Volk, S.W., et al. Gelatinase activity in synovial fluid and synovium obtained from healthy and osteoarthritic joints of dogs. *Am J Vet Res*, 2003. **64**(10): pp. 1225–33.

324. Hegemann, N., et al. Cytokine profile in canine immune-mediated polyarthritis and osteoarthritis. *Vet Comp Orthop Traumatol*, 2005. **18**(2): pp. 67–72.

325. Hegemann, N., et al. Synovial MMP-3 and TIMP-1 levels and their correlation with cytokine expression in canine rheumatoid arthritis. *Vet Immunol Immunopathol*, 2003. **91**(3–4): pp. 199–204.

326. de Bakker, E., et al. Canine synovial fluid biomarkers for early detection and monitoring of osteoarthritis. *Vet Rec*, 2017. **180**(13): pp. 328–29.

327. Pallotta, R.C., et al. Infrared (810-nm) low-level laser therapy on rat experimental knee inflammation. *Lasers Med Sci*, 2012. **27**(1): pp. 71–8.

328. Barretto, S.R., et al. Evaluation of anti-nociceptive and anti-inflammatory activity of low-level laser therapy on temporomandibular joint inflammation in rodents. *J Photochem Photobiol B*, 2013. **129**: pp. 135–42.

329. Mantineo, M., J.P. Pinheiro, and A.M. Morgado. Low-level laser therapy on skeletal muscle inflammation: evaluation of irradiation parameters. *J Biomed Opt*, 2014. **19**(9): p. 98002.

330. Aliodoust, M., et al. Evaluating the effect of low-level laser therapy on healing of tenotomized Achilles tendon in streptozotocin-induced diabetic rats by light

microscopical and gene expression examinations. *Lasers Med Sci*, 2014. **29**(4): pp. 1495–503.

331.   Cury, V., et al. Low level laser therapy increases angiogenesis in a model of ischemic skin flap in rats mediated by VEGF, HIF-1α and MMP-2. *J Photochem Photobiol B*, 2013. **125**: pp. 164–70.

332.   Carlos, F.P., et al. Protective effect of low-level laser therapy (LLLT) on acute zymosan-induced arthritis. *Lasers Med Sci*, 2014. **29**(2): pp. 757–63.

333.   Lascelles, B.D., et al. A canine-specific anti-nerve growth factor antibody alleviates pain and improves mobility and function in dogs with degenerative joint disease-associated pain. *BMC Vet Res*, 2015. **11**: p. 101.

334.   Gruen, M.E., et al. A feline-specific anti-nerve growth factor antibody improves mobility in cats with degenerative joint disease-associated pain: a pilot proof of concept study. *J Vet Intern Med*, 2016. **30**(4): pp. 1138–48.

335.   Baltzer, A.W., M.S. Ostapczuk, and D. Stosch. Positive effects of low level laser therapy (LLLT) on Bouchard's and Heberden's osteoarthritis. *Lasers Surg Med*, 2016. **48**(5): pp. 498–504.

336.   Alayat, M.S., et al. Efficacy of pulsed Nd:YAG laser in the treatment of patients with knee osteoarthritis: a randomized controlled trial. *Lasers Med Sci*, 2017. **32**(3): pp. 503–11.

337.   S, G.N., et al. Radiological and biochemical effects (CTX-II, MMP-3, 8, and 13) of low-level laser therapy (LLLT) in chronic osteoarthritis in Al-Kharj, Saudi Arabia. *Lasers Med Sci*, 2017. **32**(2): pp. 297–303.

338.   Ip, D. Does addition of low-level laser therapy (LLLT) in conservative care of knee arthritis successfully postpone the need for joint replacement? *Lasers Med Sci*, 2015. **30**(9): pp. 2335–9.

339.   Stasinopoulos, D., et al. LLLT for the management of patients with ankylosing spondylitis. *Lasers Med Sci*, 2016. **31**(3): pp. 459–69.

340.   Marini, I., M.R. Gatto, and G.A. Bonetti. Effects of superpulsed low-level laser therapy on temporomandibular joint pain. *Clin J Pain*, 2010. **26**(7): pp. 611–6.

341.   Brosseau, L., et al. Low level laser therapy (Classes I, II and III) for treating rheumatoid arthritis. *Cochrane Database Syst Rev*, 2005(4): p. CD002049.

342.   Brown, D.C., R.C. Boston, and J.T. Farrar. Comparison of force plate gait analysis and owner assessment of pain using the Canine Brief Pain Inventory in dogs with osteoarthritis. *J Vet Intern Med*, 2013. **27**(1): pp. 22–30.

343.   Hudson, J.T., et al. Assessing repeatability and validity of a visual analogue scale questionnaire for use in assessing pain and lameness in dogs. *Am J Vet Res*, 2004. **65**(12): pp. 1634–43.

344.   Hesbach, A.L. Techniques for objective outcome assessment. *Clin Tech Small Anim Pract*, 2007. **22**(4): pp. 146–54.

345.   Cachon, T., et al. Face validity of a proposed tool for staging canine osteoarthritis: Canine OsteoArthritis Staging Tool (COAST). *Vet J*, 2018. **235**: pp. 1–8.

346.   Brown, D.C. The Canine Orthopedic Index. Step 1: Devising the items. *Vet Surg*, 2014. **43**(3): pp. 232–40.

347.   Brown, D.C. The Canine Orthopedic Index. Step 2: Psychometric testing. *Vet Surg*, 2014. **43**(3): pp. 241–6.

348.   Brown, D.C. The Canine Orthopedic Index. Step 3: Responsiveness testing. *Vet Surg*, 2014. **43**(3): pp. 247–54.

349.   Reid, J., et al. Development, validation and reliability of a web-based questionnaire to measure health-related quality of life in dogs. *J Small Anim Pract*, 2013. **54**(5): pp. 227–33.

350.   Reid, J., L. Wiseman-Orr, and M. Scott. Shortening of an existing generic online health-related quality of life instrument for dogs. *J Small Anim Pract*, 2018. **59**(6): pp. 334–42.

351.   Lascelles, B.D., et al. Evaluation of client-specific outcome measures and activity monitoring to measure pain relief in cats with osteoarthritis. *J Vet Intern Med*, 2007. **21**(3): pp. 410–6.

352.   Brown, D.C., et al. Development and psychometric testing of an instrument designed to measure chronic pain in dogs with osteoarthritis. *Am J Vet Res*, 2007. **68**(6): pp. 631–7.

353.   Brown, D.C., et al. Ability of the canine brief pain inventory to detect response to treatment in dogs with osteoarthritis. *J Am Vet Med Assoc*, 2008. **233**(8): pp. 1278–83.

354.   Walton, M.B., et al. Evaluation of construct and criterion validity for the 'Liverpool Osteoarthritis in Dogs' (LOAD) clinical metrology instrument and comparison to two other instruments. *PLoS One*, 2013. **8**(3): p. e58125.

355.   Hielm-Bjorkman, A.K., et al. Evaluation of methods for assessment of pain associated with chronic osteoarthritis in dogs. *J Am Vet Med Assoc*, 2003. **222**(11): pp. 1552–8.

356.   Hielm-Bjorkman, A.K., H. Rita, and R.M. Tulamo. Psychometric testing of the Helsinki chronic pain index by completion of a questionnaire in Finnish by owners of dogs with chronic signs of pain caused by osteoarthritis. *Am J Vet Res*, 2009. **70**(6): pp. 727–34.

357.   Benito, J., et al. Reliability and discriminatory testing of a client-based metrology instrument, feline musculoskeletal pain index (FMPI) for the evaluation of degenerative joint disease-associated pain in cats. *Vet J*, 2013. **196**(3): pp. 368–73.

358.   Benito, J., et al. Feline musculoskeletal pain index: responsiveness and testing of criterion validity. *J Vet Intern Med*, 2013. **27**(3): pp. 474–82.

359.   Gruen, M.E., et al. Detection of clinically relevant pain

relief in cats with degenerative joint disease associated pain. *J Vet Intern Med*, 2014. **28**(2): pp. 346–50.

360.   Gruen, M.E., et al. Criterion validation testing of clinical metrology instruments for measuring degenerative joint disease associated mobility impairment in cats. *PLoS One*, 2015. **10**(7): p. e0131839.

361.   Jaegger, G., D.J. Marcellin-Little, and D. Levine. Reliability of goniometry in Labrador Retrievers. *Am J Vet Res*, 2002. **63**(7): pp. 979–86.

362.   Jaeger, G.H., et al. Validity of goniometric joint measurements in cats. *Am J Vet Res*, 2007. **68**(8): pp. 822–6.

363.   Mann, F.A., C. Wagner-Mann, and C.H. Tangner. Manual goniometric measurement of the canine pelvic limb. *J Am Anim Hosp Assoc*, 1988. **24**(2): pp. 189–194.

364.   Thomovsky, S.A., et al. Goniometry and limb girth in miniature dachshunds. *J Vet Med*, 2016. **2016**: p. 5846052.

365.   Millis, D. and D. Levine. Joint motions and ranges. In: Millis, D. and D. Levine (eds) *Canine Rehabilitation and Physical Therapy*, 2nd edn. 2014, Elsevier Saunders, Philadelphia, PA, Appendix 2, pp. 730–5.

366.   Cook, J.L., et al. Measurement of angles of abduction for diagnosis of shoulder instability in dogs using goniometry and digital image analysis. *Vet Surg*, 2005. **34**(5): pp. 463–8.

367.   Levine, G.J., et al. Description and repeatability of a newly developed spinal cord injury scale for dogs. *Prev Vet Med*, 2009. **89**(1–2): pp. 121–7.

368.   Draper, W.E., et al. Low-level laser therapy reduces time to ambulation in dogs after hemilaminectomy: a preliminary study. *J Small Anim Pract*, 2012. **53**(8): pp. 465–9.

369.   Tramontana, A., R. Sorge, and J.C.M. Page. Laser biostimulation effects on invertebral disks: histological evidence on intra-observer samples. Retrospective double-blind study. *Laser Ther*, 2016. **25**(4): pp. 285–90.

370.   Zdrodowska, B., et al. Comparison of the effect of laser and magnetic therapy for pain level and the range of motion of the spine of people with osteoarthritis lower back [Article in Polish]. *Pol Merkur Lekarski*, 2015. **38**(223): pp. 26–31.

371.   Takhtfooladi, M.A., et al. Effect of low-level laser therapy (685 nm, 3 J/cm(2)) on functional recovery of the sciatic nerve in rats following crushing lesion. *Lasers Med Sci*, 2015. **30**(3): pp. 1047–52.

372.   Yang, C.C., et al. Synergistic effects of low-level laser and mesenchymal stem cells on functional recovery in rats with crushed sciatic nerves. *J Tissue Eng Regen Med*, 2016. **10**(2): pp. 120–31.

373.   Santos, A.P., et al. Functional and morphometric differences between the early and delayed use of phototherapy in crushed median nerves of rats. *Lasers Med Sci*, 2012. **27**(2): pp. 479–86.

374.   Rochkind, S., et al. Laser phototherapy (780 nm), a new modality in treatment of long-term incomplete peripheral nerve injury: a randomized double-blind placebo-controlled study. *Photomed Laser Surg*, 2007. **25**(5): pp. 436–42.

375.   Yagci, I., et al. Comparison of splinting and splinting plus low-level laser therapy in idiopathic carpal tunnel syndrome. *Clin Rheumatol*, 2009. **28**(9): pp. 1059–65.

376.   Fuhrer-Valdivia, A., et al. Low-level laser effect in patients with neurosensory impairment of mandibular nerve after sagittal split ramus osteotomy. Randomized clinical trial, controlled by placebo. *Med Oral Patol Oral Cir Bucal*, 2014. **19**(4): pp. e327–34.

377.   Rochkind, S., et al. New methods of treatment of severely injured sciatic nerve and spinal cord. An experimental study. *Acta Neurochir Suppl (Wien)*, 1988. **43**: pp. 91–3.

378.   Anders, J.J., et al. *In vitro* and *in vivo* optimization of infrared laser treatment for injured peripheral nerves. *Lasers Surg Med*, 2014. **46**(1): pp. 34–45.

379.   Haeussinger, F.B., et al. Simulation of near-infrared light absorption considering individual head and prefrontal cortex anatomy: implications for optical neuroimaging. *PLoS One*, 2011. **6**(10): p. e26377.

380.   Lapchak, P.A., et al. Transcranial near-infrared laser transmission (NILT) profiles (800 nm): Systematic comparison in four common research species. *PLoS One*, 2015. **10**(6): p. e0127580.

381.   Hamblin, M.R. Shining light on the head: Photobiomodulation for brain disorders. *BBA Clin*, 2016. **6**: pp. 113–24.

382.   Moges, H., et al. Light therapy and supplementary riboflavin in the SOD1 transgenic mouse model of familial amyotrophic lateral sclerosis (FALS). *Lasers Surg Med*, 2009. **41**(1): pp. 52–9.

383.   De Taboada, L., et al. Transcranial laser therapy attenuates amyloid-beta peptide neuropathology in amyloid-beta protein precursor transgenic mice. *J Alzheimers Dis*, 2011. **23**(3): pp. 521–35.

384.   Farfara, D., et al. Low-level laser therapy ameliorates disease progression in a mouse model of Alzheimer's disease. *J Mol Neurosci*, 2015. **55**(2): pp. 430–6.

385.   Yang, X., et al. Low energy laser light (632.8 nm) suppresses amyloid-beta peptide-induced oxidative and inflammatory responses in astrocytes. *Neuroscience*, 2010. **171**(3): pp. 859–68.

386.   Meng, C., Z. He, and D. Xing. Low-level laser therapy rescues dendrite atrophy via upregulating BDNF expression: implications for Alzheimer's disease. *J Neurosci*, 2013. **33**(33): pp. 13505–17.

387.   Shaw, V.E., et al. Neuroprotection of midbrain dopaminergic cells in MPTP-treated mice after

near-infrared light treatment. *J Comp Neurol*, 2010. **518**(1): pp. 25–40.

388. Oron, A., et al. Low-level laser therapy applied transcranially to mice following traumatic brain injury significantly reduces long-term neurological deficits. *J Neurotrauma*, 2007. **24**(4): pp. 651–6.

389. Wu, Q., et al. Low-level laser therapy for closed-head traumatic brain injury in mice: effect of different wavelengths. *Lasers Surg Med*, 2012. **44**(3): pp. 218–26.

390. Xuan, W., et al. Low-level laser therapy for traumatic brain injury in mice increases brain derived neurotrophic factor (BDNF) and synaptogenesis. *J Biophotonics*, 2015. **8**(6): pp. 502–11.

391. Xuan, W., L. Huang, and M.R. Hamblin. Repeated transcranial low-level laser therapy for traumatic brain injury in mice: biphasic dose response and long-term treatment outcome. *J Biophotonics*, 2016. **9**(11–12): pp. 1263–72.

392. Naeser, M.A., et al. Improved cognitive function after transcranial, light-emitting diode treatments in chronic, traumatic brain injury: two case reports. *Photomed Laser Surg*, 2011. **29**(5): pp. 351–8.

393. Leung, M.C., et al. Treatment of experimentally induced transient cerebral ischemia with low energy laser inhibits nitric oxide synthase activity and up-regulates the expression of transforming growth factor-beta 1. *Lasers Surg Med*, 2002. **31**(4): pp. 283–8.

394. Peplow, P.V. Neuroimmunomodulatory effects of transcranial laser therapy combined with intravenous tPA administration for acute cerebral ischemic injury. *Neural Regen Res*, 2015. **10**(8): pp. 1186–90.

395. Lampl, Y., et al. Infrared laser therapy for ischemic stroke: a new treatment strategy: results of the NeuroThera Effectiveness and Safety Trial-1 (NEST-1). *Stroke*, 2007. **38**(6): pp. 1843–9.

396. Zivin, J.A., et al. Effectiveness and safety of transcranial laser therapy for acute ischemic stroke. *Stroke*, 2009. **40**(4): pp. 1359–64.

397. Huisa, B.N., et al. Transcranial laser therapy for acute ischemic stroke: a pooled analysis of NEST-1 and NEST-2. *Int J Stroke*, 2013. **8**(5): pp. 315–20.

398. Kasner, S.E., et al. Transcranial laser therapy and infarct volume. *Stroke*, 2013. **44**(7): pp. 2025–7.

399. Hacke, W., et al. Transcranial laser therapy in acute stroke treatment: results of neurothera effectiveness and safety trial 3, a phase III clinical end point device trial. *Stroke*, 2014. **45**(11): pp. 3187–93.

400. Barrett, D.W. and F. Gonzalez-Lima. Transcranial infrared laser stimulation produces beneficial cognitive and emotional effects in humans. *Neuroscience*, 2013. **230**: pp. 13–23.

401. Schiffer, F., et al. Psychological benefits 2 and 4 weeks after a single treatment with near infrared light to the forehead: a pilot study of 10 patients with major depression and anxiety. *Behav Brain Funct*, 2009. **5**: p. 46.

402. de la Torre, J.C. Treating cognitive impairment with transcranial low level laser therapy. *J Photochem Photobiol B*, 2017. **168**: pp. 149–55.

403. Myakishev-Rempel, M., et al. A preliminary study of the safety of red light phototherapy of tissues harboring cancer. *Photomed Laser Surg*, 2012. **30**(9): pp. 551–8.

404. de C. Monteiro, J.S., et al. Influence of laser phototherapy (λ660 nm) on the outcome of oral chemical carcinogenesis on the hamster cheek pouch model: histological study. *Photomed Laser Surg*, 2011. **29**(11): pp. 741–5.

405. Renno, A.C., et al. The effects of laser irradiation on osteoblast and osteosarcoma cell proliferation and differentiation *in vitro*. *Photomed Laser Surg*, 2007. **25**(4): pp. 275–80.

406. Al-Watban, F.A. and B.L. Andres. Laser biomodulation of normal and neoplastic cells. *Lasers Med Sci*, 2012. **27**(5): pp. 1039–43.

407. Werneck, C.E., et al. Laser light is capable of inducing proliferation of carcinoma cells in culture: a spectroscopic *in vitro* study. *Photomed Laser Surg*, 2005. **23**(3): pp. 300–3.

408. Kiro, N.E., M.R. Hamblin, and H. Abrahamse. Photobiomodulation of breast and cervical cancer stem cells using low-intensity laser irradiation. *Tumour Biol*, 2017. **39**(6): p. 1010428317706913.

409. Zecha, J.A., et al. Low-level laser therapy/photobiomodulation in the management of side effects of chemoradiation therapy in head and neck cancer: part 2: proposed applications and treatment protocols. *Support Care Cancer*, 2016. **24**(6): pp. 2793–805.

410. Fife, D., et al. A randomized, controlled, double-blind study of light emitting diode photomodulation for the prevention of radiation dermatitis in patients with breast cancer. *Dermatol Surg*, 2010. **36**(12): pp. 1921–7.

411. Censabella, S., et al. Photobiomodulation for the management of radiation dermatitis: the DERMIS trial, a pilot study of MLS® laser therapy in breast cancer patients. *Support Care Cancer*, 2016. **24**(9): pp. 3925–33.

412. E Lima, M.T., et al. Low-level laser therapy in secondary lymphedema after breast cancer: systematic review. *Lasers Med Sci*, 2014. **29**(3): pp. 1289–95.

413. Vaupel, P. and M. Hockel. Blood supply, oxygenation status and metabolic micromilieu of breast cancers: characterization and therapeutic relevance. *Int J Oncol*, 2000. **17**(5): pp. 869–79.

414. Ottaviani, G., et al. Laser therapy inhibits tumor growth in mice by promoting immune surveillance and vessel normalization. *EBioMedicine*, 2016. **11**: pp. 165–72.

415. Azevedo, L.H., et al. Evaluation of low intensity laser

effects on the thyroid gland of male mice. *Photomed Laser Surg*, 2005. **23**(6): pp. 567–70.

416. Parrado, C., et al. A quantitative investigation of microvascular changes in the thyroid gland after infrared (IR) laser radiation. *Histol Histopathol*, 1999. **14**(4): pp. 1067–71.

417. Zahra, A.T. Assessment of the impacts of 830 nm low power laser on triiodothyronine (T3), thyroxine (T4) and the thyroid stimulating hormone (TSH) in the rabbits. *J Med Sci Clin Res*, 2014. **2**(11): pp. 2917–29.

418. Vidal, L., M. Ortiz, and I. Perez de Vargas. Ultrastructural changes in thyroid perifollicular capillaries during normal postnatal development and after infrared laser radiation. *Lasers Med Sci*, 2002. **17**(3): pp. 187–97.

419. Hofling, D.B., et al. Low-level laser in the treatment of patients with hypothyroidism induced by chronic autoimmune thyroiditis: a randomized, placebo-controlled clinical trial. *Lasers Med Sci*, 2013. **28**(3): pp. 743–53.

420. Hofling, D.B., et al. Low-level laser therapy in chronic autoimmune thyroiditis: a pilot study. *Lasers Surg Med*, 2010. **42**(6): pp. 589–96.

421. Hofling, D.B., et al. Effects of low-level laser therapy on the serum TGF-beta1 concentrations in individuals with autoimmune thyroiditis. *Photomed Laser Surg*, 2014. **32**(8): pp. 444–9.

422. Hofling, D.B., et al. Assessment of the effects of low-level laser therapy on the thyroid vascularization of patients with autoimmune hypothyroidism by color Doppler ultrasound. *ISRN Endocrinol*, 2012. **2012**: p. 126720.

423. Fronza, B., et al. Assessment of the systemic effects of low-level laser therapy (LLLT) on thyroid hormone function in a rabbit model. *Int J Oral Maxillofac Surg*, 2013. **42**(1): pp. 26–30.

424. Weber, J.B., et al. Effect of three different protocols of low-level laser therapy on thyroid hormone production after dental implant placement in an experimental rabbit model. *Photomed Laser Surg*, 2014. **32**(11): pp. 612–7.

425. Kerstein, R.L., T. Lister, and R. Cole. Laser therapy and photosensitive medication: a review of the evidence. *Lasers Med Sci*, 2014. **29**(4): pp. 1449–52.

426. Navratil, L. and J. Kymplova. Contraindications in noninvasive laser therapy: truth and fiction. *J Clin Laser Med Surg*, 2002. **20**(6): pp. 341–3.

427. Pomba, C., et al. Public health risk of antimicrobial resistance transfer from companion animals. *J Antimicrob Chemother*, 2017. **72**(4): pp. 957–68.

428. He, W., et al. Effectiveness of interstitial laser acupuncture depends upon dosage: Experimental results from electrocardiographic and electrocorticographic recordings. *Evid Based Complement Alternat Med*, 2013. **2013**: p. 934783.

429. Jiang, W.L., et al. Effects of different intensity laser acupuncture at two adjacent same-meridian acupoints on nitric oxide and soluble guanylate cyclase releases in human. *Microcirculation*, 2017. **24**(7): p. e12390.

430. Quah-Smith, I., et al. The brain effects of laser acupuncture in healthy individuals: an FMRI investigation. *PLoS One*, 2010. **5**(9): p. e12619.

431. Litscher, G., et al. Acupuncture using laser needles modulates brain function: first evidence from functional transcranial Doppler sonography and functional magnetic resonance imaging. *Lasers Med Sci*, 2004. **19**(1): pp. 6–11.

432. Erthal, V., et al. ST36 laser acupuncture reduces pain-related behavior in rats: involvement of the opioidergic and serotonergic systems. *Lasers Med Sci*, 2013. **28**(5): pp. 1345–51.

433. Lorenzini, L., et al. Laser acupuncture for acute inflammatory, visceral and neuropathic pain relief: An experimental study in the laboratory rat. *Res Vet Sci*, 2010. **88**(1): pp. 159–65.

434. Al Rashoud, A.S., et al. Efficacy of low-level laser therapy applied at acupuncture points in knee osteoarthritis: a randomised double-blind comparative trial. *Physiotherapy*, 2014. **100**(3): pp. 242–8.

435. Kibar, S., et al. Laser acupuncture treatment improves pain and functional status in patients with subacromial impingement syndrome: a randomized, double-blind, sham-controlled study. *Pain Med*, 2017. **18**(5): pp. 980–7.

436. Adly, A.S., et al. Laser acupuncture versus reflexology therapy in elderly with rheumatoid arthritis. *Lasers Med Sci*, 2017. **32**(5): pp. 1097–103.

437. Oates, A., et al. Laser acupuncture reduces pain in pediatric kidney biopsies: a randomized controlled trial. *Pain*, 2017. **158**(1): pp. 103–9.

438. Marques, V.I., et al. Laser Acupuncture for postoperative pain management in cats. *Evid Based Complement Alternat Med*, 2015. **2015**: p. 653270.

439. Attia, A.M., et al. Therapeutic antioxidant and anti-inflammatory effects of laser acupuncture on patients with rheumatoid arthritis. *Lasers Surg Med*, 2016. **48**(5): pp. 490–7.

440. Yurtkuran, M., et al. Laser acupuncture in knee osteoarthritis: a double-blind, randomized controlled study. *Photomed Laser Surg*, 2007. **25**(1): pp. 14–20.

441. Naeser, M.A., et al. Laser acupuncture in the treatment of paralysis in stroke patients: a CT scan lesion site study. *Am J Acupuncture*, 1995. **23**(1): pp. 13–28.

442. Raith, W., et al. Laser acupuncture for neonatal abstinence syndrome: a randomized controlled trial. *Pediatrics*, 2015. **136**(5): pp. 876–84.

443. Cafaro, A., et al. Effect of laser acupuncture on salivary flow rate in patients with Sjogren's syndrome. *Lasers Med Sci*, 2015. **30**(6): pp. 1805–9.

444. Yang, Z.K., et al. Manual acupuncture and laser

acupuncture for autonomic regulations in rats: observation on heart rate variability and gastric motility. *Evid Based Complement Alternat Med*, 2013. **2013**: p. 276320.

445.   Radmayr, C., et al. Prospective randomized trial using laser acupuncture versus desmopressin in the treatment of nocturnal enuresis. *Eur Urol*, 2001. **40**(2): pp. 201–5.

446.   Schlager, A., T. Offer, and I. Baldissera. Laser stimulation of acupuncture point P6 reduces postoperative vomiting in children undergoing strabismus surgery. *Br J Anaesth*, 1998. **81**(4): pp. 529–32.

447.   Dabbous, O.A., et al. Evaluation of the improvement effect of laser acupuncture biostimulation in asthmatic children by exhaled inflammatory biomarker level of nitric oxide. *Lasers Med Sci*, 2017. **32**(1): pp. 53–9.

448.   Baxter, G.D., C. Bleakley, and S. McDonough. Clinical effectiveness of laser acupuncture: a systematic review. *J Acupunct Meridian Stud*, 2008. **1**(2): pp. 65–82.

449.   Law, D., et al. Laser acupuncture for treating musculoskeletal pain: a systematic review with meta-analysis. *J Acupunct Meridian Stud*, 2015. **8**(1): pp. 2–16.

450.   Wang, L., et al. Patterns of traditional chinese medicine diagnosis in thermal laser acupuncture treatment of knee osteoarthritis. *Evid Based Complement Alternat Med*, 2013. **2013**: p. 870305.

451.   Mao, H., et al. Effects of infrared laser moxibustion on cancer-related fatigue: A randomized, double-blind, placebo-controlled trial. *Cancer*, 2016. **122**(23): pp. 3667–72.

452.   Petermann, U. Laser acupuncture and local laser therapy in veterinary medicine with overview of applied laser types and clinical uses. *AJTCVM*, 2017. **12**(1): pp. 89–101.

453.   Robinson, N.G. Laser acupuncture: keep it scientific. *Photomed Laser Surg*, 2014. **32**(12): pp. 647–8.

454.   WALT. Recommended treatment doses for low level laser therapy laser class 3 B, 780–860nm GaAlAs lasers. 2010. Available at: http://waltza.co.za/wp-content/uploads/2012/08/Dose_table_780-860nm_for_Low_Level_Laser_Therapy_WALT-2010.pdf (accessed September 2018).

455.   WALT. Recommended treatment doses for low level laser therapy laser class 3B, 904 nm GaAs lasers. 2010. Available at: http://waltza.co.za/wp-content/uploads/2012/08/Dose_table_904nm_for_Low_Level_Laser_Therapy_WALT-2010.pdf (accessed September 2018).

456.   Xie, H. and V. Preast. *Xie´s Veterinary Acupuncture*, 1st edn. 2007, Blackwell Publishing, Ames, Iowa.

457.   Schoen, A.M. *Veterinary Acupuncture*, 2nd edn. 2001, Mosby, Inc., Maryland Heights, Missouri.

458.   Haslerud, S., et al. Achilles tendon penetration for continuous 810 nm and superpulsed 904 nm lasers before and after ice application: an *in situ* study on healthy young adults. *Photomed Laser Surg*, 2017. **35**(10): pp. 567–75.

459.   Haslerud, S., et al. Low-level laser therapy and cryotherapy as mono- and adjunctive therapies for achilles tendinopathy in rats. *Photomed Laser Surg*, 2017. **35**(1): pp. 32–42.

460.   Ulusoy, A., L. Cerrahoglu, and S. Orguc. Magnetic resonance imaging and clinical outcomes of laser therapy, ultrasound therapy, and extracorporeal shock wave therapy for treatment of plantar fasciitis: a randomized controlled trial. *J Foot Ankle Surg*, 2017. **56**(4): pp. 762–7.

461.   Paolillo, A.R., et al. Synergic effects of ultrasound and laser on the pain relief in women with hand osteoarthritis. *Lasers Med Sci*, 2015. **30**(1): pp. 279–86.

462.   Agrawal, T., et al. Pre-conditioning with low-level laser (light) therapy: light before the storm. *Dose Response*, 2014. **12**(4): pp. 619–49.

463.   Canapp, D.A. Select modalities. *Clin Tech Small Anim Pract*, 2007. **22**(4): pp. 160–5.

464.   Saayman, L., C. Hay, and H. Abrahamse. Chiropractic manipulative therapy and low-level laser therapy in the management of cervical facet dysfunction: a randomized controlled study. *J Manipulative Physiol Ther*, 2011. **34**(3): pp. 153–63.

465.   de Villiers, J.A., N.N. Houreld, and H. Abrahamse. Influence of low intensity laser irradiation on isolated human adipose derived stem cells over 72 hours and their differentiation potential into smooth muscle cells using retinoic acid. *Stem Cell Rev*, 2011. **7**(4): pp. 869–82.

466.   Fallahnezhad, S., et al. Effect of low-level laser therapy and oxytocin on osteoporotic bone marrow-derived mesenchymal stem cells. *J Cell Biochem*, 2018. **119**(1): pp. 983–97.

467.   Yin, K., et al. Low level laser (LLL) attenuate LPS-induced inflammatory responses in mesenchymal stem cells via the suppression of NF-kappaB signaling pathway *in vitro*. *PLoS One*, 2017. **12**(6): p. e0179175.

468.   Soleimani, M., et al. The effects of low-level laser irradiation on differentiation and proliferation of human bone marrow mesenchymal stem cells into neurons and osteoblasts—an *in vitro* study. *Lasers Med Sci*, 2012. **27**(2): pp. 423–30.

469.   Nagata, M.J., et al. Bone marrow aspirate combined with low-level laser therapy: a new therapeutic approach to enhance bone healing. *J Photochem Photobiol B*, 2013. **121**: pp. 6–14.

470.   Emelyanov, A.N., and Kiryanov, V.V. Photomodulation of proliferation and differentiation of stem cells by the visible and infrared light. *Photomedicine and Laser Surgery*, 2015. **33**(3): pp. 164–74.

471.   Black, L.L., et al. Effect of adipose-derived

mesenchymal stem and regenerative cells on lameness in dogs with chronic osteoarthritis of the coxofemoral joints: a randomized, double-blinded, multicenter, controlled trial. *Vet Ther*, 2007. **8**(4): pp. 272–84.

472.   Vilar, J.M., et al. Controlled, blinded force platform analysis of the effect of intraarticular injection of autologous adipose-derived mesenchymal stem cells associated to PRGF-Endoret in osteoarthritic dogs. *BMC Vet Res*, 2013. **9**: p. 131.

473.   Zeira, O., et al. Adult autologous mesenchymal stem cells for the treatment of suspected non-infectious inflammatory diseases of the canine central nervous system: safety, feasibility and preliminary clinical findings. *J Neuroinflammation*, 2015. **12**: p. 181.

474.   Granger, N., et al. Autologous olfactory mucosal cell transplants in clinical spinal cord injury: a randomized double-blinded trial in a canine translational model. *Brain*, 2012. **135**(Pt 11): pp. 3227–37.

475.   Perez-Merino, E.M., et al. Safety and efficacy of allogeneic adipose tissue-derived mesenchymal stem cells for treatment of dogs with inflammatory bowel disease: Clinical and laboratory outcomes. *Vet J*, 2015. **206**(3): pp. 385–90.

476.   Pinheiro, C.C.G., et al. Low laser therapy: a strategy to promote the osteogenic differentiation of deciduous dental pulp stem cells from cleft lip and palate patients. *Tissue Eng Part A*, 2018. **24**(7–8): pp. 569–75.

477.   El Gammal, Z.H., A.M. Zaher, and N. El-Badri. Effect of low-level laser-treated mesenchymal stem cells on myocardial infarction. *Lasers Med Sci*, 2017. **32**(7): pp. 1637–46.

478.   Park, I.S., P.S. Chung, and J.C. Ahn. Adipose-derived stem cell spheroid treated with low-level light irradiation accelerates spontaneous angiogenesis in mouse model of hindlimb ischemia. *Cytotherapy*, 2017. **19**(9): pp. 1070–8.

479.   Ginani, F., et al. Effect of low-level laser therapy on mesenchymal stem cell proliferation: a systematic review. *Lasers Med Sci*, 2015. **30**(8): pp. 2189–94.

480.   Fahie, M.A., et al. A randomized controlled trial of the efficacy of autologous platelet therapy for the treatment of osteoarthritis in dogs. *J Am Vet Med Assoc*, 2013. **243**(9): pp. 1291–7.

481.   Franklin, S.P., E.E. Burke, and S.P. Holmes. The effect of platelet-rich plasma on osseous healing in dogs undergoing high tibial osteotomy. *PLoS One*, 2017. **12**(5): p. e0177597.

482.   Barbosa, D., et al. Low-level laser therapy combined with platelet-rich plasma on the healing calcaneal tendon: a histological study in a rat model. *Lasers Med Sci*, 2013. **28**(6): pp. 1489–94.

483.   Garcia, T.A., et al. Histological analysis of the association of low level laser therapy and platelet-rich plasma in regeneration of muscle injury in rats. *Braz J Phys Ther*, 2017. **21**(6): pp. 425–33.

484.   Ozaki, G.A., et al. Analysis of photobiomodulation associated or not with platelet-rich plasma on repair of muscle tissue by Raman spectroscopy. *Lasers Med Sci*, 2016. **31**(9): pp. 1891–8.

485.   Nagata, M.J., et al. Platelet-rich plasma, low-level laser therapy, or their combination promotes periodontal regeneration in fenestration defects: a preliminary *in vivo* study. *J Periodontol*, 2014. **85**(6): pp. 770–8.

Index